Addiction Medicine: A Multidisciplinary Approach

Editorial Advisor

JOEL J. HEIDELBAUGH

ELSEVIER

1600 John F. Kennedy Boulevard • Suite 1800 • Philadelphia, Pennsylvania, 19103-2899

http://www.theclinics.com

CLINICS COLLECTIONS
ISSN 2352-7986, ISBN-13: 978-0-323-78945-5

Editor: John Vassallo (j.vassallo@elsevier.com)

Clinics Collections (ISSN 2352-7986) is published by Elsevier Inc., 360 Park Avenue South, New York, NY 10010-1710. Business and editorial offices: 1600 John F. Kennedy Boulevard, Suite 1800, Philadelphia, PA 19103-2899. **POSTMASTER:** Send address changes to *Clinics Collections*, Elsevier Health Sciences Division, Subscription Customer Service, 3251 Riverport Lane, Maryland Heights, MO 63043. **Customer Service: Telephone: 1-800-654-2452** (U.S. and Canada); **1-314-447-8871** (outside U.S. and Canada). **Fax: 314-447-8029. E-mail: journalscustomerserviceusa@elsevier.com** (for print support); **journalsonlinesupport-usa@ elsevier.com** (for online support).

Reprints. For copies of 100 or more of articles in this publication, please contact the Commercial Reprints Department, Elsevier Inc., 360 Park Avenue South, New York, NY 10010-1710. Tel.: 212-633-3874; Fax: 212-633-3820; E-mail: reprints@elsevier.com.

Contributors

EDITOR

JOEL J. HEIDELBAUGH, MD, FAAFP, FACG
Clinical Professor, Departments of Family Medicine and Urology, University of Michigan Medical School, Ann Arbor, Michigan, USA

AUTHORS

ANA ABRANTES, PhD
Butler Hospital, Behavioral Medicine and Addictions Research, Butler, Pennsylvania, USA; Department of Psychiatry and Human Behavior, The Warren Alpert Medical School of Brown University, Providence, Rhode Island, USA

JOSEPH ARTHUR, MD
Assistant Professor, Department of Palliative Care, Rehabilitation and Integrative Medicine, The University of Texas MD Anderson Cancer Center, Houston, Texas, USA

PAGE D. AXLEY, MD
Resident in Internal Medicine, Department of Medicine, The University of Alabama at Birmingham, Birmingham, Alabama, USA

WILLIAM C. BECKER, MD
Core Investigator, Opioid Reassessment Clinic, VA Connecticut Healthcare System, Pain Research, Informatics, Multimorbidities and Education (PRIME) Center, West Haven, Connecticut, USA; Assistant Professor, Department of Medicine, Yale School of Medicine, New Haven, Connecticut, USA

INGRID A. BINSWANGER, MD, MPH, MS
Senior Investigator, Institute for Health Research, Kaiser Permanente Colorado, Associate Professor, Department of Medicine, Division of General Internal Medicine, University of Colorado, Aurora, Colorado, USA

REBECCA BUDISH, MS
Medical Student, Department of Anesthesiology, LSU Health Shreveport, Shreveport, Louisiana, USA

ALAN J. BUDNEY, PhD
Professor, Department of Psychiatry, Center for Technology and Behavioral Health, Geisel School of Medicine at Dartmouth, Lebanon, New Hampshire, USA

MEGAN E. BURESH, MD
Division of Chemical Dependence, Johns Hopkins University School of Medicine, Baltimore, Maryland, USA

DEEPA R. CAMENGA, MD, MHS
Assistant Professor of Emergency Medicine, Yale School of Medicine, New Haven, Connecticut, USA

MICHELLE CANGIANO, MD
Physician Site Leader, Assistant Professor, Department of Family Medicine, The Robert Larner, M.D. College of Medicine, University of Vermont, Burlington, Vermont, USA

SUBHAJIT CHAKRAVORTY, MD
Assistant Professor of Psychiatry, Perelman School of Medicine, Corporal Michael J. Crescenz VA Medical Center, Philadelphia, Pennsylvania, USA

LEE S. COHEN, MD
Perinatal and Reproductive Psychiatry Program, Director, Massachusetts General Hospital Center for Women's Mental Health, Professor of Psychiatry, Harvard Medical School, Boston, Massachusetts, USA

ELYSE M. CORNETT, PhD
Assistant Professor, Department of Anesthesiology, LSU Health Shreveport, Shreveport, Louisiana, USA

KAREN J. DEREFINKO, PhD
Assistant Professor, The University of Tennessee Health Science Center, Memphis, Tennessee, USA

JEFFREY L. DEREVENSKY, PhD
James McGill Professor, Director, International Centre for Youth Gambling Problems and High-Risk Behaviors, McGill University, Montreal, Quebec, Canada

E. JENNIFER EDELMAN, MD, MHS
Yale University School of Medicine and Public Health, New Haven, Connecticut, USA

FRANCISCO I. SALGADO GARCÍA, PhD
The University of Tennessee Health Science Center, Memphis, Tennessee, USA

LYNETTE GILBEAU, BEd
International Centre for Youth Gambling Problems and High-Risk Behaviors, McGill University, Montreal, Quebec, Canada

RYAN GRADDY, MD
Division of Chemical Dependence, Johns Hopkins University School of Medicine, Baltimore, Maryland, USA

BRENDON HART, DO
Resident, Department of Anesthesiology, LSU Health Shreveport, Shreveport, Louisiana, USA

VICTORIA HAYMAN, BSc
International Centre for Youth Gambling Problems and High-Risk Behaviors, McGill University, Montreal, Quebec, Canada

SEAN HE, BS
Student, Post-baccalaureate Studies Program, College of Liberal Arts and Professional Studies, University of Pennsylvania, Corporal Michael J. Crescenz VA Medical Center, Philadelphia, Pennsylvania, USA

DAVID HUI, MD, MSc
Associate Professor, Departments of Palliative Care, Rehabilitation and Integrative Medicine and General Oncology, The University of Texas MD Anderson Cancer Center, Houston, Texas, USA

ALICIA A. JACOBS, MD
Vice Chair of Clinical Operations, Associate Professor, Department of Family Medicine, The Robert Larner, M.D. College of Medicine at the University of Vermont, Burlington, Vermont, USA

AMANDA J. JOHNSON, MD
Department of Obstetrics and Gynecology, Division of Maternal-Fetal Medicine, Medical College of Wisconsin, Milwaukee, Wisconsin, USA

CRESTA W. JONES, MD
Department of Obstetrics, Gynecology and Women's Health, Division of Maternal-Fetal Medicine, University of Minnesota Medical School, Minneapolis, Minnesota, USA

HENDRÉE E. JONES, PhD
Professor, Department of Obstetrics and Gynecology, University of North Carolina at Chapel Hill, Executive Director, UNC Horizons, Chapel Hill, North Carolina, USA; Adjunct Professor, Departments of Psychiatry and Behavioral Sciences, and Obstetrics and Gynecology, School of Medicine, Johns Hopkins University, Baltimore, Maryland, USA

TAMAR ARIT KAMINSKI, BS
Clinical Research Coordinator, Pediatric Psychopharmacology Program, Division of Child Psychiatry, Massachusetts General Hospital, Boston, Massachusetts, USA

ALAN DAVID KAYE, MD, PhD
Chairman, Program Director, Professor, Departments of Anesthesiology and Pharmacology, LSU School of Medicine, LSU Health Science Center, New Orleans, Louisiana, USA

WALTER K. KRAFT, MD
Professor of Pharmacology, Medicine and Surgery, Director, Clinical Research Unit, Department of Pharmacology and Experimental Therapeutics, Thomas Jefferson University, Philadelphia, Pennsylvania, USA

DUSTIN LATIMER, BS
Medical Student, Department of Anesthesiology, LSU Health Shreveport, Shreveport, Louisiana, USA

BERNARD LE FOLL, MD, PhD
Head, Translational Addiction Research Laboratory, Medical Head of Addiction Medicine Service, Addiction Division, Centre for Addiction and Mental Health (CAMH), Professor, Departments of Pharmacology and Toxicology, Psychiatry, Family and Community Medicine, Institute of Medical Sciences, University of Toronto, Toronto, Ontario, Canada

ANNIE LÉVESQUE, MD, MSc
Assistant Professor, Icahn School of Medicine at Mount Sinai, Department of Psychiatry, Mount Sinai West Hospital, New York, New York, USA

AJAY MANHAPRA, MD
Research Scientist, Veteran Affairs New England Mental Illness Research, Education and Clinical Center (MIRECC), West Haven, Connecticut, USA; Lead Physician, Advanced PACT Pain Clinic, VA Hampton Medical Center, Hampton, Virginia, USA; Lecturer, Department of Psychiatry, Yale School of Medicine, New Haven, Connecticut, USA

RUTA NONACS, MD, PhD
Perinatal and Reproductive Psychiatrist, Perinatal and Reproductive Psychiatry Program, Massachusetts General Hospital Center for Women's Mental Health, Instructor in Psychiatry, Harvard Medical School, Boston, Massachusetts, USA

BENJAMIN J. OLDFIELD, MD
National Clinician Scholars Program, Yale University School of Medicine, New Haven, Connecticut, USA

STEPHANIE LEE PEGLOW, DO, MPH
Assistant Professor, Department of Psychiatry and Behavioral Sciences, Norfolk, Virginia, USA

EDWIN R. RAFFI, MD, MPH
Perinatal and Reproductive Psychiatrist, Perinatal and Reproductive Psychiatry Program, Massachusetts General Hospital Center for Women's Mental Health, Instructor in Psychiatry, Harvard Medical School, Boston, Massachusetts, USA

DARIUS A. RASTEGAR, MD
Division of Chemical Dependence, Johns Hopkins University School of Medicine, Baltimore, Maryland, USA

CRIT TAYLOR RICHARDSON, MD
Fellow in Gastroenterology, Division of Gastroenterology and Hepatology, University of Alabama at Birmingham, Birmingham, Alabama, USA

SHERYL A. RYAN, MD
Professor of Pediatrics, Chief, Division of Adolescent Medicine, Department of Pediatrics, Milton S. Hershey Medical Center, Penn State Hershey Children's Hospital, Hershey, Pennsylvania, USA

ASHWANI K. SINGAL, MD, MS, FACG, FAASLD
Associate Professor of Medicine, Director, Porphyria Center, Division of Gastroenterology and Hepatology, University of Alabama at Birmingham, Birmingham, Alabama, USA

CATHERINE STANGER, PhD
Associate Professor, Department of Psychiatry, Center for Technology and Behavioral Health, Geisel School of Medicine at Dartmouth, Lebanon, New Hampshire, USA

MICHAEL D. STEIN, MD
Professor and Chair, Department of Health Law, Policy and Management, Boston University School of Public Health, Boston, Massachusetts, USA

DANIEL D. SUMROK, MD, FAAFP, DABAM, DFASAM
Assistant Professor, The University of Tennessee Health Science Center, Memphis, Tennessee, USA

JEANETTE M. TETRAULT, MD
Department of Internal Medicine, Yale University School of Medicine, New Haven, Connecticut, USA

HILARY A. TINDLE, MD, MPH
Associate Professor of Medicine, Vanderbilt University Medical Center, Nashville, Tennessee, USA

BABAK TOFIGHI, MD, MSc
Assistant Professor, Department of Population Health, Division of General Internal Medicine, New York University School of Medicine, New York, New York, USA

RICHARD D. URMAN, MD, MBA, CPE, FASA
Associate Professor, Department of Anesthesiology, Perioperative and Pain Medicine, Center for Perioperative Research, Brigham and Women's Hospital, Harvard Medical School, Boston, Massachusetts, USA

RYAN G. VANDREY, PhD
Associate Professor of Psychiatry and Behavioral Sciences, Behavioral Pharmacology Research Unit, Johns Hopkins University School of Medicine, Baltimore, Maryland, USA

TIMOTHY E. WILENS, MD
Chief, Child & Adolescent Psychiatry, Massachusetts General Hospital, Professor of Psychiatry, Harvard Medical School, Boston, Massachusetts, USA

Contents

Primary care is an important setting for delivering evidence-based treatment to address substance use disorders. To date, effective approaches to treat, care largely incorporate pharmacotherapy with counselingbased interventions and rely on multidisciplinary teams. There is strong support for primary care–based approaches to address alcohol and opioid use disorder, with growing data focused on people living with human immunodeficiency virus and those experiencing incarceration. Future work should focus on the implementation of these effective approaches to decrease health disparities among people with substance use and to identify optimal approaches to address substance use in primary care and specialty settings.

The burden of alcohol and drug use disorders (substance use disorders [SUDs]) has intensified efforts to expand access to cost-effective psychosocial interventions and pharmacotherapies. This article provides an overview of technology-based interventions (eg, computer-based and Web-based interventions, text messaging, interactive voice recognition, smartphone apps, and emerging technologies) that are extending the reach of effective addiction treatments both in substance use treatment and primary care settings. It discusses the efficacy of existing technology-based interventions for SUDs, prospects for emerging technologies, and special considerations when integrating technologies in primary care (eg, privacy and regulatory protocols) to enhance the management of SUDs.

The current opioid crisis highlights an urgent need for better paradigms for prevention and treatment of chronic pain and addiction. Although many approach this complex clinical condition with the question "Is this pain or is this addiction?" it is more than the sum of its parts. Chronic pain among those with dependence and addiction often evolves into a complex disabling condition with pain at multiple sites, psychosocial dysfunctions, medical and psychiatric disorders, polypharmacy, and polysubstance use, all interacting with each other in complex ways (multimorbidity). The

stimulants, and medication-assisted treatment of substance use disorders. Early screening, diagnosis, and intervention prior to and/or during pregnancy often reduce morbidity and mortality of mental health disorders for mothers and infants.

treatment, focusing on methods, timing, and breadth of intervention strategies, is also presented. Common methodologies that may be used across tobacco use and alcohol and substance use disorder to prevent lapse and relapse are discussed. Physicians can and should adhere to the policy that tobacco use is a common and dangerous comorbid condition that demands concomitant treatment.

This article reviews the current evidence on electronic cigarette (e-cigarette) safety and efficacy for smoking cessation, with a focus on smokers with cardiovascular disease, pulmonary disease, or serious mental illness. In the United States, adult smokers use e-cigarettes primarily to quit or reduce cigarette smoking. An understanding of the potential risks and benefits of e-cigarette use may help clinicians counsel smokers about the potential impact of e-cigarettes on health.

Cannabis (marijuana) is a drug product derived from the plant Cannabis sativa. Cannabinoid is a general term for all chemical constituents of the cannabis plant. Legalization of marijuana in numerous US states, the availability of cannabis of higher potency, and the emergence of synthetic cannabinoids may have contributed to the increased demand for related medical services. The most effective available treatments for cannabis use disorder are psychosocial approaches. There is no pharmacotherapyapproved treatment. This article reviews the current state of knowledge regarding effective treatments for cannabis use disorder.

Alcohol abuse is a major determinant of public health outcomes. Worldwide data from 2016 indicate that alcohol is the seventh leading risk factor in terms of disability-adjusted life years, an increase of more than 25% from 1990 to 2016. Understanding the epidemiology of alcoholic liver disease, including the regional variations in consumption and public policy, is an area of active research. In countries where the per capita consumption of alcohol decreases, there appears to be an associated decrease in disease burden. Given alcohol's health burden, an increased focus on alcohol control policies is needed.

The introduction of behavioral addictions is a relatively new concept in psychiatry. It was not until 2010 that the term behavioral addictions was added to the official classification of psychiatric diagnoses in the

Diagnostic and Statistical Manual of Mental Disorders, Fifth Edition. Gambling, typically thought to be an adult behavior, has become commonplace among adolescents. Although technological advances have made accessing information and communication easier, excessive use of the Internet and smartphones can result in multiple mental and physical health issues. Gambling disorders, gaming disorders, Internet use disorder, and excessive smartphone use often begin during childhood and adolescence.

Catherine Stanger and Alan J. Budney

Multiple interventions for treating adolescents with substance use disorders have demonstrated efficacy, but most teens do not show an enduring positive response to these treatments. Contingency management (CM)-based strategies provide a promising alternative, and clinical research focused on the development and testing of innovative CM models continues to grow. This article provides information on the principles that underlie CM interventions, key metrics that define their development and implementation, a brief review of studies that have tested these approaches, and some clinical CM tools. As with other interventions to help youth with substance use problems, there is much to learn about CM approaches.

Timothy E. Wilens and Tamar Arit Kaminski

The nonmedical use of prescription stimulants has become increasingly pervasive among transitional age youth (TAY), aged 16 years to 26 years. Although therapeutically administered stimulants are regarded as safe and effective in TAY with attention-deficit/hyperactivity syndrome (ADHD), stimulant misuse is of concern due to prevalence, behavioral health and substance use correlates, and negative short-term and long-term outcomes. Although academic motivations primarily drive misuse, it is unclear whether prescription ADHD stimulants enhance cognition. Providers are advised to exercise precautions when prescribing ADHD medications, enhance surveillance for misuse, and screen those with misuse for ADHD and other psychopathology, executive dysfunction, and substance use disorders.

Sheryl A. Ryan

Cocaine use by adolescents and young adults continues to be a significant public health issue and the cause of medical and psychological morbidity and mortality. Although use rates are lower than those seen with alcohol, tobacco, and other illicit substances such as marijuana, cocaine is highly addictive and presents significant acute and longterm medical and psychological effects. This article reviews the epidemiology of cocaine use among adolescents and young adults, discusses the pharmacology and neurobiology of cocaine use and dependence, provides information

Preface

Clinics Review Articles have been a part of the physicians', nurses', and residents' library for nearly 100 years. This trusted resource covers more than 50 medical disciplines every year, producing thousands of articles focused on the most current concepts and techniques in medicine. This collection of articles, devoted to addiction management, draws from this *Clinics* database to provide multidisciplinary teams with practical clinical advice on treatments and interventions for many common substance abuse disorders.

A multidisciplinary perspective is key to effective team-based management. Featured articles from the *Medical Clinics*, *Primary Care: Clinics in Office Practice*, *Anesthesiology Clinics*, *Pediatric Clinics*, *Clinics in Liver Disease*, and *Clinics in Perinatology* reflect the wide range of clinicians who manage patients with substance abuse disorders.

I encourage you to share this issue with your colleagues in hopes that it may promote more collaboration, new perspectives, and informed effective care for your patients.

Joel J. Heidelbaugh, MD, FAAFP, FACG
Departments of Family Medicine and Urology
University of Michigan Medical School
Ann Arbor, MI 48103, USA

Ypsilanti Health Center
200 Arnet, Suite 200
Ypsilanti, MI 48198, USA

E-mail address:
jheidel@umich.edu

https://doi.org/10.1016/j.ccol.2020.07.042
2352-7986/20/© 2020 Published by Elsevier Inc.

Office-Based Addiction Treatment in Primary Care

Approaches That Work

E. Jennifer Edelman, MD, MHS[a],*, Benjamin J. Oldfield, MD[b],
Jeanette M. Tetrault, MD[c]

KEYWORDS

- Primary health care • Opioid use disorder • Alcohol use disorder • Buprenorphine
- Naltrexone

KEY POINTS

- Primary care practices are well-suited for implementing evidence-based treatments to address alcohol and other substance use disorders.
- Effective approaches to treatment largely focus on provision of pharmacotherapy (eg, buprenorphine, naltrexone) in conjunction with counseling-based treatments.
- Studies to identify effective approaches for treating vulnerable populations are needed.

INTRODUCTION

Of the roughly 22 million individuals in the United States suffering from addiction, only 11% receive specialty care.[1] Reasons cited for the treatment gap include lack of provider education with regard to substance use and substance use disorders, perceived lack of need for treatment on the part of the patient, and lack of access to evidence-based treatment.[1,2] Integrating addiction treatment into office-based primary care is an important approach to improving access to care.[3] Primary care settings, including those providing primary care to special populations, offer several advantages to

This article originally appeared in *Medical Clinics*, Volume 102, Issue 4, July 2018.

Disclosure Statement: The authors have no conflicts of interest. Dr B.J. Oldfield was supported as a Yale National Clinician Scholar with additional support from the Veterans Health Administration during the conduct of this work. Dr J.M. Tetrault was supported as a Macy Foundation Faculty Scholar during the conduct of this work.

[a] Department of Medicine, Yale University School of Medicine and Public Health, 367 Cedar Street, E.S. Harkness Memorial Hall, Building A, Suite 401, New Haven, CT 06510, USA;
[b] National Clinician Scholars Program, Yale University School of Medicine, PO Box 208088, New Haven, CT 06520, USA; [c] Department of Internal Medicine, Yale University School of Medicine, 367 Cedar Street, Suite 305, New Haven, CT 06510, USA

* Corresponding author.

E-mail address: ejennifer.edelman@yale.edu

treatment of substance use disorder over specialty settings. These advantages include accessibility to patients, ability to tailor services to patient need, reduction of stigma associated with accessing treatment, and the ability to provide many services in one location. Additionally, clinical preventive services are an integral part of primary care medicine, with screening and provision of brief counseling for alcohol use and treatment of tobacco use among the top priorities for the provision of high-quality care.[4]

Through primary care settings, patients may receive a range of evidence-based addiction treatment services, in addition to treatment for tobacco use. These services include US Food and Drug Administration (FDA)-approved medications for alcohol (ie, disulfiram, acamprosate and oral and extended-release [XR] naltrexone) and opioid use disorder (ie, buprenorphine alone or coformulated with naloxone by a certified provider; and oral and XR naltrexone; **Table 1**). Additionally, primary care settings may lend themselves well to the implementation of counseling-based strategies. Specifically, brief counseling may be provided and the Affordable Care Act has supported the integration of additional behavioral health services into primary care. Efforts at treatment expansion have resulted in several proposed approaches for office-based addiction treatment in primary care.

Based on a PubMed and Ovid MEDLINE search designed to identify articles published since 2007 that reported on behavioral and/or medical treatments used in outpatient settings to address alcohol, opioid, and/or stimulant (cocaine, amphetamine) use, we identified office-based approaches to addiction treatment. Herein, we highlight office-based treatment approaches within primary care and a specialty treatment setting (**Box 1**) to address alcohol, opioid, and other substance use.

PRIMARY CARE-BASED APPROACHES
Alcohol

The prevalence of alcohol use disorder in the US population is increasing and has been termed a public health crisis. Certain groups, such as women, older adults,

Table 1
Pharmacotherapy options for alcohol use disorder and opioid use disorder

Generic Name	Usual Daily Dose
FDA approved for alcohol use disorder	
Acamprosate	666 mg orally 3 times daily
Disulfiram	250–500 mg orally daily
Naltrexone	50 mg orally daily
Extended-release Naltrexone	380 mg intramuscularly every 4 wk
Not FDA approved for alcohol use disorder	
Gabapentin	300–600 mg orally 3 times daily
Topiramate	100 mg orally twice daily
FDA approved for opioid use disorder	
Buprenorphine (with and without naloxone)	2–24 mg sublingually daily
Methadone	60–80 mg orally daily
Naltrexone	50 mg orally daily
Extended-release Naltrexone	380 mg intramuscularly every 4 wk

Abbreviation: FDA, US Food and Drug Administration.

Box 1
Approaches to care for addiction treatment

Primary care settings

- Alcohol
  - Brief intervention
  - Clinic-based counseling
  - Pharmacotherapy
  - Technological interventions

- Opioids
  - Pharmacotherapy with variable levels of counseling
  - Primary care based treatment
  - FQHC based treatment
  - Midlevel practitioner models
  - Hub and spoke models
  - Shared medical appointments
  - Improved provider education through Internet-based audiovisual networks to improve care access

- Stimulants
  - Contingency management
  - Cognitive–behavioral therapy with harm reduction framework

Specialty settings

- HIV clinics
  - Alcohol
    - Pharmacotherapy
    - Stepped care
  - Opioids
    - Pharmacotherapy
    - Rapid treatment access programs
  - Stimulants

- Transitions clinics
  - Alcohol
    - Pharmacotherapy
  - Opioids
    - Pharmacotherapy

Abbreviations: FQHC, federally qualified health center; HIV, human immunodeficiency virus.

---

racial/ethnic minorities, and the socioeconomically disadvantaged, are particularly affected.[5] For decades, primary care settings have been considered important sites for the delivery of care to people with alcohol use and related disorders.[6] However, uptake of these treatments remains low: overall only 7.8% of US adults with alcohol use disorder received treatment in 2013.[7] A menu of evidence-based treatments are available in the office setting, including brief interventions by primary providers and other clinicians, clinic-based counseling, pharmacotherapy, referral for specialized treatment, or combinations thereof.

Screening and brief intervention (SBI) is widely recommended for prevention and early intervention of unhealthy alcohol use[8] in primary care settings based on high-quality evidence.[9] SBI, designed to suit the time constraints of primary care, consists of alcohol screening with a validated instrument[10,11] followed by a brief intervention[12] for those who exceed recommended drinking limits. For those who drink alcohol, the National Institute on Alcohol Abuse and Alcoholism recommends screening for unhealthy alcohol use with a single question: "How many times in the past year have you had five or more drinks in a day (for men) or four or more drinks in a day (for women)?"[13] Weekly average (in drinks per week) alcohol intake should be calculated and documented in the medical record. Those who screen positive for at-risk drinking but do not meet criteria for an alcohol use disorder should undergo a brief intervention (**Table 2**). The sequence of Screening, Brief Intervention, and Referral to Treatment (SBIRT) is associated with improvements in alcohol use severity, clinical efficiency, cost, and also is associated with a reduction of disparities in treatment of alcohol use disorder.[14] These interventions can be performed effectively by nurses[15] and other nonphysician clinicians in primary care settings.[16]

The Substance Abuse and Mental Health Services Administration (SAMHSA) allocated significant resources into expanding the continuum of care for unhealthy alcohol and other substance use through demonstration projects and cooperative agreements. Over 5 years, these SAMHSA–funded projects screened more than 1 million patients. Although decreases in substance use were observed, this effort also raised questions about the optimal ways to proceed with SBIRT as a public health intervention. Assessment of another SBIRT implementation project within 5 Veterans Administration Hospital Primary Care clinics found that key informants and stakeholders thought that further training or academic detailing of providers may address SBIRT implementation barriers.[17] Additional data further questions the usefulness of widespread SBIRT implementation for substances other than unhealthy alcohol use, including data suggesting that SBIRT did not improve engagement in specialty treatment.[18,19] Which elements of the counseling provided may be efficacious remains unknown, however,[20,21] and recent evidence suggests SBIRT may not be effective in certain populations (such as people living with human immunodeficiency virus [HIV, PLWH]), or delivered in certain settings.[22] Repeated brief counseling by a registered nurse has been shown to engage patients in alcohol-related care (including the use of pharmacotherapy for alcohol use disorder), but not to improve drinking outcomes at 12 months.[23]

Pharmacotherapy for alcohol use disorder does not require specialized training to prescribe, is efficacious, and is grossly underused,[24–28] and can be prescribed as part of a standard medical management approach (**Table 3**).[29] Naltrexone (in oral and XR forms), acamprosate, and disulfiram are FDA approved for the treatment of alcohol use disorder,[25] and topiramate[24,30,31] and gabapentin[32] have shown efficacy in randomized clinical trials (see **Table 1**). Pharmacotherapy need not be combined with intensive behavioral interventions to be efficacious.[29,33] In medical management, a patient attends office visits with a licensed health professional (physician, nurse, physician assistant, or clinical pharmacist) weekly at first, then spacing to monthly visits. These sessions include a review of drinking, overall level of functioning, medication adherence, and adverse effects. External supports, such as group treatment, can be offered within this approach.[29] The clinician should be prepared to make appropriate counseling referrals if the patient requires a greater intensity of services. With alcohol pharmacotherapy grossly underprescribed, especially by primary care providers, expanding access to these medications will add to the nationwide efforts to address a critical unmet need with an evidence-based approach and further decrease stigma related to treatment.

Technology-delivered interventions can also be incorporated into outpatient practices and have demonstrated feasibility for those with unhealthy alcohol use. Emerging digital technologies (eg, treatment-based digital kiosk) show promise for helping to both hone therapies to patients' individual needs and to support them in settings beyond the clinic, but how to integrate them successfully into outpatient treatment settings remains unknown.[34]

Table 2
How to conduct a brief intervention for unhealthy alcohol use

1. Raise subject	• Hello, I am _____. Would you mind taking a few minutes to talk with me about your alcohol/drug use? <<PAUSE>>
2. Provide feedback	
Review screen	• From what I understand you are drinking/using [insert screening data]... We know that drinking above certain levels or using... can cause problems, such as [insert facts]... I am concerned about your drinking/drug use.
Make connection	• What connection, if any, do you see between your drinking/drug use and this medical visit or other medical issue? **If patient sees connection**: reflect/reiterate what patient has said. **If patient does not see connection**: make one using facts.
Show NIAAA guidelines	• These are what we consider the upper limits of low risk drinking for your age and sex. You would be less likely to experience illness or injury if you stayed within these guidelines.
3. Enhance motivation	
Readiness to change	• **[Show readiness ruler]** On a scale from 1 to 10, how ready are you to change any aspect of your drinking or drug use... Or seek treatment?
Develop discrepancy	• **If patient says:** ≥2 ask: Why did you choose that number and not a lower one? ≤1 or unwilling ask: What would it take for you to become a "2"? What would make this a problem for you? How important would it be for you to prevent that from happening? Have you ever done anything you wish you hadn't while drinking?
Reflective listening	• Reflect/reiterate patients reasons for making a change
4. Negotiate and advise	
Negotiate goal	• What's the next step? *(If a positive next step, reflect it; if not, suggest one.)*
Give advice	• If you can stay within these limits...or reduce or abstain from your drug use... you will be less likely to experience illness/injury related to your use of...
Summarize	• Overall, this is what I've heard you say... *(reflect on reasons for change)*... You have agreed to... *(state actual amounts of reduction of drinking/drug use or to seek treatment.)* I have included this in your discharge instructions that you are signing. This is an agreement between you and yourself.
Suggest follow-up with primary care	• **Suggest follow-up to discuss drinking/drug use.**
Thank patient	• **Thank patient for their time.**

Abbreviation: NIAAA, National Institute on Alcohol Abuse and Alcoholism.
Adapted from D'Onofrio G, Pantalon MV, Degutis LC, et al. Development and implementation of an emergency practitioner-performed brief intervention for hazardous and harmful drinkers in the emergency department. Acad Emerg Med 2005;12(3):252; with permission.

Table 3
Counseling and adjunctive considerations in the provision of pharmacotherapy for AUD and OUD in office-based settings

Pharmacotherapy for AUD	Office-Based Pharmacotherapy for OUD
Counseling	
Medical management	Addiction counseling
• Weekly to monthly 20-min visits with licensed health care professional (physician, nurse, physician assistant, clinical pharmacist)	• Weekly 15- to 30-min visits with licensed health care professional or behavioral health specialist with periodic, longer counseling sessions (30–60 min)
• Review drinking, overall functioning, medication adherence, and adverse effects	• Individual or group therapies that may include elements of cognitive, behavioral, insight-oriented, and/or supportive psychotherapies
• Encourage attendance at support groups and other community resources	Cognitive–behavioral therapy
Combined behavioral intervention	• Weekly to biweekly 50-min visits with licensed behavioral health specialist
• Weekly to biweekly 50-min visits with licensed behavioral health specialist	
• Integrates aspects of cognitive behavioral therapy, 12-step facilitation, motivational interviewing, and support system involvement	
Patient education	
Medication interactions	Medication interactions
• Naltrexone should not be used concurrently with opioids	• Concurrent use of alcohol, benzodiazepines, or gabapentin with buprenorphine may increase risk of sedation, respiratory depression, and death
	• Naltrexone should not be used concurrently with opioids
	Pain syndromes
	• Strategies should be offered regarding how to manage pain syndromes without misusing opioids or other drugs
Laboratory testing	
Hepatic aminotransferases	Urine toxicology
• For patients receiving naltrexone, aspartate aminotransferase and alanine aminotransferase should be checked before initiation and periodically; elevations >3–5 times the upper limit of normal should prompt discontinuation or transition to another option	• Periodic urine drug testing to assess risk of medication interaction (eg, risk of overdose with buprenorphine and concurrent benzodiazepine use)
	Hepatic aminotransferases
	• For patients receiving naltrexone, aspartate aminotransferase and alanine aminotransferase should be checked before initiation and periodically; elevations >3–5 times the upper limit of normal should prompt discontinuation or transition to another option

Abbreviations: AUD, alcohol use disorder; OUD, opioid use disorder.

Opioids

The cornerstone of treatment for opioid use disorder is pharmacotherapy[35,36] and models for integrating pharmacotherapy into office-based settings vary in structure.[37] FDA-approved medications include a full opioid agonist (methadone), which can be only delivered in specialty treatment settings for treatment of opioid use disorder; partial opioid agonists (buprenorphine sublingual, buprenorphine-naloxone sublingual or buccal, and implantable buprenorphine); and opioid antagonists (oral and XR naltrexone).[37] Naltrexone may be an attractive option for patients with mild opioid use disorder, those in situations where medication administration can be supervised, and those with occupations that do not permit opioid agonist treatment. However, data to compare the efficacy of opioid agonists versus naltrexone are just beginning to emerge.[38,39] These pharmacotherapies more effectively reduce opioid use than behavioral treatment alone, translating into improved health outcomes and survival, and the Office of National Drug Control Policy and the US Department of Health and Human Services have recently prioritized increasing access to pharmacotherapy for opioid use disorder, with a focus on primary care providers.[40] With the goal of initiating treatment for opioid use disorder as soon as possible, patients are increasingly initiated on pharmacotherapy in emergency department and inpatient settings.[41–44] Additionally, new treatment options now include XR buprenorphine.

The advent of buprenorphine and the passage of the Drug Addiction Treatment Act in 2000 transformed the opioid use disorder delivery system by granting physicians the ability to administer office-based opioid agonist treatment.[45] Although fixed-dose buprenorphine, in most studies, is considered noninferior to moderate doses of methadone in terms of retention in treatment and illicit opioid use,[36] buprenorphine is generally considered a safer alternative to methadone.[46] In primary care settings, ongoing maintenance treatment in patients with prescription opioid use disorder who receive buprenorphine is more efficacious than tapering.[47] Concurrent counseling along with buprenorphine pharmacotherapy need not be extensive: brief, once-weekly counseling with once-weekly medication dispensing is no less efficacious than extended weekly counseling and more frequent dispensing.[48] Primary care-based options are available for counseling provided concurrently with buprenorphine (see **Table 3**). Patients who also take benzodiazepines, have severe alcohol use disorder, or have severe respiratory diseases are at risk of respiratory depression with buprenorphine[49] and, therefore, may benefit from specialist referral for a higher level of monitoring.

Given that a great deal of additional resources are not needed to provide buprenorphine in primary care, Federally Qualified Health Centers are an ideal clinical setting to offer office-based addiction treatment.[50] Buprenorphine may be successfully initiated by primary providers, but approaches in which a specialist performs initial psychological evaluation and initiates buprenorphine, then transitions patients once stabilized to community health centers, also show efficacy.[51] Collaborative care consisting of generalist clinicians working alongside nurse care managers, who perform patient education, obtain informed consent, develop treatment plans, oversee medication management, refer to specialty care, and monitor adherence, provides successful treatment to most patients with opioid and/or alcohol use disorder and makes effective use of time for physicians who prescribe buprenorphine.[52–54] The recent passage of legislation allowing advance practice nurse practitioners and physician assistants the ability to provide buprenorphine after 24 hours of training will open the door for the development of new and innovative models of care delivery. On a health systems level, hub-and-spoke models allow for centralized intake at a "hub," and then patients are connected to "spokes" in primary care settings for ongoing management.[55,56]

Group visit models (ie, shared medical appointments) can be important and efficient sites of primary care for patients with opioid use disorder, including pharmacotherapy with buprenorphine. Group visit models allow providers to see many patients at once, decrease relapse rates and craving, and increase treatment retention rates.[57,58] They may also foster group-specific communication behaviors that uniquely support patients through treatment.[59] Groups, described and offered to patients during individual visits, are typically hour-long sessions that occur weekly with rolling enrollment, and thus continually welcome new patients in varying stages of treatment. Urine drug testing samples are taken weekly, and the previous week's results may be posted for the group to see if all consent. Patients check in about their week and engage in psychoeducation related to addiction self-management skills.[59] Internet-based, audiovisual networks for provider education can increase access to buprenorphine in rural areas, and can emphasize and empower the physician assistants and nurse practitioners in the primary care of those with opioid use disorder. In the Project Extension for Community Healthcare Outcomes model (ECHO), an MD/DO primary care provider, nurse practitioner, or physician assistant performs an initial evaluation and screening and then refers to a collaborating physician for mentored buprenorphine prescribing.[60] Telemedicine models, in which a patient presents at a secure videoconferencing site under the supervision of a nurse and videoconferences with a buprenorphine provider, have successfully increased access to buprenorphine in Canada.[61] Text message interventions can foster patients' self-efficacy and facilitate unobserved, home initiation of buprenorphine.[62]

XR naltrexone can be successfully integrated into some of the models of care described herein, including the collaborative care between generalists and nurse care managers.[52,53] One-stop shop models, or integrated centers in mental health clinics that provide psychosocial services, primary care, care for comorbid conditions such as HIV and hepatitis C virus, and harm reduction services such as syringe exchange, are well-suited to offer naltrexone and other pharmacotherapies as treatment options.[63]

As with treatment of alcohol use disorder, approaches focusing on the movement of the treatment of opioid use disorder out of specialty settings and into office-based care, with delivery of a medical model by an interdisciplinary team, offers the greatest potential for patient success. Additionally, this approach increases treatment access and decreases treatment-related stigma. Based on resources, alternative models such as those that rely on a hub-and-spoke model or telemedicine may also be appropriate.

Other Drugs

There is limited evidence for effective treatment of cocaine and other stimulants, as well as other drug use disorders in office-based settings. Current data do not support the use of anticonvulsants,[64] dopamine agonists,[65] antipsychotics,[66] or antidepressants[67] in the management of cocaine use disorder. Some evidence supports the effectiveness of disulfiram for cocaine use disorder, but large-scale, randomized trials are lacking.[68] Contingency management (CM), a psychosocial treatment that offers rewards and incentives for demonstration of reduced use or abstinence, show positive but short-lived efficacy and likely represents the best currently available treatment option (**Table 4**).[69,70]

Methamphetamine use disorder presents a similar conundrum to office-based providers. No pharmacotherapies are currently FDA approved for methamphetamine use disorder.[71–73] CM again may be an efficacious option.[73–76] In addition, community-based cognitive–behavioral therapy that uses a harm reduction framework has been effective in the treatment of methamphetamine use disorder in men who have sex with men, but large or randomized studies of these interventions are lacking.[77,78]

Given the limited evidence for managing these disorders in primary care settings, patients with these disorders, particularly those with complex withdrawal, psychiatric comorbidity, or medical comorbidity, should be considered for referral to higher levels of care.

Table 4	
Prize-based contingency management: Rewarded behaviors	
Behavior	**Comments/Examples**
Health-related activities	• Scheduling a medical or nutritionist appointment • Obtaining medications • Recording medication or food consumption daily • Exercising.
General goal-related activities	Activities that focused on • Abstinence • Recreation • Transportation • Housing • Legal • Education or employment • Psychiatric or personal improvement
Submission of a test to assess for abstinence	• Submission of urine and breath samples to assess for drug and alcohol use, respectively
Evidence of abstinence	• Negative urine and breath samples, with potential for increased earnings if abstinence from both drugs and alcohol demonstrated and over time

Data from Petry NM, Weinstock J, Alessi SM, et al. Group-based randomized trial of contingencies for health and abstinence in HIV patients. J Consult Clin Psychol 2010;78(1):89–97.

SPECIALTY SETTINGS AND POPULATIONS
Human Immunodeficiency Virus Clinics

Among PLWH, alcohol and other substance use adversely impacts care along the HIV care continuum, resulting in uncontrolled HIV with negative consequences for the individual and public health. To address this problem, the integration of addiction treatment and HIV care is recommended by national and international organizations.[79,80] Several approaches have been developed and evaluated to promote addiction treatment in HIV clinics, and others are actively being investigated.

Alcohol

XR naltrexone decreases heavy drinking days among those with alcohol use disorder[33] and is safe for use in PLWH, including those on antiretroviral therapy.[81,82] The availability of an injectable formulation with monthly administration avoids adding to pill burden, an important consideration for this population. A recent study demonstrated the feasibility and acceptability of XR naltrexone for alcohol use disorder in combination with medical management when delivered in HIV clinics.[83] These findings were supported by a separate randomized clinical trial that evaluated the impact of XR naltrexone versus placebo on HIV-related and drinking outcomes among PLWH with heavy alcohol use and suboptimal antiretroviral therapy adherence.[84] In this study, participants in both treatment groups also received counseling, which incorporated medical management and medication coaching.[29,85] By combining these 2 efficacious behavioral treatments, participants received counseling and advice to decrease alcohol use by health care practitioners with referral to mutual help groups (eg, Alcoholics Anonymous) and education regarding the importance of and strategies to promote antiretroviral medication adherence. Compared with the placebo group, those randomized to XR naltrexone demonstrated a decrease in heavy alcohol use; this result, however, did not translate into improved antiretroviral therapy adherence or other HIV-related outcomes (ie, HIV viral load, CD4 cell count, and VACS Index score [a validated measure of morbidity and mortality based on routinely collected laboratory data]).[84]

In the STEP Trials (Starting Treatment for Ethanol in Primary Care), the effectiveness of integrated stepped care to address unhealthy alcohol use among PLWH when delivered in HIV clinics is being evaluated.[86] In this approach to care and consistent with approaches used for the treatment of medical conditions routinely treated in office-based settings (eg, depression, diabetes mellitus, and hypertension), individuals receive an increasing intensity of services depending on their treatment response and level of alcohol use, including a social worker-delivered brief negotiation interview with a follow-up telephone booster at 2 weeks, 4 sessions of psychologist-delivered motivational enhancement therapy, addiction physician management with consideration of alcohol pharmacotherapy, and/or referral to a higher level of care (eg, detoxification, intensive outpatient program). This approach holds promise for addressing unhealthy alcohol use among patients with moderate alcohol and liver disease[87]; however, the impact of this approach on addressing at-risk drinking and alcohol use disorder is actively being studied.

Findings that PLWH are 14% less likely than uninfected patients to receive evidence-based alcohol-related care after a positive screen for unhealthy alcohol use[88] underscore the need for ongoing research and implementation efforts. Given the lack of training and comfort with delivering alcohol-related care among HIV providers,[89] approaches that include multidisciplinary care as applied in the STEP Trials or include targeted training, are likely to be most effective in specialty settings.

Opioids

The BHIVES Collaborative (Buprenorphine HIV Evaluation and Support), a 10-site demonstration project, led to the implementation and evaluation of integration HIV care and buprenorphine/naloxone for opioid use disorder. Before patient enrollment, physicians and clinical staff participated in an 8-hour training on buprenorphine, which was followed by the opportunity for sites to participate in monthly 1-hour-long technical assistance conference calls to discuss issues related to clinical management and access to a restricted access listserv to allow for discussion of clinical issues via email and dissemination of appropriate clinical support material. In addition, technical assistance was provided as needed during annual meetings, site visits, and individually via phone and email.[90] This demonstration project revealed the importance of multidisciplinary teams for implementing buprenorphine/naloxone in HIV clinics. Specifically, these programs had multiple prescribers (ie, 2–5 depending on patient census) to ensure sufficient coverage coupled with a nonphysician "buprenorphine/naloxone coordinator." This coordinator, who had varying credentials across sites (ie, licensed practice nurse, registered nurse, nurse practitioner, certified substance use counselor, health educator, or pharmacist) was essential and offered counseling and case management services, and served as a link between the patients and providers; in some clinics, this individual also performed outreach services.[91] This approach to care is associated with improvements in HIV and substance use-related outcomes, as well as other important outcomes.[90,92–96]

In the FAST PATH program (Facilitated Access to Substance abuse Treatment with Prevention And Treatment for HIV), which has been implemented in both HIV and general medical clinics, a physician, nurse care manager, and licensed addiction counselor together deliver care to address addiction treatment needs to people living with and at increased risk for HIV. Physicians provided addiction care along with primary care (if primary care was not already provided by another provider). FAST PATH included the following services: an initial multidisciplinary team visit including the physician, nurse, and addiction counselor, addiction pharmacotherapy with medication monitoring with treatment agreements, urine drug testing and pill counts, weekly individual and group addiction counseling with the addiction counselor, HIV risk reduction and overdose prevention counseling, case management and facilitated referral for higher level of services as needed, and ongoing coordination with the primary care team. On-site face-to-face buprenorphine inductions were conducted by the nurse. Counseling provided by addiction counselors included cognitive behavioral therapy, with the addition of motivational interviewing–based therapy for those with ongoing substance use, plus encouragement of engagement in 12-step programs. In this approach to care, buprenorphine receipt was associated with improved treatment engagement and qualitative data revealed patient endorsement of this approach.[97,98]

In addition to the provision of buprenorphine, XR naltrexone may offer a future potential treatment option to address opioid use disorder in isolation or in combination with comorbid alcohol use disorder. However, larger studies are first needed to evaluate its efficacy and effectiveness in HIV treatment settings.[83]

In specialty HIV settings, on-site addiction treatment provided by a multidisciplinary team and linkage to enhanced clinical services offers the best approach for patient success. Other public health benefits of this approach include improvement in access to care and destigmatization of opioid use disorder and its treatment.

Other substances

Similar to primary care settings, few treatment approaches have shown efficacy for the treatment of other substance use disorders in specialty treatment settings. CM is an effective intervention to address stimulant use with similar benefits in individuals with and without HIV.[99] Offered through a HIV drop-in center and involving a sample of PLWH in which the majority had cocaine dependence, prize-based CM increased the number of consecutive drug-free urine specimens, and decreased HIV viral load and HIV risk behaviors during the treatment period when compared with a 12-step treatment approach.[100] In this study, specific behaviors were reinforced (see **Table 4**). These findings complement other studies in HIV treatment settings that use CM and rewards-based interventions to promote antiretroviral therapy adherence and decrease HIV viral load.[101]

Lesbian, Gay, Bisexual, and Transgender Populations

Substance use is more common among men who have sex with men and associated with increased HIV risk behaviors and health disparities. However, there are few high-quality studies to guide how to best implement an approach to care to address tobacco, alcohol, or opioid use among MSM in primary-care based settings.[73] Although a recent review demonstrates support for use of motivational interviewing/motivational enhancement therapy and CBT-based approaches to address alcohol use, future work is needed to address this critical area to generate evidence to guide best practices.[102]

People Transitioning Out of Incarceration

An increasing number of studies have evaluated treatment strategies to address substance use, including alcohol and opioid use, among people transitioning out of incarceration. These approaches include the initiation of pharmacotherapy before release into the community. In post hoc analyses, 1 such study found that, among PLWH, XR naltrexone decreased the time to relapse to heavy drinking.[103] Given the particularly high risk of opioid-related overdose after release from incarceration,[104] there have been a number of studies to address this problem. These studies have largely focused on evaluating use of XR naltrexone before release into the community and demonstrated decreased rates of relapse to opioid use.[105,106]

SUMMARY AND FUTURE CONSIDERATIONS

There are a range of approaches to care, incorporating both medications and behaviorally based interventions, that may be applied to primary care and specialty settings, such as HIV clinics, to address alcohol, opioid, and other substance use. Given the pressing need to address the treatment gap, efforts to design and evaluate interventions that promote implementation of these approaches to care are critical and are underway. Future work should also aim to refine quality metrics for assessing quality of addiction treatment services in primary care-based settings and in coordination with other community-based and addiction specialty settings. Last, the importance of ongoing provider education to the implementation and maintenance of effective approaches to care for patients with substance use disorder is vital.

ACKNOWLEDGMENTS

The editors thank P. Todd Korthuis, Oregon Health and Science University, for providing a critical review of this article. The authors acknowledge Janis Glover for her assistance with conducting the literature review.

REFERENCES

1. Lipari RN, Park-Lee E, Van Horn S. America's need for and receipt of substance use treatment in 2015. The CBHSQ report. Rockville (MD): Substance Abuse and Mental Health Services Administration (US); 2013.
2. Tetrault JM, Petrakis IL. Partnering with psychiatry to close the education gap: an approach to the addiction epidemic. J Gen Intern Med 2017;32(12):1387–9.
3. Saitz R, Daaleman TP. Now is the time to address substance use disorders in primary care. Ann Fam Med 2017;15(4):306–8.
4. Maciosek MV, LaFrance AB, Dehmer SP, et al. Updated priorities among effective clinical preventive services. Ann Fam Med 2017;15(1):14–22.
5. Grant BF, Chou SP, Saha TD, et al. Prevalence of 12-month alcohol use, high-risk drinking, and DSM-IV alcohol use disorder in the United States, 2001-2002 to 2012-2013: results from the national epidemiologic survey on alcohol and related conditions. JAMA Psychiatry 2017;74(9):911–23.
6. Babor TF, Ritson EB, Hodgson RJ. Alcohol-related problems in the primary health care setting: a review of early intervention strategies. Br J Addict 1986; 81(1):23–46.
7. Substance Abuse and Mental Health Services Administration (SAMHSA). Results from the 2013 National survey on drug use and health: summary of national findings. Rockville (MD): Substance Abuse and Mental Health Services Administration; 2014. NSDUH Series H-48, DHHS Publication No. (SMA) 04-4863.
8. U.S. Preventive Services Task Force. Final recommendation statement: alcohol misuse: screening and behavioral counseling interventions in primary care. 2013. Available at: https://www.uspreventiveservicestaskforce.org/Page/

Document/RecommendationStatementFinal/alcohol-misuse-screening-and-behavioral-counseling-interventions-in-primary-care. Accessed March 26, 2018.

9. Jonas DE, Garbutt JC, Amick HR, et al. Behavioral counseling after screening for alcohol misuse in primary care: a systematic review and meta-analysis for the U.S. Preventive Services Task Force. Ann Intern Med 2012;157(9):645–54.

10. Bush K, Kivlahan DR, McDonell MB, et al. The AUDIT alcohol consumption questions (AUDIT-C): an effective brief screening test for problem drinking. Ambulatory Care Quality Improvement Project (ACQUIP). Alcohol use disorders identification test. Arch Intern Med 1998;158(16):1789–95.

11. Saitz R. Lost in translation: the perils of implementing alcohol brief intervention when there are gaps in evidence and its interpretation. Addiction 2014;109(7):1060–2.

12. Moyer VA, Preventive Services Task Force. Screening and behavioral counseling interventions in primary care to reduce alcohol misuse: U.S. preventive services task force recommendation statement. Ann Intern Med 2013;159(3):210–8.

13. National Institute on Alcohol Abuse and Alcoholism (NIAAA). Helping patients who drink too much: a clinician's guide. U.S. Department of Health & Human Services; 2005. Available at: https://pubs.niaaa.nih.gov/publications/Practitioner/CliniciansGuide2005/guide.pdf. Accessed March 26, 2018.

14. Babor TF, Del Boca F, Bray JW. Screening, brief intervention and referral to treatment: implications of SAMHSA's SBIRT initiative for substance abuse policy and practice. Addiction 2017;112(Suppl 2):110–7.

15. Joseph J, Basu D, Dandapani M, et al. Are nurse-conducted brief interventions (NCBIs) efficacious for hazardous or harmful alcohol use? A systematic review. Int Nurs Rev 2014;61(2):203–10.

16. Sullivan LE, Tetrault JM, Braithwaite RS, et al. A meta-analysis of the efficacy of nonphysician brief interventions for unhealthy alcohol use: implications for the patient-centered medical home. Am J Addict 2011;20(4):343–56.

17. Williams EC, Achtmeyer CE, Young JP, et al. Local implementation of alcohol screening and brief intervention at five veterans health administration primary care clinics: perspectives of clinical and administrative staff. J Subst Abuse Treat 2016;60:27–35.

18. Aldridge A, Dowd W, Bray J. The relative impact of brief treatment versus brief intervention in primary health-care screening programs for substance use disorders. Addiction 2017;112(Suppl 2):54–64.

19. Kim TW, Bernstein J, Cheng DM, et al. Receipt of addiction treatment as a consequence of a brief intervention for drug use in primary care: a randomized trial. Addiction 2017;112(5):818–27.

20. McCambridge J, Rollnick S. Should brief interventions in primary care address alcohol problems more strongly? Addiction 2014;109(7):1054–8.

21. McCambridge J, Saitz R. Rethinking brief interventions for alcohol in general practice. BMJ 2017;356:j116.

22. Williams EC, Lapham GT, Bobb JF, et al. Documented brief intervention not associated with resolution of unhealthy alcohol use one year later among VA patients living with HIV. J Subst Abuse Treat 2017;78:8–14.

23. Bradley KA, Bobb JF, Ludman EJ, et al. Alcohol-Related Nurse Care Management in Primary Care: A Randomized Clinical Trial. JAMA Intern Med 2018;178(5):613–21.

24. Del Re AC, Gordon AJ, Lembke A, et al. Prescription of topiramate to treat alcohol use disorders in the Veterans Health Administration. Addict Sci Clin Pract 2013;8:12.
25. Harris AH, Kivlahan DR, Bowe T, et al. Pharmacotherapy of alcohol use disorders in the Veterans Health Administration. Psychiatr Serv 2010;61(4):392–8.
26. Harris AH, Oliva E, Bowe T, et al. Pharmacotherapy of alcohol use disorders by the Veterans Health Administration: patterns of receipt and persistence. Psychiatr Serv 2012;63(7):679–85.
27. Marienfeld C, Iheanacho T, Issa M, et al. Long-acting injectable depot naltrexone use in the Veterans' Health Administration: a national study. Addict Behav 2014;39(2):434–8.
28. Petrakis IL, Leslie D, Rosenheck R. Use of naltrexone in the treatment of alcoholism nationally in the Department of Veterans Affairs. Alcohol Clin Exp Res 2003;27(11):1780–4.
29. Anton RF, O'Malley SS, Ciraulo DA, et al. Combined pharmacotherapies and behavioral interventions for alcohol dependence: the COMBINE study: a randomized controlled trial. JAMA 2006;295(17):2003–17.
30. Arbaizar B, Diersen-Sotos T, Gomez-Acebo I, et al. Topiramate in the treatment of alcohol dependence: a meta-analysis. Actas Esp Psiquiatr 2010;38(1):8–12.
31. Johnson BA, Rosenthal N, Capece JA, et al. Topiramate for treating alcohol dependence: a randomized controlled trial. JAMA 2007;298(14):1641–51.
32. Mason BJ, Quello S, Goodell V, et al. Gabapentin treatment for alcohol dependence: a randomized clinical trial. JAMA Intern Med 2014;174(1):70–7.
33. Jonas DE, Amick HR, Feltner C, et al. Pharmacotherapy for adults with alcohol use disorders in outpatient settings: a systematic review and meta-analysis. JAMA 2014;311(18):1889–900.
34. Muench F. The promises and pitfalls of digital technology in its application to alcohol treatment. Alcohol Res 2014;36(1):131–42.
35. Mattick RP, Breen C, Kimber J, et al. Methadone maintenance therapy versus no opioid replacement therapy for opioid dependence. Cochrane Database Syst Rev 2009;(3):CD002209.
36. Mattick RP, Breen C, Kimber J, et al. Buprenorphine maintenance versus placebo or methadone maintenance for opioid dependence. Cochrane Database Syst Rev 2014;(2):CD002207.
37. Korthuis PT, McCarty D, Weimer M, et al. Primary care-based models for the treatment of opioid use disorder: a scoping review. Ann Intern Med 2017; 166(4):268–78.
38. Tanum L, Solli KK, Latif ZE, et al. Effectiveness of injectable extended-release naltrexone vs daily buprenorphine-naloxone for opioid dependence: a randomized clinical noninferiority trial. JAMA Psychiatry 2017;74(12):1197–205.
39. Lee JD, Nunes EV Jr, Novo P, et al. Comparative effectiveness of extended-release naltrexone versus buprenorphine-naloxone for opioid relapse prevention (X: BOT): a multicentre, open-label, randomised controlled trial. Lancet 2017; 391(10118):309–18.
40. Macrae J, Hyde P, Slavitt A. HHS launches multi-pronged effort to combat opioid abuse, vol. 2017. HHS Blog; 2015. Available at: https://blog.samhsa.gov/2015/07/27/hhs-launches-multi-pronged-effort-to-combat-opioid-abuse/#.Wrj_3OzwbIU. Accessed March 26, 2018.
41. D'Onofrio G, O'Connor PG, Pantalon MV, et al. Emergency department-initiated buprenorphine/naloxone treatment for opioid dependence: a randomized clinical trial. JAMA 2015;313(16):1636–44.

42. Liebschutz JM, Crooks D, Herman D, et al. Buprenorphine treatment for hospitalized, opioid-dependent patients: a randomized clinical trial. JAMA Intern Med 2014;174(8):1369–76.
43. Wakeman SE, Metlay JP, Chang Y, et al. Inpatient addiction consultation for hospitalized patients increases post-discharge abstinence and reduces addiction severity. J Gen Intern Med 2017;32(8):909–16.
44. Englander H, Weimer M, Solotaroff R, et al. Planning and designing the improving addiction care team (IMPACT) for hospitalized adults with substance use disorder. J Hosp Med 2017;12(5):339–42.
45. Kraus ML, Alford DP, Kotz MM, et al. Statement of the American Society Of Addiction Medicine Consensus Panel on the use of buprenorphine in office-based treatment of opioid addiction. J Addict Med 2011;5(4):254–63.
46. Bell JR, Butler B, Lawrance A, et al. Comparing overdose mortality associated with methadone and buprenorphine treatment. Drug Alcohol Depend 2009;104(1–2):73–7.
47. Fiellin DA, Schottenfeld RS, Cutter CJ, et al. Primary care-based buprenorphine taper vs maintenance therapy for prescription opioid dependence: a randomized clinical trial. JAMA Intern Med 2014;174(12):1947–54.
48. Fiellin DA, Pantalon MV, Chawarski MC, et al. Counseling plus buprenorphine-naloxone maintenance therapy for opioid dependence. N Engl J Med 2006;355(4):365–74.
49. Tracqui A, Kintz P, Ludes B. Buprenorphine-related deaths among drug addicts in France: a report on 20 fatalities. J Anal Toxicol 1998;22(6):430–4.
50. Haddad MS, Zelenev A, Altice FL. Buprenorphine maintenance treatment retention improves nationally recommended preventive primary care screenings when integrated into urban federally qualified health centers. J Urban Health 2015;92(1):193–213.
51. Stoller KB. A collaborative opioid prescribing (CoOP) model linking opioid treatment programs with office-based buprenorphine providers. Addict Sci Clin Pract 2015;10(Suppl 1):A63.
52. Alford DP, LaBelle CT, Kretsch N, et al. Collaborative care of opioid-addicted patients in primary care using buprenorphine: five-year experience. Arch Intern Med 2011;171(5):425–31.
53. LaBelle CT, Han SC, Bergeron A, et al. Office-based opioid treatment with buprenorphine (OBOT-B): statewide implementation of the Massachusetts collaborative care model in community health centers. J Subst Abuse Treat 2016;60:6–13.
54. Watkins KE, Ober AJ, Lamp K, et al. Collaborative care for opioid and alcohol use disorders in primary care: the SUMMIT randomized clinical trial. JAMA Intern Med 2017;177(10):1480–8.
55. Patient-Centered Primary Care Collaborative. Vermont hub and spokes health homes statewide. Available at: www.pcpcc.org/initiate/vermont-hub-and-spokes-health-homes. Accessed September 22, 2017.
56. Brooklyn JR, Sigmon SC. Vermont hub-and-spoke model of care for opioid use disorder: development, implementation, and impact. J Addict Med 2017;11(4):286–92.
57. Berger R, Pulido C, Lacro J, et al. Group medication management for buprenorphine/naloxone in opioid-dependent veterans. J Addict Med 2014;8(6):415–20.
58. Suzuki J, Zinser J, Klaiber B, et al. Feasibility of implementing shared medical appointments (SMAs) for office-based opioid treatment with buprenorphine: a pilot study. Subst Abus 2015;36(2):166–9.

59. Sokol R, Albanese C, Chaponis D, et al. Why use group visits for opioid use disorder treatment in primary care? A patient-centered qualitative study. Subst Abus 2018;39(1):52–8.

60. Komaromy M, Duhigg D, Metcalf A, et al. Project ECHO (Extension for Community Healthcare Outcomes): a new model for educating primary care providers about treatment of substance use disorders. Subst Abus 2016;37(1):20–4.

61. Eibl JK, Gauthier G, Pellegrini D, et al. The effectiveness of telemedicine-delivered opioid agonist therapy in a supervised clinical setting. Drug Alcohol Depend 2017;176:133–8.

62. Tofighi B, Grossman E, Bereket S, et al. Text message content preferences to improve buprenorphine maintenance treatment in primary care. J Addict Dis 2016;35(2):92–100.

63. LifeSpring Health Systems. About us: locations. 2016. Available at: www.lifespringhealthsystems.org/about-us/locations. Accessed September 22, 2017.

64. Minozzi S, Cinquini M, Amato L, et al. Anticonvulsants for cocaine dependence. Cochrane Database Syst Rev 2015;(4):CD006754.

65. Minozzi S, Amato L, Pani PP, et al. Dopamine agonists for the treatment of cocaine dependence. Cochrane Database Syst Rev 2015;(5):CD003352.

66. Indave BI, Minozzi S, Pani PP, et al. Antipsychotic medications for cocaine dependence. Cochrane Database Syst Rev 2016;(3):CD006306.

67. Pani PP, Trogu E, Vecchi S, et al. Antidepressants for cocaine dependence and problematic cocaine use. Cochrane Database Syst Rev 2011;(12):CD002950.

68. Pani PP, Trogu E, Vacca R, et al. Disulfiram for the treatment of cocaine dependence. Cochrane Database Syst Rev 2010;(1):CD007024.

69. Fischer B, Blanken P, Da Silveira D, et al. Effectiveness of secondary prevention and treatment interventions for crack-cocaine abuse: a comprehensive narrative overview of English-language studies. Int J Drug Policy 2015;26(4):352–63.

70. Dutra L, Stathopoulou G, Basden SL, et al. A meta-analytic review of psychosocial interventions for substance use disorders. Am J Psychiatry 2008;165(2):179–87.

71. Kampman KM. The search for medications to treat stimulant dependence. Addict Sci Clin Pract 2008;4(2):28–35.

72. Karila L, Weinstein A, Aubin HJ, et al. Pharmacological approaches to methamphetamine dependence: a focused review. Br J Clin Pharmacol 2010;69(6):578–92.

73. Coffin PO, Santos GM, Hern J, et al. Extended-release naltrexone for methamphetamine dependence among men who have sex with men: a randomized placebo-controlled trial. Addiction 2018;113(2):268–78.

74. Roll JM. Contingency management: an evidence-based component of methamphetamine use disorder treatments. Addiction 2007;102(Suppl 1):114–20.

75. Roll JM, Petry NM, Stitzer ML, et al. Contingency management for the treatment of methamphetamine use disorders. Am J Psychiatry 2006;163(11):1993–9.

76. Shoptaw S, Huber A, Peck J, et al. Randomized, placebo-controlled trial of sertraline and contingency management for the treatment of methamphetamine dependence. Drug Alcohol Depend 2006;85(1):12–8.

77. Carrico AW, Flentje A, Gruber VA, et al. Community-based harm reduction substance abuse treatment with methamphetamine-using men who have sex with men. J Urban Health 2014;91(3):555–67.

78. Reback CJ, Veniegas R, Shoptaw S. Getting Off: development of a model program for gay and bisexual male methamphetamine users. J Homosex 2014;61(4):540–53.

79. Office of National AIDS Policy. The national HIV/AIDS strategy: updated to 2020. Washington, DC: The White House; 2015.

80. United Nations Office on Drugs and Crime, International Network of People Who Use Drugs, Joint United Nations Programme on HIV/AIDS, United Nations Development Programme, United Nations Population Fund, World Health Organization, United States Agency for International Development. Implementing comprehensive HIV and HCV programmes with people who inject drugs: practical guidance for collaborative interventions. Vienna (Austria): United Nations Office on Drugs and Crime; 2017.

81. Tetrault JM, Tate JP, McGinnis KA, et al. Hepatic safety and antiretroviral effectiveness in HIV-infected patients receiving naltrexone. Alcohol Clin Exp Res 2012;36(2):318–24.

82. Vagenas P, Di Paola A, Herme M, et al. An evaluation of hepatic enzyme elevations among HIV-infected released prisoners enrolled in two randomized placebo-controlled trials of extended release naltrexone. J Subst Abuse Treat 2014;47(1):35–40.

83. Korthuis PT, Lum PJ, Vergara-Rodriguez P, et al. Feasibility and safety of extended-release naltrexone treatment of opioid and alcohol use disorder in HIV clinics: a pilot/feasibility randomized trial. Addiction 2017;112(6):1036–44.

84. Edelman EJ, Moore B, Holt S, et al. The impact of injectable naltrexone on antiretroviral therapy adherence, HIV viral load, and drinking in HIV-positive heavy drinkers. Paper presented at: Research Society on Alcoholism. Denver, CO, June 26, 2017.

85. Haug NA, Sorensen JL, Gruber VA, et al. HAART adherence strategies for methadone clients who are HIV-positive: a treatment manual for implementing contingency management and medication coaching. Behav Modif 2006;30(6):752–81.

86. Edelman EJ, Maisto SA, Hansen NB, et al. The Starting Treatment for Ethanol in Primary care Trials (STEP Trials): Protocol for Three Parallel Multi-Site Stepped Care Effectiveness Studies for Unhealthy Alcohol Use in HIV-Positive Patients. Contemp Clin Trials 2017;52:80–90.

87. Edelman EJ, Maisto SA, Hansen NB, et al. Integrated stepped care to address moderate alcohol use among HIV-positive patients with liver disease: Results from a randomized controlled clinical trial. Presented as an oral presentation at INEBRIA, September 15, 2017, New York, New York.

88. Williams EC, Lapham GT, Shortreed SM, et al. Among patients with unhealthy alcohol use, those with HIV are less likely than those without to receive evidence-based alcohol-related care: a national VA study. Drug Alcohol Depend 2017;174:113–20.

89. Chander G, Monroe AK, Crane HM, et al. HIV primary care providers–Screening, knowledge, attitudes and behaviors related to alcohol interventions. Drug Alcohol Depend 2016;161:59–66.

90. Fiellin DA, Weiss L, Botsko M, et al. Drug treatment outcomes among HIV-infected opioid-dependent patients receiving buprenorphine/naloxone. J Acquir Immune Defic Syndr 2011;56(Suppl 1):S33–8.

91. Weiss L, Netherland J, Egan JE, et al. Integration of buprenorphine/naloxone treatment into HIV clinical care: lessons from the BHIVES collaborative. J Acquir Immune Defic Syndr 2011;56(Suppl 1):S68–75.

92. Altice FL, Bruce RD, Lucas GM, et al. HIV treatment outcomes among HIV-infected, opioid-dependent patients receiving buprenorphine/naloxone treatment within HIV clinical care settings: results from a multisite study. J Acquir Immune Defic Syndr 2011;56(Suppl 1):S22–32.

93. Edelman EJ, Chantarat T, Caffrey S, et al. The impact of buprenorphine/naloxone treatment on HIV risk behaviors among HIV-infected, opioid-dependent patients. Drug Alcohol Depend 2014;139:79–85.

94. Tetrault JM, Moore BA, Barry DT, et al. Brief versus extended counseling along with buprenorphine/naloxone for HIV-infected opioid dependent patients. J Subst Abuse Treat 2012;43(4):433–9.

95. Korthuis PT, Tozzi MJ, Nandi V, et al. Improved quality of life for opioid-dependent patients receiving buprenorphine treatment in HIV clinics. J Acquir Immune Defic Syndr 2011;56(Suppl 1):S39–45.

96. Korthuis PT, Fiellin DA, Fu R, et al. Improving adherence to HIV quality of care indicators in persons with opioid dependence: the role of buprenorphine. J Acquir Immune Defic Syndr 2011;56(Suppl 1):S83–90.

97. Drainoni ML, Farrell C, Sorensen-Alawad A, et al. Patient perspectives of an integrated program of medical care and substance use treatment. AIDS Patient Care STDS 2014;28(2):71–81.

98. Walley AY, Palmisano J, Sorensen-Alawad A, et al. Engagement and substance dependence in a primary care-based addiction treatment program for people infected with HIV and people at high-risk for HIV infection. J Subst Abuse Treat 2015;59:59–66.

99. Burch AE, Rash CJ, Petry NM. Cocaine-using substance abuse treatment patients with and without HIV respond well to contingency management treatment. J Subst Abuse Treat 2017;77:21–5.

100. Petry NM, Weinstock J, Alessi SM, et al. Group-based randomized trial of contingencies for health and abstinence in HIV patients. J Consult Clin Psychol 2010;78(1):89–97.

101. Farber S, Tate J, Frank C, et al. A study of financial incentives to reduce plasma HIV RNA among patients in care. AIDS Behav 2013;17(7):2293–300.

102. Wray TB, Grin B, Dorfman L, et al. Systematic review of interventions to reduce problematic alcohol use in men who have sex with men. Drug Alcohol Rev 2016;35(2):148–57.

103. Springer SA, Di Paola A, Azar MM, et al. Extended-release naltrexone reduces alcohol consumption among released prisoners with HIV disease as they transition to the community. Drug Alcohol Depend 2017;174:158–70.

104. Binswanger IA, Blatchford PJ, Mueller SR, et al. Mortality after prison release: opioid overdose and other causes of death, risk factors, and time trends from 1999 to 2009. Ann Intern Med 2013;159(9):592–600.

105. Lincoln T, Johnson BD, McCarthy P, et al. Extended-release naltrexone for opioid use disorder started during or following incarceration. J Subst Abuse Treat 2018;85:97–100.

106. Lee JD, Friedmann PD, Kinlock TW, et al. Extended-release naltrexone to prevent opioid relapse in criminal justice offenders. N Engl J Med 2016;374(13):1232–42.

The Role of Technology-Based Interventions for Substance Use Disorders in Primary Care

A Review of the Literature

Babak Tofighi, MD, MSc[a,b,]*, Ana Abrantes, PhD[c,d],
Michael D. Stein, MD[e]

KEYWORDS

• Technology • Addiction • Mobile • Substance-related disorders

KEY POINTS

• The burden of alcohol and drug use disorders (substance use disorders [SUDs]) has intensified efforts to expand access to cost-effective psychosocial interventions and pharmacotherapies.

• This article provides an overview of technology-based interventions (eg, computer-based and Web-based interventions, text messaging, interactive voice recognition, smartphone apps, and emerging technologies) that are extending the reach of effective addiction treatments both in substance use treatment and primary care settings.

• This article discusses the efficacy of existing technology-based interventions for SUDs, prospects for emerging technologies, and special considerations when integrating technologies in primary care (eg, privacy and regulatory protocols) to enhance the management of SUDs.

This article originally appeared in *Medical Clinics*, Volume 102, Issue 4, July 2018.
Disclosure: B. Tofighi is supported by an NIH Mentored Patient-oriented Research Career Development Award (NIDA K23DA042140 - 01A1).
[a] Department of Population Health, New York University School of Medicine, 227 East 30th Street 7th Floor, New York, NY 10016, USA; [b] Division of General Internal Medicine, New York University School of Medicine, New York, NY 10016, USA; [c] Butler Hospital, Department of Psychiatry and Human Behavior, Behavioral Medicine and Addictions Research, Butler, PA, USA; [d] Department of Psychiatry and Human Behavior, Alpert Medical School of Brown University, 345 Blackstone Boulevard, Providence, RI 02906, USA; [e] Department of Health Law, Policy and Management, Boston University School of Public Health, 715 Albany Street, Talbot Building, Boston, MA 02118, USA
* Corresponding author. 227 East 30th Street 7th Floor, New York, NY 10016.
E-mail address: babak.tofighi@nyumc.org

Clinics Collections 9 (2020) 19–35
https://doi.org/10.1016/j.ccol.2020.07.022

INTRODUCTION

The burden of alcohol and substance use disorders (SUDs) is significant. For example, costs associated with opioid use disorder in 2013 were estimated at $78.5 billion and opioid-related overdose deaths have increased by 200% in the last 15 years.[1] Excessive alcohol use remains a leading modifiable cause of death and cost an estimated $250 billion in 2010.[2,3] However, nearly 50 years after the introduction of pharmacotherapies for SUDs, fewer than 10% of individuals with SUD are linked to treatment.[4]

Primary care settings are optimally positioned to reduce the burden of SUDs by providing a patient-centered care model for addiction treatment and related comorbidities (prescribing pharmacotherapies, patient education, and access to specialty care).[5,6] Costs of expanding addiction treatment to office-based settings are offset by reductions in emergency department visits and hospitalizations, and improved addiction and medical outcomes.[6,7] However, effective management of SUDs is seldom delivered in primary care. Patient-level barriers to office-based management of SUDs include cost, insurance limitations, stigma, and transportation.[8,9] Among physicians trained in SUD care, lack of adequate administrative and clinical support impede the delivery of effective medication-assisted therapies and psychosocial interventions targeting SUDs.[10,11]

The integration of innovative technology-based interventions (eg, computer-based and Web-based interventions, text messaging, interactive voice recognition, smartphone apps, and emerging technologies) in primary care has the potential to address gaps in care for individuals with SUDs (**Table 1**).[12-14] This pairing of effective technology-based interventions (TBIs) with primary care has already shown improvements in appointment adherence, diabetes self-management, smoking cessation, and human immunodeficiency virus (HIV) care.[15-17] Importantly, TBIs readily enhance between-visit patient engagement with their care by easing patient-physician communication, point of service data gathering, and adherence management, and offering the delivery of evidence-based psychosocial interventions with high fidelity.[12,13,16,18]

Advances in emerging technologies have also accelerated the development and delivery of effective TBIs targeting SUDs in specialty addiction treatment settings.[12,13,18,19] Patient surveys in primary care signal high acceptability and uptake of TBIs to enhance the management of SUDs.[20,21] Although primary care often constitutes the mainstay of medical care for populations with SUDs,[22] efforts to expand TBIs in primary care for the treatment of SUDs have yet to be fully realized. Adoption of evidence-based interventions targeting SUDs in primary care may produce positive outcomes comparable with those observed in specialty addiction treatment settings.[14,19,23,24]

This article describes the rapidly evolving nature of TBIs targeting alcohol and illicit substance use in community and outpatient addiction treatment settings and implications for integrating TBIs in primary care to reduce the burden of SUDs. It primarily focuses on computer-based and Web-based interventions, text messaging, interactive voice recognition, and smartphone applications supported by randomized controlled trials and evidence-based behavior change models (eg, cognitive behavior therapy [CBT], community reinforcement approach [CRA], therapeutic education system).[18]

Computer and Web-Based Interventions

Recent reviews and meta-analyses suggest that computer-based and Web-based interventions are a cost-effective approach to expand the reach of evidence-based psychotherapeutic interventions, reduce the burden of SUDs in community and specialty addiction treatment settings, and show clinical outcomes (improved cognitive

Table 1 Published data on technology-based interventions for substance use disorders				
Reference	Device	Target Substances	Target Behaviors or Behavior Change Model	Contact Information
Carroll, et al,[34] 2008	Internet/Web	Alcohol, cocaine, opioid, cannabis	CBT	http://www.cbt4cbt.com/
Marsch et al,[36] 2014	Internet/Web	Opioids	CRA, CBT	http://www.c4tbh.org/
Postel et al,[37] 2010	Internet/Web	Alcohol	CBT, biopsychosocial model	www.lookatyourdrinking.com
Campbell, et al,[38] 2014	Internet/Web	Alcohol, cocaine, cannabis, opiates, stimulants	CRA	http://sudtech.org/
Stoner et al,[43] 2015	Text message	Alcohol	Adherence to oral naltrexone	sastoner@uw.edu
Dulin et al,[56] 2013	Smartphone app	Alcohol		http://stepaway.biz/
Gustafson et al,[23] 2014	Smartphone app	Alcohol	Self-determination theory, cognitive-behavioral relapse prevention	https://chess.wisc.edu
Kay-Lambkin et al,[82] 2011	Internet/Web	Alcohol	Depression	http://www.shadetreatment.com/

Abbreviations: CBT, cognitive behavior therapy; CRA, community reinforcement approach.

functioning, retention of behavior change techniques, treatment engagement, and abstinence) comparable with studies evaluating the impact of individual counseling.[13,25,26] Web-based interventions are available to patients remotely through any Internet browser and may consist of a home page linking participants to addiction treatment services, self-selected modules, and peer discussion forums. In a meta-analysis by Riper and colleagues,[27] Web-based interventions used by participants in community settings (eg, home, employment) targeting alcohol use showed a small but significant effect (g = 0.20; 95% confidence interval [CI], 0.13–0.27; $P<.001$).

The effect of Web-based interventions is potentiated when delivered in multiple sessions at home or in specialty addiction treatment settings.[28,29] Findings in a systematic review by Riper and colleagues[28] reported higher effect sizes in multi-session modularized Web-based interventions (g = 0.61, 95% CI 0.33–0.90) targeting alcohol use in community settings (eg, home, library, work) compared with single-session personalized feedback programs (g = 0.27, 95% CI 0.11–0.43, P = .04). Kay-Lambkin and colleagues[30] described equivalent treatment outcomes among participants recruited from primary care and mental health settings with major depressive disorder and problematic alcohol use (>4 drinks per day for men or >2 drinks per day for women) or at least weekly marijuana use randomized to a computer-based motivational interviewing (MI)/CBT intervention (SHADE [self-help for alcohol and other drug use and depression] therapy) versus therapist-delivered MI/CBT sessions.

Bickel and colleagues[31] also reported comparable weeks of continuous opioid and cocaine abstinence and significantly greater weeks of abstinence among patients enrolled in buprenorphine maintenance treatment in a university-based research clinic receiving a computer-assisted intervention grounded in the CRA combined with contingency management versus standard treatment (CRA-based in-person counseling plus contingency management). CRA reinforces the client's motivation and coping strategies to reduce substance use and integrate social, recreational, and vocational reinforcers to avoid substance use.[32] CM is based on operant conditioning and offers a system of incentives to enhance patient motivation for abstinence.[33] Carroll and colleagues[34] reported that individuals recruited from a community-based outpatient addiction treatment program who met Diagnostic and Statistical Manual of Mental Disorders, Fourth Edition criteria for alcohol, cocaine, opioid, or marijuana dependence randomized to a CBT-based computer intervention (CBT4CBT) showed similar rates of treatment retention compared with standard treatment; further, participants assigned to the CBT4CBT program provided significantly more negative urine drug screen tests and longer continuous durations of abstinence.[35]

Subsequent studies assessed the impact of substituting portions of in-person counseling with Web-based interventions to reduce the burden on health care personnel while ensuring improved therapeutic support and clinical outcomes. Marsch and colleagues[36] evaluated the effectiveness of the Therapeutic Education System (TES), a Web-based psychosocial intervention constituted of modules grounded in the CRA and CBT models among methadone maintenance treatment patients (N = 160) randomized to standard treatment or TES partially substituting for in-person counseling. Findings showed significantly higher rates of abstinence among participants receiving the TES (48%) compared with standard treatment (37%) across all study weeks ($P<.05$). Notably, participants exposed to the TES system showed less dropout compared with patients receiving only clinician-delivered treatment (log-rank $P = .017$) and were exposed to a higher "dose" of the psychosocial intervention.[36] Postal and colleagues[37] assessed the effectiveness of the Alcohol de Baas intervention, a Web-based platform integrating CBT to reduce alcohol use and problem drinking behavior, and improve health status. Participants were recruited from the community and showed significantly improved health status and abstinence, reduced problem drinking, and higher readiness to initiate alcohol treatment compared with the control group. At 6 and 9 months, weekly consumption was less than baseline and participants showed significant improvements in depression, anxiety, and stress scores.[38]

Campbell and colleagues[39] evaluated the effectiveness of the TES, consisting of 62 interactive multimedia modules (eg, basic cognitive-behavioral relapse prevention skills; improving psychosocial functioning; and prevention of HIV, hepatitis, and sexually transmitted infections) requiring approximately 30 minutes each to complete. Interactive modules substituted for 2 hours of standard clinician-led group therapy sessions per week. Incentives were earned by participants for negative urine or alcohol breathalyzer screens and TES module completion, and redeemed using the TES platform to reduce high dropout and relapse rates in the early stages of treatment. Nearly half of the draws consisted of supportive content (eg, "Good job"), and the remaining draws rewarded participants with prizes worth $1, $20, or $80 to $100 in decreasing probability. Participants in the TES group had a significantly greater abstinence rate (odds ratio, 1.62; 95% CI, 1.12, 2.35), and improved retention in treatment (log-rank $P = .017$).[39]

Findings from these trials show the effectiveness of Web-based TES interventions targeting SUDs while overcoming administrative and clinical barriers limiting the reach of evidence-based psychotherapeutic interventions in diverse specialty addiction treatment settings.[39] The applicability of similar Web-based TES interventions across traditional primary care settings remains promising and requires further implementation studies to inform TES integration into service delivery.

Text Message–Based Interventions

Less technologically complex compared with computer-based, Internet-based, or smartphone-based interventions, text messaging (TM) remains a cost-effective platform for improving chronic disease management in primary care (eg, smoking cessation, appointment adherence, and adherence to antiretroviral therapies).[19,40,41] It is the most popular mobile phone feature nationally among patients in addiction treatment and in primary care.[12,42] TM may deliver multimedia content (eg, images, videos, audio) and incorporate behavior change approaches, including CBT, and motivational interventions, with high fidelity.[12]

Recent systematic reviews have described the feasibility and preliminary efficacy of TM interventions to reduce the burden of alcohol and illicit substance use in primary care and university-based research clinic settings. Studies indicate improved retention in treatment; medication adherence; and reduced alcohol, methamphetamine, and opioid use.[12,18,35,36] Stoner and colleagues[43] randomized participants with alcohol use disorder to a text-based tool providing medication reminders for oral naltrexone, adherence support, and prompts eliciting potential side effects, cravings, and alcohol use versus the control condition (i.e., receipt of a prepaid phone and prompts for alcohol use and related side effects). Although adherence to naltrexone did not predict drinking outcomes, the intervention group reported significantly longer periods of adherence to naltrexone (mean = 19 days; 95% CI, 0.0–44.0) than those in the control group (mean = 3 days; 95% CI, 0.0–8.1) during the first month of treatment ($P = .04$).

Researchers have also leveraged TM to enhance appointment adherence,[44] self-efficacy, relapse prevention, social support, and linkage with peer support groups.[45] Gonzales and colleagues[46] described significantly improved participation in extracurricular recovery activities, rates of abstinence, and reduced substance use problem severity among young adults (aged 12–24 years) recruited from outpatient and residential treatment programs randomized to TM-based self-monitoring prompts, educational content, and information regarding social support resources. TM tools may also enhance access to health care providers in real time to reduce the risk of relapse or other adverse events. Lucht and colleagues[47] randomized participants completing inpatient detoxification for alcohol and scheduled to follow-up in outpatient addiction treatment with a TM intervention offering as-needed counselor telephone support and showed significantly improved rates of low-risk alcohol use, treatment retention, and later episodes of relapse compared with standard care.

TM interventions have also addressed clinical barriers to managing SUDs in primary care, including the management of comorbidities prevalent in patients with SUDs (ie, HIV, depression).[48,49] Agyapong and colleagues[48] randomized dual-diagnosis participants with alcohol use and major depressive disorder to a twice-daily supportive TM tool in combination with primary care. TM content was designed to reduce cravings, stress, relapse, and nonadherence to medications, and to provide general support. Although there were no significant improvements in depression symptoms, participants randomized to the TM tool showed increased days to first drink.

Interactive Voice Recognition

Outpatient management of SUDs requires close monitoring of daily substance use, medication adherence, cravings, and adverse events. Similar to TM, Interactive voice response (IVR) offers a seamless approach to enhance between-visit patient engagement with care. IVR technology uses a telephone-delivered system of recorded scripts to persons seeking substance use treatment. IVR automatizes scheduled phone calls to elicit participant responses in real time using telephone keypad responses or voice recognition, which is preferable for certain patient subgroups that are less comfortable with TM or with limited literacy skills.[50] More dynamic IVR systems include automatic logical skipping or branching sequences to offer more user-centered feedback. Notably, some patients report increased comfort reporting sensitive information to the IVR system than to their clinician.[51] IVR has also shown an impact on chronic illness management outcomes (blood pressure and glycemic control),[51] but the clinical efficacy of IVR in reducing substance use (other than cigarette use)[52] remains unclear.[53–55]

Smartphone Applications

The near ubiquity of mobile phones and increasing popularity of smartphone ownership has hastened the development and study of mobile phone–based health interventions to reduce the burden of SUDs. Smartphone applications offer a diverse range of functions with advanced software capabilities to enhance chronic illness management. The effectiveness of smartphone applications has been supported in recent trials among participants with alcohol use disorder in specialty addiction treatment settings. Dulin and colleagues[56] conducted a pilot randomized controlled trial to evaluate the clinical impact of a stand-alone, self-administered smartphone-delivered intervention for participants recruited from the community with alcohol use disorder (ie, drinking a minimum of $\geq$14 drinks for women or $\geq$21 drinks for men per week over a consecutive 30-day period and $\geq$2 heavy drinking days consisting of 4 or more drinks for women and 5 or more drinks for men in the same 30-day period) who were not enrolled in specialty addiction treatment. The intervention modules enhanced patient awareness of their drinking problems, assessment of daily alcohol use, triggers, personalized weekly feedback reports, and reinforcement of users' social support networks. These features were coupled with offering users coping strategies to reduce cravings and psychological distress to reduce the risk of drinking. The intervention reduced the number of hazardous drinking days and numbers of drinks per day. These preliminary findings suggest clinical benefit for stand-alone evidence-based interventions for individuals unable to access specialty treatment and require further study for potential adoption in primary care.

More recently, Gustafson and colleagues[23] examined the effectiveness of A-CHESS (Alcohol – Comprehensive Health Enhancement Support System) among participants transitioning from residential alcohol treatment to outpatient treatment. A-CHESS is based on self-determination theory[57] and cognitive-behavioral relapse prevention[58] to enhance perceived competence, social relatedness, and motivation to reduce alcohol use. This multifeatured smartphone intervention offers self-assessments, discussion groups, counselor support, links to online resources on addiction management, GPS (global positioning system) tracking to prompt patients if they approach a high-risk location that may lead to relapse, and personalized therapeutic goals. Patients randomized to A-CHESS showed significantly fewer risky drinking days (mean difference, 1.37; 95% CI, 0.46–2.27; $P = .003$), and increased abstinence in the previous 30 days at months 8 and 12 ($P = .04$ and .02), compared with patients receiving treatment as usual, and sustained engagement with the application.[23]

Online Forums and Social Media

Online platforms (eg, discussion/chat rooms, e-mail threads, social media) offer anonymous and socially supportive communication that reinforces self-management, self-esteem, and assistance linking with treatment.[59] Twelve-step–based online sites remain the most popular among participants with SUDs. In addition, an increasing number of sites offer alternatives to the 12-step approach (eg, Women For Sobriety, Rational Recovery Center, SMART [Self-Management and Recovery Training] recovery, Rational Emotive Behavior Therapy). The popularity, quality of information, and clinical impact of such online forums as yet remains unclear.[20] However, given the effectiveness of in-person peer support as an adjunct to primary care–based approaches to managing SUDs,[60] similar online forums based on the 12-step or SMART recovery model have the potential to also enhance clinician-delivered interventions in primary care for SUDs. There are also hundreds of commercial online sites and social media pages promising access to therapists, peer support networks, and motivational and informational content. Sites accredited by the Joint Commission on Accreditation of Healthcare Organizations (eg, soberrecovery.com) may assist some patients in accessing potentially beneficial content (**Table 2**). Recent National Institutes of Health funding of research that leverages social media and online forums promises to reveal important insights into these diversifying platforms facilitating recovery.[61]

Emerging Technologies

In addition to the TBIs reviewed earlier, there are also several emerging technologies that are likely to have an impact on SUD treatment in the years ahead. Technological advances have been rapid over the last decade, resulting in smaller, faster devices with increased computing power. In addition, wireless communication between devices can allow real-time information gathering and transfer between patients and providers. Further, relevant data that extend beyond alcohol and drug use (eg, heart rate, tone of voice) can be processed with machine learning approaches that can ultimately lead to the ability to predict patient behaviors. These novel technological approaches coupled with existing theoretically informed TBIs have the potential to increase the reach and efficacy of SUD treatment (**Table 3**).

Advances in biosensor technology have contributed to the emergence of novel interventional approaches. To date, the most work has been conducted with transdermal alcohol sensors such as the commercially available Secure Continuous Remote Alcohol Monitoring device (SCRAM; Alcohol Monitoring Systems, Inc, Littleton, CO). SCRAM takes measurements every 30 minutes and is able to wirelessly convey transdermal readings to a remote server. Although frequently used in the criminal justice system, SCRAM, especially in conjunction with contingency management interventions, has resulted in promising drinking outcomes among outpatients engaged in alcohol treatment.[62–64] Other transdermal sensors include the WrisTAS

Table 2 Online support forums	
Program	**Web Site**
Sober Recovery	www.soberrecovery.com/forums/
12 Step Recovery Forums	www.12stepforums.net
Women for Sobriety	womenforsobriety.org
Rational Recovery	rational.org
SMART Recovery	https://www.smartrecovery.org/community/forums/6-Tools-and-Discussions

Abbreviation: SMART, Self-Management and Recovery Training.

Table 3 Emerging technologies			
Secure Continuous Remote Alcohol Monitoring Device (Alcohol Monitoring Systems, Inc)	Sensor	(1) Alcohol	www.scramsystems.com/
WrisTAS (Giner, Inc)	Sensor	(1) Alcohol	www.ginerinc.com/ wrist-transdermal-alcohol-sensor
Wisepill device (Wisepill Technologies)	Pillbox plus smartphone app	(1) Medication adherence	www.wisepill.com
Soberlink device (Soberlink, Inc)	Portable breathalyzer	(1) Alcohol	www.soberlink.com/

(Giner, Inc, Newton, MA). The WrisTAS, unlike the SCRAM, is worn on the wrist and takes measurements every minute and has shown high sensitivity and specificity.[65]

Other emerging technologies have focused on the ability to obtain real-time feedback, thereby increasing the potential to intervene more promptly. Examples of this include technological approaches for monitoring medication adherence. The Wisepill device (Wisepill Technologies, Cape Town, South Africa), the size of a pack of cards, stores pills, tracks when the device has been opened, and wirelessly sends information to an external server (eg, to a researcher or clinician). In addition, the Wisepill device can also be paired with text message reminders to help facilitate patient adherence. The Wisepill device and messages have been used successfully to increase adherence to antiretroviral therapy in patients with HIV and has been used to monitor naltrexone adherence in methamphetamine users and binge drinkers.[66,67] Because of concerns about whether patients actually ingest a medication when opening such monitoring devices, researchers have explored the use of inert radiofrequency emitters attached to the medication to create an ingestible digital pill that communicates with a cloud-based server while in the stomach.[68,69] Another real-time monitoring approach involves the use of a Soberlink device (Soberlink, Inc, CA), equipped with facial recognition software to verify identity, that allows patients to provide breath sample data on breath alcohol levels, which are wirelessly sent to treating providers.[70] The clinician is then able to promptly respond to positive results and provide the patient who continues to drink with appropriate intervention. Alternatively, others have explored pairing breathalyzer results with a smartphone app to provide feedback and encourage skill building.[71]

Although the technologies described earlier involve obtaining objective information on alcohol and drug use from patients, there are several emerging technologies that can be used to predict potentially risky behaviors before they happen. For example, Boyer and colleagues[72] (2012) argued that, in concert, technologies including artificial intelligence, continuous physiologic monitoring, wireless connectivity, and smartphone computation would be able to detect when an individual is experiencing craving for alcohol or drug use and could receive a just-in-time intervention to prevent substance use. Acute changes in negative affect and craving (known risk factors for relapse) are associated with concomitant changes in physiologic arousal; namely, heart rate and electrodermal activity (EDA).[73–76] Both research-grade devices and commercially available smartwatches that communicate wirelessly with smartphones are equipped with medical-grade biosensors that provide continuous monitoring of heart rate, temperature, and EDA. Physiologic data that include EDA and temperature, measured by a portable biosensor wristwatch (Q sensor; Affectiva, Waltham, MA), have been shown to be associated with cocaine and opiate use in both laboratory and ambulatory environments.[77,78] Work is currently underway to identify drug use cravings and, through machine learning approaches, develop algorithms for predicting drug use so that personalized relapse prevention interventions can be delivered during the time of greatest need.[72]

Machine learning approaches have also been proposed to aid in the prediction of whether an individual is intoxicated. For example, Arnold and colleagues[79] argue that data collected from the smartphone accelerometer and gyroscope (called Alcogait) coupled with information on how much an individual has consumed alcohol could, through machine learning, reliably predict blood alcohol levels. In doing so, when this information can be used to deliver feedback to an individual about their ability to drive, for example, alcohol-related risk behaviors may be decreased or avoided.

These emerging technologies can be integrated into individuals' everyday lives, with passive collection of data that can be computationally processed for available feedback to the at-risk individual, without much additional effort from the individual. As these technologies enter the next stage of experimental investigation and efficacy testing, clinicians will have a greater understanding of their impact on reducing the overall public health risk associated with SUDs.

IMPORTANT CONSIDERATIONS RELATED TO TECHNOLOGY-BASED INTERVENTIONS FOR SUBSTANCE USE DISORDERS
Technology-Based Interventions for Dual-Diagnosis Populations

Comorbid SUD and psychiatric disorder is common. Although efforts have been made to address psychiatric comorbidity in patients with SUD, few treatments exist that effectively address multiple comorbidities. Because individuals with comorbid disorders experience more treatment access barriers, including social deficits and stigma,[80] the use of TBIs in dual-diagnosis populations may be a particularly effective strategy.

In a recent systematic review of TBIs for substance use and comorbid disorders, Sugarman and colleagues[81] (2017) identified only 9 studies, with the largest number being for depression comorbidity. The TBI with the most empirical testing has been the SHADE, a 9-session MI plus CBT computer-delivered intervention that has shown reduction in alcohol and cannabis use as well as decreases in depressive symptoms.[82] An abbreviated version of SHADE has been developed for young adults with alcohol and depressive comorbidity, called DEAL.[83] Short-term decreases in drinking and depression were found but not sustained, and adherence to the intervention was challenging. There is an ongoing study of DEAL that adds a social networking component for depressed, binge drinking young adults.[84] There are also several studies examining TBIs for individuals with comorbid trauma experiences and SUDs, with or without a diagnosis of posttraumatic stress disorder. In a recent review of these studies, Gilmore and colleagues[85] (2016) found that TBIs are feasible for this population and are likely to be efficacious in reducing either trauma symptoms or substance use.

As reported by Sugarman and colleagues[81] (2017), there are several special considerations when developing and testing TBIs for a dual-diagnosis population. First, the more effective interventions tend to be longer and more intensive. Adherence to the intervention is therefore a challenge and the investigators suggested that financial incentives, gamification of TBIs, and some clinical involvement may be necessary to increase engagement with the intervention. Also, because there is always a concern for clinical deterioration and suicidal ideation, there is a need to consider strategies for incorporating clinical monitoring in the delivery of TBIs in dual-diagnosis patients.

Factors Influencing the Fidelity of Technology-Based Interventions

If well-designed, TBIs can minimize the burden on delivery systems and reduce net spending for SUDs while expanding the use of underused addiction pharmacotherapies and psychosocial interventions. Translating evidence-based TBIs into mainstream health care settings will rely on a reorganization of clinical practices that consider patient-level factors to sustained engagement with emerging platforms (eg, socioeconomic and clinical barriers to care), privacy and regulatory concerns, on-boarding delivery systems and providers that have limited experience with TBIs, and reimbursement mechanisms.[24,86]

Patient-level barriers to treatment entry for SUDs (eg, race/ethnicity, socioeconomic status, less education, impaired cognition, severe mental illness)[8,80] mirror the barriers to access to mobile phones, computers, and Internet.[19,87,88] However, offering free mobile phones or in-clinic access to computers ensures open access to evidence-based interventions and improved clinical outcomes (eg, cognitive functioning, abstinence, and treatment retention).[12,23,49,89,90] Additional strategies for dissemination of evidence-based TBIs include subsidizing Internet or mobile phone plans, offering instructions on intervention use, and tailoring intervention content and design features to user preferences.

The spread of unvalidated, commercially driven smartphone applications, social media pages, and Web-based interventions has dampened the dissemination of effective TBIs. Developers often claim medical expertise and offer unsubstantiated claims of intervention efficacy, and may sell user data to third parties for commercial use.[91] The monetization of digital data and risks for compromised patient health information require clinicians to caution patients regarding commercially driven TBIs. The US Food and Drug Administration (FDA) has increased oversight of emerging TBIs, including mobile medical applications but may have difficulties in regulating product claims unrelated to specific medical conditions (eg, promotes reduced stress, concentration, behavior control).[92] Nonetheless, clinicians should help patients navigate the marketplace by confirming device approval via the FDA (eg, https://www.accessdata.fda.gov/scripts/cdrh/cfdocs/cfRL/rl.cfm) and existing literature.

Privacy and Regulatory Considerations to Technology-Based Intervention Integration

Adoption of effective TBIs in mainstream and addiction treatment settings remains slow because concerns over social, legal, and ethical implications remain unanswered. Potential issues for patients and providers include:

1. Open access to indefinitely stored content in mobile phones, emails, IVR platforms, online forums, or mobile sensors requires protocols for deletion
2. Inability for physicians or patients to confirm the authenticity of authorship of content transmitted between one another
3. Interception of content exchanged between providers and patients
4. Lack of familiarity with the Health Insurance Portability and Accountability Act (HIPAA)[93]

Risk management of compromising patient health information includes the removal of any patient's identifiers or stigmatizing content (eg, HIV, addict, methadone), restricting patient contact to only 1 provider or software, password protecting all mobile phones and devices, obtaining security certifications from mobile phone service providers, using encryption technologies for transmitted content, and regularly deleting transmitted content.[24,93]

Clarifying Intervention Design and Clinical Impact

Interventions that are overly complex, contain redundant or ineffective components, and seem homogenous can lead to a reduction in treatment efficacy with every type of intervention. To preempt such problems, software that incorporates graded approaches, such as adjusting the frequency of TM prompts based on the patient's clinical condition and level of responsiveness with the intervention, sustains engagement during the different stages of recovery.[12,49] In addition, intervention development based on mixed-methods research and usability testing (eg, intervention mapping approach, multiphase optimization strategy testing) improves the reach, long-term engagement, and effectiveness of newly introduced platforms.[12,94,95] Meta-analysis and recent reviews have also found that integrating patient-tailored design features and effective psychosocial interventions enhances engagement with the TBI, is associated with greater effect sizes, and optimizes behavior change and clinical outcomes.[12,13,18,96] In addition, linking TBIs with immediate access to health care providers or supportive peers is preferable to interventions that lack any human contact because of the demotivating nature of some automated interactions.[12,18,21]

Although TBIs may be tailored to the patient's clinical needs, studies are needed to assess the appropriate level of exposure or dose of TBIs versus clinician-delivered psychosocial interventions, the effectiveness of computer-based versus mobile phone–based interventions, and smartphone-based compared with TM-based platforms. In addition, the clinical effectiveness of adding TBI-delivered psychosocial interventions to existing addiction pharmacotherapies (eg, buprenorphine, naltrexone) in traditional primary care settings remains limited.

SUMMARY

In the last 2 decades, advances in TBIs addressing SUDs, most often in addiction treatment settings, have made possible effective point of service data gathering, adherence management, reinforcement of evidence-based psychosocial interventions, improved patient-physician communication, retention in office-based treatment, and increased abstinence with minimal disruption to health care personnel and clinical workflow. For TBIs to reach their full potential to reduce the burden of SUDs, strategies are needed to facilitate their dissemination and implementation in primary care: addressing clinician adoption of TBIs, financial reimbursement, adaptability of hardware in primary care, integration and interoperability, and user engagement.[97]

ACKNOWLEDGMENTS

The authors wish to thank Sarah Lord, Geisel School of Medicine at Dartmouth College, and Christopher W. Shanahan, Boston Medical Center/Boston University, for providing a critical review of this article.

REFERENCES

1. Florence CS, Zhou C, Luo F, et al. The economic burden of prescription opioid overdose, abuse, and dependence in the United States, 2013. Med Care 2016; 54(10):901–6.

2. Bauer UE, Briss PA, Goodman RA, et al. Prevention of chronic disease in the 21st century: elimination of the leading preventable causes of premature death and disability in the USA. Lancet 2014;384(9937):45–52.
3. Sacks JJ, Gonzales KR, Bouchery EE, et al. 2010 national and state costs of excessive alcohol consumption. Am J Prev Med 2015;49(5):e73–9.
4. Nosyk B, Anglin MD, Brissette S, et al. A call for evidence-based medical treatment of opioid dependence in the United States and Canada. Health Aff 2013; 32(8):1462–9.
5. Anton RF, O'Malley SS, Ciraulo DA, et al. Combined pharmacotherapies and behavioral interventions for alcohol dependence: the COMBINE study: a randomized controlled trial. Jama 2006;295(17):2003–17.
6. Bhatraju EP, Grossman E, Tofighi B, et al. Public sector low threshold office-based buprenorphine treatment: outcomes at year 7. Addict Sci Clin Pract 2017;12(1):7.
7. Saitz R, Horton NJ, Larson MJ, et al. Primary medical care and reductions in addiction severity: a prospective cohort study. Addiction 2005;100(1):70–8.
8. Hansen HB, Siegel CE, Case BG, et al. Variation in use of buprenorphine and methadone treatment by racial, ethnic, and income characteristics of residential social areas in New York City. J Behav Health Serv Res 2013;40(3):367–77.
9. Teruya C, Schwartz RP, Mitchell SG, et al. Patient perspectives on buprenorphine/naloxone: a qualitative study of retention during the Starting Treatment with Agonist Replacement Therapies (START) study. J Psychoactive Drugs 2014; 46(5):412–26.
10. Kermack A, Flannery M, Tofighi B, et al. Buprenorphine prescribing practice trends and attitudes among New York providers. J Subst Abuse Treat 2017; 74:1–6.
11. Duncan LG, Mendoza S, Hansen H. Buprenorphine maintenance for opioid dependence in public sector healthcare: benefits and barriers. J Addict Med Ther Sci 2015;1(2):31.
12. Tofighi B, Nicholson JM, McNeely J, et al. Mobile phone messaging for illicit drug and alcohol dependence: a systematic review of the literature. Drug Alcohol Rev 2017;36(4):477–91.
13. Bickel WK, Christensen DR, Marsch LA. A review of computer-based interventions used in the assessment, treatment, and research of drug addiction. Subst Use Misuse 2011;46(1):4–9.
14. Copeland J, Martin G. Web-based interventions for substance use disorders: a qualitative review. J Subst Abuse Treat 2004;26(2):109–16.
15. Free C, Phillips G, Galli L, et al. The effectiveness of mobile-health technology-based health behaviour change or disease management interventions for health care consumers: a systematic review. PLoS Med 2013;10(1):e1001362.
16. Muessig KE, Nekkanti M, Bauermeister J, et al. A systematic review of recent smartphone, Internet and Web 2.0 interventions to address the HIV continuum of care. Curr HIV/AIDS Rep 2015;12(1):173–90.
17. Buller DB, Borland R, Bettinghaus EP, et al. Randomized trial of a smartphone mobile application compared to text messaging to support smoking cessation. Telemed J E Health 2014;20(3):206–14.
18. Litvin EB, Abrantes AM, Brown RA. Computer and mobile technology-based interventions for substance use disorders: an organizing framework. Addict Behav 2013;38(3):1747–56.
19. Cole-Lewis H, Kershaw T. Text messaging as a tool for behavior change in disease prevention and management. Epidemiol Rev 2010;32(1):56–69.

20. Hall MJ, Tidwell WC. Internet recovery for substance abuse and alcoholism: an exploratory study of service users. J Substance Abuse Treat 2003;24(2):161–7.
21. Tofighi B, Grossman E, Buirkle E, et al. Mobile phone use patterns and preferences in safety net office-based buprenorphine patients. J Addict Med 2015; 9(3):217.
22. Reid MC, Fiellin DA, O'Connor PG. Hazardous and harmful alcohol consumption in primary care. Arch Intern Med 1999;159(15):1681–9.
23. Gustafson DH, McTavish FM, Chih M-Y, et al. A smartphone application to support recovery from alcoholism: a randomized clinical trial. JAMA Psychiatry 2014;71(5):566–72.
24. Tofighi B, Grossman E, Sherman S, et al. Mobile phone messaging during unobserved "home" induction to buprenorphine. J Addict Med 2016;10(5):309–13.
25. Rooke S, Thorsteinsson E, Karpin A, et al. Computer-delivered interventions for alcohol and tobacco use: a meta-analysis. Addiction 2010;105(8):1381–90.
26. Moore BA, Fazzino T, Garnet B, et al. Computer-based interventions for drug use disorders: a systematic review. J substance abuse Treat 2011;40(3):215–23.
27. Riper H, Blankers M, Hadiwijaya H, et al. Effectiveness of guided and unguided low-intensity internet interventions for adult alcohol misuse: a meta-analysis. PLoS One 2014;9(6):e99912.
28. Riper H, Spek V, Boon B, et al. Effectiveness of E-self-help interventions for curbing adult problem drinking: a meta-analysis. J Med Internet Res 2011; 13(2):e42.
29. White A, Kavanagh D, Stallman H, et al. Online alcohol interventions: a systematic review. J Med Internet Res 2010;12(5):e62.
30. Kay-Lambkin FJ, Baker AL, Lewin TJ, et al. Computer-based psychological treatment for comorbid depression and problematic alcohol and/or cannabis use: a randomized controlled trial of clinical efficacy. Addiction 2009;104(3):378–88.
31. Bickel WK, Marsch LA, Buchhalter AR, et al. Computerized behavior therapy for opioid-dependent outpatients: a randomized controlled trial. Exp Clin Psychopharmacol 2008;16(2):132.
32. Roozen HG, Boulogne JJ, van Tulder MW, et al. A systematic review of the effectiveness of the community reinforcement approach in alcohol, cocaine and opioid addiction. Drug and alcohol dependence 2004;74(1):1–13.
33. Stitzer ML, Bigelow GE, Liebson I. Reinforcement of drug abstinence: a behavioral approach to drug abuse treatment. Behavioral analysis and treatment of substance abuse 1979;25(68).
34. Carroll KM, Ball SA, Martino S, et al. Computer-assisted delivery of cognitive-behavioral therapy for addiction: a randomized trial of CBT4CBT. Am J Psychiatry 2008;165(7):881–8.
35. Olmstead TA, Ostrow CD, Carroll KM. Cost-effectiveness of computer-assisted training in cognitive-behavioral therapy as an adjunct to standard care for addiction. Drug and alcohol dependence 2010;110(3):200–7.
36. Marsch LA, Guarino H, Acosta M, et al. Web-based behavioral treatment for substance use disorders as a partial replacement of standard methadone maintenance treatment. J Substance Abuse Treat 2014;46(1):43–51.
37. Postel MG, de Haan HA, ter Huurne ED, et al. Effectiveness of a web-based intervention for problem drinkers and reasons for dropout: randomized controlled trial. J Med Internet Res 2010;12(4):e68.
38. Postel MG, ter Huurne ED, de Haan HA, et al. A 9-month follow-up of a 3-month web-based alcohol treatment program using intensive asynchronous therapeutic support. Am J Drug Alcohol Abuse 2015;41(4):309–16.

39. Campbell AN, Nunes EV, Matthews AG, et al. Internet-delivered treatment for substance abuse: a multisite randomized controlled trial. Am J Psychiatry 2014;171(6):683–90.
40. Whittaker R, McRobbie H, Bullen C, et al. Mobile phone-based interventions for smoking cessation. Cochrane Database Syst Rev 2016;(4):CD006611.
41. Guerriero C, Cairns J, Roberts I, et al. The cost-effectiveness of smoking cessation support delivered by mobile phone text messaging: Txt2stop. Eur J Health Econ 2013;14(5):789–97.
42. Rainie L. Internet, broadband, and cell phone statistics. Pew Internet & American Life Project 2010;5:3–8.
43. Stoner SA, Arenella PB, Hendershot CS. Randomized controlled trial of a mobile phone intervention for improving adherence to naltrexone for alcohol use disorders. PLoS One 2015;10(4):e0124613.
44. Tofighi B, Grazioli F, Bereket S, et al. Text message reminders for improving patient appointment adherence in an office-based buprenorphine program: a feasibility study. Am J Addict 2017;26(6):581–6.
45. Keoleian V, Polcin D, Galloway GP. Text messaging for addiction: a review. J psychoactive Drugs 2015;47(2):158–76.
46. Gonzales R, Ang A, Murphy DA, et al. Substance use recovery outcomes among a cohort of youth participating in a mobile-based texting aftercare pilot program. J substance abuse Treat 2014;47(1):20–6.
47. Lucht MJ, Hoffman L, Haug S, et al. A surveillance tool using mobile phone short message service to reduce alcohol consumption among alcohol-dependent patients. Alcohol Clin Exp Res 2014;38(6):1728–36.
48. Agyapong VI, McLoughlin DM, Farren CK. Six-months outcomes of a randomised trial of supportive text messaging for depression and comorbid alcohol use disorder. J Affect Disord 2013;151(1):100–4.
49. Reback CJ, Fletcher JB, Shoptaw S, et al. Exposure to theory-driven text messages is associated with HIV risk reduction among methamphetamine-using men who have sex with men. AIDS Behav 2015;19(2):130–41.
50. Abu-Hasaballah K, James A, Aseltine RH. Lessons and pitfalls of interactive voice response in medical research. Contemp Clin Trials 2007;28(5):593–602.
51. Piette JD. Interactive voice response systems in the diagnosis and management of chronic disease. Am J Manag Care 2000;6(7):817–27.
52. Regan S, Reyen M, Lockhart AC, et al. An interactive voice response system to continue a hospital-based smoking cessation intervention after discharge. Nicotine Tob Res 2011;13(4):255–60.
53. Toll BA, Cooney NL, McKee SA, et al. Correspondence between Interactive Voice Response (IVR) and Timeline Followback (TLFB) reports of drinking behavior. Addict behaviors 2006;31(4):726–31.
54. Mundt JC, Moore HK, Bean P. An interactive voice response program to reduce drinking relapse: a feasibility study. J substance abuse Treat 2006;30(1):21–9.
55. Andersson C, Öjehagen A, Olsson MO, et al. Interactive voice response with feedback intervention in outpatient treatment of substance use problems in adolescents and young adults: a randomized controlled trial. Int J Behav Med 2017;24(5):789–97.
56. Dulin PL, Gonzalez VM, King DK, et al. Development of a smartphone-based, self-administered intervention system for alcohol use disorders. Alcohol Treat Q 2013;31(3):321–36.

57. Patrick H, Williams GC. Self-determination theory: its application to health behavior and complementarity with motivational interviewing. Int J Behav Nutr Phys Act 2012;9:18.
58. Larimer ME, Palmer RS, Marlatt GA. Relapse prevention. An overview of Marlatt's cognitive-behavioral model. Alcohol Res Health 1999;23(2):151–60.
59. Barak A, Klein B, Proudfoot JG. Defining internet-supported therapeutic interventions. Ann Behav Med 2009;38(1):4–17.
60. Monico LB, Gryczynski J, Mitchell SG, et al. Buprenorphine treatment and 12-step meeting attendance: conflicts, compatibilities, and patient outcomes. J substance abuse Treat 2015;57:89–95.
61. NIDA. Using social media to better understand, prevent, and treat substance use. In: NIDA, editor. Bethesda (MD): National Institute on Drug Abuse; 2014. Available at: https://www.drugabuse.gov/news-events/news-releases/2014/10/using-social-media-to-better-understand-prevent-treat-substance-use. Accessed October 1, 2017.
62. Alessi SM, Barnett NP, Petry NM. Experiences with SCRAMx alcohol monitoring technology in 100 alcohol treatment outpatients. Drug and Alcohol Dependence 2017;178:417–24.
63. Barnett NP, Celio MA, Tidey JW, et al. A preliminary randomized controlled trial of contingency management for alcohol use reduction using a transdermal alcohol sensor. Addiction 2017;112:1025–35.
64. Dougherty DM, Hill-Kapturczak N, Liang Y, et al. Use of continuous transdermal alcohol monitoring during a contingency management procedure to reduce excessive alcohol use. Drug Alcohol Depend 2014;142:301–6.
65. Greenfield TK, Bond J, Kerr WC. Biomonitoring for improving alcohol consumption surveys: the new gold standard? Alcohol Res 2014;36:39–45.
66. Orrell C, Cohen K, Mauff K, et al. A randomized controlled trial of real-time electronic adherence monitoring with text message dosing reminders in people starting first-line antiretroviral therapy. J Acquir Immune Defic Syndr 2015;70:495–502.
67. Santos G, Coffin P, Santos D, et al. Feasibility, acceptability and tolerability of targeted naltrexone for non-dependent methamphetamine-using and binge drinking men who have sex with men. JAIDS J Acquired Immune Deficiency Syndromes 2016;72:21–30.
68. Carreiro S, Chai PR, Carey J, et al. Integrating personalized technology in toxicology: sensors, smart glass, and social media applications in toxicology research. J Med Toxicol 2017;13:166–72.
69. Chai PR, Rosen RK, Boyer EW, et al. Ingestible biosensors for real-time medical adherence monitoring: MyTMed. Proc Annu Hawaii Int Conf Syst Sci 2016;2016:3416–23.
70. Gordon A, Jaffe A, McLellan AT, et al. How should remote clinical monitoring be used to treat alcohol use disorders? J Addict Med 2017;11:145–53.
71. You CW, Chen YC, Chen CH, et al. Smartphone-based support system (SoberDiary) coupled with a Bluetooth breathalyser for treatment-seeking alcohol-dependent patients. Addict Behaviors 2017;65:174–8.
72. Boyer EW, Fletcher R, Fay RJ, et al. Preliminary efforts directed toward the detection of craving of illicit substances: the iHeal project. J Med Toxicol 2012;8:5–9.
73. Ebner-Priemer UW, Kuo J, Schlotz W, et al. Distress and affective dysregulation in patients with borderline personality disorder: a psychophysiological ambulatory monitoring study. J Nerv Ment Dis 2008;196(4):314–20.

74. Feldman G, Dunn E, Stemke C, et al. Mindfulness and rumination as predictors of persistence with a distress tolerance task. Pers Individ Dif 2014;56:154–8.
75. Herrero N, Gadea M, Rodriguez-Alarcon G, et al. What happens when we get angry? Hormonal, cardiovascular and asymmetrical brain responses. Horm Behav 2010;57(3):276–83.
76. Kobele R, Koschke M, Schulz S, et al. The influence of negative mood on heart rate complexity measures and baroreflex sensitivity in healthy subjects. Indian J Psychiatry 2010;52(1):42–7.
77. Carreiro S, Fang H, Zhang J, et al. iMStrong: deployment of a biosensor system to detect cocaine use. J Med Syst 2015;39:1–14.
78. Carreiro S, Wittbold K, Indic P, et al. Wearable biosensors to detect physiologic change during opioid use. J Med Toxicol 2016;12:255–62.
79. Arnold Z, LaRose D, Agu E. Smartphone inference of alcohol consumption levels from gait. Proceedings - 2015 IEEE International Conference on Healthcare Informatics, ICHI 2015 2015. Verona, Italy, September 15 – 17, 2014. p. 417–26.
80. Priester MA, Browne T, Iachini A, et al. Treatment access barriers and disparities among individuals with co-occurring mental health and substance use disorders: an integrative literature review. J Substance Abuse Treat 2016;61:47–59.
81. Sugarman DE, Campbell ANC, Iles BR, et al. Technology-based interventions for substance use and comorbid disorders. Harv Rev Psychiatry 2017;25:123–34.
82. Kay-Lambkin FJ, Simpson AL, Bowman J, et al. Dissemination of a computer-based psychological treatment in a drug and alcohol clinical service: an observational study. Addict Sci Clin Pract 2014;9(1):15.
83. Deady M, Mills KL, Teesson M, et al. An online intervention for co-occurring depression and problematic alcohol use in young people: primary outcomes from a randomized controlled trial. J Med Internet Res 2016;18:1–12.
84. Kay-Lambkin F, Baker A, Geddes J, et al. The iTreAD project: a study protocol for a randomised controlled clinical trial of online treatment and social networking for binge drinking and depression in young people. BMC Public Health 2015;15(1):1025.
85. Gilmore AK, Wilson SM, Skopp NA, et al. A systematic review of technology-based interventions for co-occurring substance use and trauma symptoms. J Telemed Telecare 2017;23(8):701–9.
86. Buntin MB, Burke MF, Hoaglin MC, et al. The benefits of health information technology: a review of the recent literature shows predominantly positive results. Health Aff 2011;30(3):464–71.
87. Eyrich-Garg KM. Mobile phone technology: a new paradigm for the prevention, treatment, and research of the non-sheltered "street" homeless? J Urban Health 2010;87(3):365–80.
88. Tofighi B, Campbell A, Pavlicova M, et al. Recent internet use and associations with clinical outcomes among patients entering addiction treatment involved in a web-delivered psychosocial intervention study. J Urban Health 2016;93(5):871–83.
89. Acosta MC, Marsch LA, Xie H, et al. A web-based behavior therapy program influences the association between cognitive functioning and retention and abstinence in clients receiving methadone maintenance treatment. J Dual Diagn 2012;8(4):283–93.
90. Bates ME, Buckman JF, Nguyen TT. A role for cognitive rehabilitation in increasing the effectiveness of treatment for alcohol use disorders. Neuropsychol Rev 2013;23(1):27–47.

91. Lupton D, Jutel A. 'It's like having a physician in your pocket!' A critical analysis of self-diagnosis smartphone apps. Social Sci Med 2015;133:128–35.
92. Administration USFD. Mobile medical applications. 2017. Available at: https://www.fda.gov/MedicalDevices/DigitalHealth/MobileMedicalApplications/default.htm. Accessed September 8, 2017.
93. Karasz HN, Eiden A, Bogan S. Text messaging to communicate with public health audiences: how the HIPAA Security Rule affects practice. Am J Public Health 2013;103(4):617–22.
94. Bartholomew LK, Parcel GS, Kok G. Intervention mapping: a process for developing theory and evidence-based health education programs. Health Educ Behav 1998;25(5):545–63.
95. Collins LM, Murphy SA, Strecher V. The Multiphase Optimization Strategy (MOST) and the Sequential Multiple Assignment Randomized Trial (SMART): new methods for more potent eHealth interventions. Am J Prev Med 2007;32(5): S112–8.
96. Webb TL, Joseph J, Yardley L, et al. Using the internet to promote health behavior change: a systematic review and meta-analysis of the impact of theoretical basis, use of behavior change techniques, and mode of delivery on efficacy. J Med Internet Res 2010;12(1):e4.
97. Bates DW, Bitton A. The future of health information technology in the patient-centered medical home. Health Aff 2010;29(4):614–21.

Pain and Addiction

An Integrative Therapeutic Approach

Ajay Manhapra, MD[a,b,c],*, William C. Becker, MD[d,e,f]

KEYWORDS

- Substance use disorder • Addiction • Opioid use disorder • Pain • Chronic pain
- Multimorbidity • Treatment • Management

KEY POINTS

- Treating "pain and addiction" as 2 separate problems is often unsuccessful, because this clinical condition is often more than the sum of its parts.
- Patients with pain and addiction often have multiple psychological, psychiatric, and medical comorbidities with associated polypharmacy, all interacting with each other in complex ways (multimorbidity).
- Multimorbidity appears to be the key driver of "chronification" of pain (evolution of acute pain to severely disabling chronic pain) and associated adverse outcomes, rather than the persistence of injuries.
- The authors suggest an integrative approach that involves reexplaining the pain based on multimorbidity as the driver, followed by concurrent coordinated management of addiction/dependence, comorbidities, and chronic pain, and polypharmacy reduction.

INTRODUCTION

The current opioid crisis, partly fueled by the excess availability of prescription opioids for pain management, has highlighted the enormous challenge of managing disabling chronic pain intertwined with physiologic dependence to medications (here forward

This article originally appeared in *Medical Clinics*, Volume 102, Issue 4, July 2018.

Funding: A. Manhapra was supported by the Research in Addiction Medicine Scholars Research in Addiction Medicine Scholars (RAMS) Program, Grant number R25DA033211 from the National Institute on Drug Abuse, and VA/OAA Interprofessional Advanced Fellowship in Addiction Treatment. The funding organizations had no role in the design and conduct of the study; collection, management, analysis, and interpretation of the data; preparation, review, or approval of the article; and decision to submit the article for publication.

[a] Veteran Affairs New England Mental Illness Research, Education and Clinical Center (MIRECC), West Haven, CT, USA; [b] Advanced PACT Pain Clinic, VA Hampton Medical Center, 100 Emancipation Drive, PRIME 5, Hampton, VA 23667, USA; [c] Department of Psychiatry, Yale School of Medicine, New Haven, CT, USA; [d] Opioid Reassessment Clinic, VA Connecticut Healthcare System, 950 Campbell Avenue, Mailstop 151B, West Haven, CT 06516, USA; [e] Pain Research, Informatics, Multimorbidities and Education (PRIME) Center, West Haven, CT, USA; [f] Department of Medicine, Yale School of Medicine, New Haven, CT, USA

* Corresponding author. 100 Emancipation Drive, PRIME 5, Hampton, VA 23667.

E-mail address: ajay.manhapra@yale.edu

termed "medication dependence") and substance use disorders (SUDs) and other medical and psychiatric disorders.[1,2] It is also now clear that long-term opioid therapy (LTOT), especially at high doses, is neither as safe nor as effective for treating chronic pain as once considered.[3] Many patients continue to have disabling pain despite high-dose LTOT and yet may be unable to discontinue opioids without major challenges.[4] Also, the prevalence of prior SUDs and psychiatric and medical comorbidities is high among these patients.[5,6] Given this complex context, there is an urgent need for better paradigms for the clinical conceptualization of disabling chronic pain among patients with dependence and addiction to opioids and other substances.[1]

Clinicians evaluating patients with the dual problem of pain and addiction often face the question, "Is this pain or is this addiction?" However, constricted focus on chronic pain and SUD as separate treatment entities often misses the complexity of the whole individual who suffers from the 2 maladies. These patients may also have high psychiatric and medical illness burden and may also use multiple substances or medications to manage their symptoms. These coexisting multiple problems interact with each other and pain and addiction in complex ways (multimorbidity), making clinical management challenging. In a nutshell, the problem of "pain and addiction" is more than the sum of its parts and thus necessitates an integrated, multidimensional therapeutic approach.

In this article, the authors first describe the complex interconnections of pain with dependence, opioid use disorder (OUD), and other SUDs. They then seek to draw attention to the critical role of multimorbidity (multiple illnesses existing together and interacting with each other in complex ways).[7] In light of the complexity of the current opioid epidemic, the authors propose an integrative multidimensional pharmacobehavioral model to manage these complex, commonly cooccurring conditions.

PAIN AND ADDICTION, A COMPLEX PROBLEM
Prevalence of Pain, Opioid Use Disorder, and Other Substance Use Disorders

Pain and SUD, including OUD, have a complicated reciprocal relationship with a myriad of interconnections (**Fig. 1**). Although a large proportion of patients with SUD have chronic pain compared with those without SUD, a smaller, nonetheless significant proportion of patients with chronic pain tends to report SUD.[8] In the National

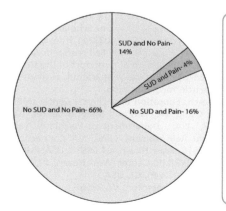

NESARC wave 1 data (2001–2002)- US Adults
- 20% reported significant pain interference, and 25% of them had SUD (including tobacco)
- 18% reported SUD, and 22% of them have significant Pain interference
- 2-year prescription OUD incidence: 0.62% among those with significant pain interference compared to 0.44% among those without PI

NCS-R data (2001–2002)- US Adults in past year
- About 5% of those with chronic spinal pain (40 million, 23% of adults) had alcohol or drug use disorders
- 40% of those with AUD/DUD (5 million, 4.8% of adults) had chronic spinal pain (2 million with both).

Pertinent results from other studies
- Up to 75% of those on Opioid Agonist Treatment for OUD can have chronic pain or pain interference
- Current OUD (DSM-5) prevalence was 8%–12% among those on LTOT for chronic pain, but studies vary dramatically in methodology.
- Between 2005 and 2013, among those using heroin, opioid initiation with prescription opioid decreased from 84% to 52%, and initiation with heroin increased from 8.7% to 33% with no signs of stabilization.
- In patients with SUD and pain, SUD preceded pain in 58.2%, pain preceded SUD in 35.4% and simultaneous onset in 6.4%

Fig. 1. Key information regarding pain and SUD including OUD. AUD/DUD, Alcohol use disorder and drug use disorder; NESARC, National Epidemiologic Survey on Alcohol and Related Conditions; PI, pain interference. (*Data from* Refs.[2,9,12–24,116])

Comorbidity Survey Replication (NCS-R), 35% of those with lifetime SUD reported chronic spinal pain, whereas only 4.8% of those with chronic spinal pain had SUD in the past year.[2] Although 38% of those with prescription OUD (pOUD) reported pain to the level that it interferes with life (pain interference) in a US national sample, only 18.9% of those without pOUD reported pain interference. Among those reporting pain interference, approximately 20% reported any SUD and 0.6% reported pOUD.[9] The prevalence of chronic pain and pain interference is even higher among those engaging in treatment of SUD,[10–18] with rates as high as 75% among patients with OUD treated with methadone or buprenorphine.[11,14,16,19–27]

Opioid Use Disorder, Pain, and Prescription Opioid Use

An estimated 12.5% of the 91.8 million US adults who used prescription opioids in 2015 misused them, with substantially higher misuse rates among those with pOUD and other SUDs.[28] Although those without pOUD reported pain as the most common reason for misuse (63%), more than half of those with pOUD and other SUDs reported other reasons, such as relaxing and getting high. Prescription opioid misuse among patients entering treatment for SUD appears to be largely for withdrawal prevention and getting high,[29,30] with slightly higher misuse for pain relief among those using heroin.[30,31]

The demographics of heroin use have changed over time. Those who started heroin use in the 1960s were mostly racially heterogeneous young people who initiated with heroin, whereas those who used heroin use in subsequent decades tended to be mostly older Caucasian men who started with prescription opioids.[32,33] More recently, this trend seems to be reversing because of decreased availability and increased cost of prescription opioids and increased availability of the often cheaper option of heroin. Between 2005 and 2013, opioid initiation with prescription opioids among treatment-seeking heroin users decreased from 84% to 52%, whereas opioid initiation with heroin increased from 8.7% to 33%.[34,35] Because the use of prescription opioids alone is waning among those with OUD, their concurrent use with heroin is steadily increasing.[34]

Pain and Substance Use Disorders: Which Starts First?

Although it is often assumed that chronic pain precedes onset of SUDs, it appears that SUD typically precedes the onset of chronic pain among those with both. However, the less common pathway, pain before SUD, is by no means rare. Among those with pain and SUD in the NCS-R, SUD preceded pain in 58.2%, and pain preceded SUD in 35.4%.[36] A similar temporal pattern of OUD more often preceding chronic pain is also seen among those using prescription opioids, in both clinical trial data and epidemiologic studies.[9–11]

Pain, a Driver of Opioid Use Disorder in Individuals

Pain drives increased craving for opioids[37] and use of multiple substances for pain relief among individuals engaged in SUD treatment.[38,39] Although a higher intensity of pain has only shown limited association with OUD outcomes,[25,26,30] higher variability in pain fluctuations (pain volatility) is associated with higher relapse rates and poor outcomes after detoxification.[14,40,41] A high level of persistent pain is often observed after opioid use cessation among patients with OUD and predicts a high level of craving and substance use.[13,14,42] Also, those with a history of SUD show lower improvement with pain treatments.[43]

These data suggest that although persistent pain and its volatility could be a symptom reflective of the severity of ongoing opioid use and OUD, it could also be a symptom of protracted abstinence syndrome after opioid cessation or dose reduction.[4,44] This dual role of pain in different treatment phases of OUD can often be perplexing to patients and providers.[4] Other SUDs also show a similar relationship to pain as seen with OUD.[38,45–48]

Opioid Use Disorder in Long-Term Opioid Therapy for Pain

The data regarding OUD among patients on LTOT are somewhat confusing because of the nonuniform methodologies in studies. The prevalence of current OUD (Diagnostic and Statistical Manual of Mental Disorders, 5th Edition [DSM-5]) among those on LTOT was 8% to 12% in a recent systematic review.[49] An earlier review with stricter inclusion criteria reported that the median incidence of opioid dependence (DSM-IV) was only 0.5% (range 0%–24%) and the median prevalence was 4.5% (range 0%–32%).[50] Both studies reported substantial methodological heterogeneity among individual studies as a serious limitation. The influential 2016 Centers for Disease Control and Prevention Guideline for Prescribing Opioids for Chronic Pain[3] reported that the rates of opioid abuse or dependence diagnoses (DSM-IV) were 0.7% with a low daily dose of opioids and 6.1% with a higher daily dose versus 0.004% among those without LTOT.

LONG-TERM OPIOID THERAPY, OPIOID USE DISORDER DIAGNOSIS, AND COMPLEX PERSISTENT OPIOID DEPENDENCE

OUD diagnosis among patients on LTOT for pain can be clinically challenging for 2 main reasons:

1. Many of the DSM-5 criteria for OUD can also be attributed to pain
2. The procurement of opioids is within a therapeutic context

One study on LTOT reported 31% prevalence of DSM-IV opioid dependence when pain-related symptoms were included in the criteria-based diagnosis and 2% when they were excluded.[51] Ballantyne and colleagues[52,53] have suggested that despite lacking a DSM-5 diagnosis of OUD, many patients with pain on LTOT have complex persistent dependence (CPD), which is qualitatively more severe than simple physical dependence. One of the clinical hallmarks of this condition is that the patients are unwilling or unable to taper LTOT despite medical or functional deterioration, and classic OUD-like behaviors often emerge with opioid dose reduction or cessation.[4,52,53] About 20% of patients on LTOT in a primary care practice who tend to have high pain interference, addictive behaviors, high daily opioid doses, and significant psychiatric comorbidity[6] can be characterized as having significant CPD, the gray area between the uncomplicated physical dependence and full opioid addiction (**Fig. 2**).[4,52,53] The management principles in the gray area of CPD is currently being clarified.[4]

CHRONIC PAIN AND SUBSTANCE USE DISORDERS: THE MULTIMORBIDITY UNDERNEATH

Multimorbidity in Chronic Pain and Substance Use Disorders

As pointed out before, patients with pain and addiction are often suffering many other maladies, too. For example, in an analysis of NCS-R, 87.1% of the people with chronic spinal pain reported that at least one other comorbid condition, including other chronic pain conditions (68.6%), chronic physical conditions (55.3%), and mental disorders (35.0%). In a study of patients with OUD, pain, physical illness, psychiatric disorders, and polysubstance use were frequent even among younger patients, but the severity of these grew with age, with 75% of those older than 45 years of age having significant

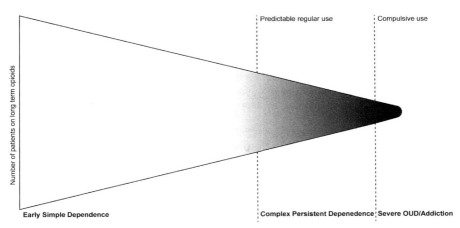

Fig. 2. A pictorial representation of the continuum of opioid dependence among LTOT patients.

pain and psychiatric problems.[54] Similar high levels of comorbidities and polypharmacy/polysubstance use have been reported by many other studies related to SUD, including OUD,[8,45,55–61] and among patients on LTOT for chronic pain.[62–65] A higher level of comorbidity and polypharmacy has been linked with higher frequency of pain, too.[66] In summary, the presence of significant chronic pain with SUD in an individual often reveals a complex, multifaceted clinical scenario involving multiple other illnesses: a multimorbid disease state underneath.

Consequences of Multimorbidity in Chronic Pain and Substance Use Disorder (Including Opioid Use Disorder)

The multimorbidity seen in association with chronic pain and substance use has significant consequences. Two separate analyses from NCS-R suggested that the excess risk of suicidal ideations, plans, and attempts among those with chronic pain is substantially mediated by comorbidities, including SUDs, mental illness, and medical illness.[67,68] Recently, Oliva and colleagues[5] reported that SUDs, mental health disorders, medical comorbidity, and nonopioid psycho-polypharmacy are more predictive of the increased risk of overdose, suicide, and suicide-related event associated with opioids than the higher opioid dose level.

Although heroin overdose deaths are often conceptualized as the consumption of a quantity or purity of opioid in excess of the person's tolerance, most overdose deaths occur among experienced users with low levels of heroin detected at autopsy,[69] but in combination with multiple substances and medications.[69–71] The recent fentanyl-related overdose deaths also largely seem to be among experienced users with polysubstance use and polypharmacy.[72–74]

Autopsy examination of heroin deaths has revealed a growing pattern of systemic disease burden, especially among older individuals.[69,75] Chronic medical illness–related morbidity and mortality are substantially higher among individuals with long-term heroin use compared with the general population, and more than half of the years of potential life lost before 65 years of age among them is due to chronic diseases,[76] with only about a third of the deaths due to overdose and accidents.[77,78]

The impact of chronic medical diseases also seems to compound with increasing age. Overdose declines as a cause of death, and chronic diseases become the more common cause for death among those with OUD those older than 45 years of age. Indeed, the median age of death among persons with OUD is steadily increasing over time.[75,76,78–80] Suicide also increases with age, but at a lower rate.[78,79]

Patients on LTOT for chronic pain also seem to experience substantially higher all-cause mortalities and chronic disease mortality than those who are not on opioids, with only a small portion of the excess mortality (about 20%) due to direct opioid-related causes.[81–83] LTOT is also associated with poor overall physical health on long-term follow-up.[84,85]

On a larger scale, Case and Deaton[86,87] have reported that midlife mortality is selectively increasing among white non-Hispanics in the United States because of a significant contribution from drug and alcohol poisoning, suicide, liver disease, and a slowing of the historic decline in cardiovascular mortality. They also reported a parallel increase in disabling chronic pain and the self-reported decline in mental and physical health in this subpopulation.

In summary, there is ample evidence that multimorbidity involving chronic pain, SUD, psychiatric illness, and medical comorbidities is associated with declining overall health and increasing mortality due to suicide, overdose, and systemic causes.

Multimorbidity and Evolution from Acute to Chronic to Disabling Chronic Pain (Chronification of Pain)

Acute pain is defined by a peripheral injurious or inflammatory focus initiating the neural processing of nociceptive stimuli by the central nervous system resulting in the perception of pain with assigned severity and salience; **Box 1** provides a definition of pain and chronic pain. Although many patients and practitioners view and manage chronic pain as persistent or recurrent acute pain, modern neurobiological research suggests this is a flawed approach. Chronic pain is by definition a pain that persists beyond tissue repair following an injury and has no known adaptive utility with regards to preservation of life and prevention of injury (see **Box 1** for definition).

Chronification of Pain

The progression from acute pain to disabling chronic pain, the "chronification" of pain, is a complex process. Only a small proportion of the patients progress from an acute injury to established chronic pain with normal function and even fewer to disabling chronic pain (**Fig. 3**). Neurobiologically, pain chronification involves neuroplasticity (central nervous system learning and adapting) in pain-processing central nervous pathways and downward pain-inhibition pathways. Such neuroplasticity causes changes in several domains related to pain, including perception, cognition, attention, emotion, learning, memory, and motivation. The pain processing also shows an overall shift from pain pathways to emotional pathways.[88–90] These neurobiological changes drive the chronic pain experience through various mechanisms. The threshold for nociception at the site of pain is often reduced, and the severity and the extent of pain sensation are amplified as it ascends the pain pathways. The endogenous pain

---

Box 1
Definition of pain and chronic pain

Pain: An unpleasant sensory and emotional experience associated with actual or potential tissue damage, or described in terms of such damage.

Chronic pain: A pain without apparent biological value that has persisted beyond the normal tissue healing time (usually taken to be 3 months).

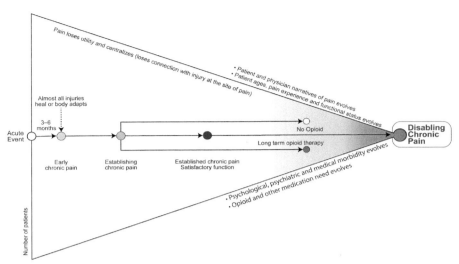

Fig. 3. Progression from persistent pain in many to disabling chronic pain among few.

inhibition through the downward pathways is also altered. At the cognitive level, there are maladaptive modifications of the assigned salience of pain, associated negative affect, and behavioral response.

Multimorbidity and Pain Chronification

A multitude of factors influence pain chronification,[91] and for clinical utility, this complex array of factors can be categorized into 3 main groups (**Fig. 4, Box 2**):

1. Psychosocial factors
2. Comorbidities with psychological impact (psychiatric and medical)
3. Dependencies (SUD, SUD recovery, and medication dependence)

Decades of research have established that several demographic, social, and psychological factors (see **Box 2**) can drive chronification of pain, and many of them are amenable to psychological treatment.[91,92] Although the severity of initial pain and associated disability play a role in chronification, it is confined to the early part of chronification.[91,93]

Extensive available literature supports the notion that preexisting psychiatric comorbidities (see **Box 2**) are key drivers of pain chronification, and pain, in turn, worsens psychiatric status.[8,91,92,94–96] It is less appreciated that medical comorbidities (see **Box 2**) also greatly influence pain chronification, especially among older individuals.[91,94,97–101] Recently, there is also growing recognition of the increased burden of chronic pain and opioid use following recovery from life-threatening medical illness,[102] traumatic brain injury and concussions,[103,104] and cancer.[105] As the population, including those with SUD, ages, multimorbidity and chronic pain prevalence are simultaneously increasing.[99–101] In addition, several infectious and noninfectious sequelae like hepatitis C, HIV, liver disease, pancreatitis, and infectious arthritis can all lead to chronic pain. Multiple painful conditions due to different initiating abnormalities are also common among those with chronic pain.[2,100]

As detailed in prior sections, regular use of substances that can cause dependence is a key driver in the development of disabling chronic pain. Often, those substances

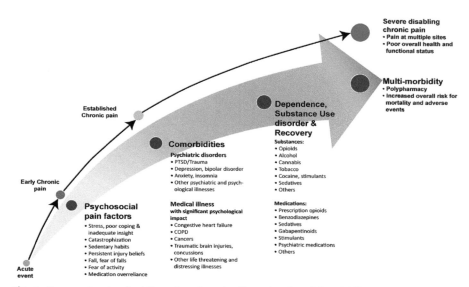

Fig. 4. Progression to disabling chronic pain: the role of multimorbidity.

are medications for pain and accompanying symptoms like insomnia, lack of focus, anxiety and mood disorders, and other medical comorbidities, often leading to a dizzying array of polypharmacy. This, in turn, can adversely affect pain and disability.[5,30,54,64–66,106,107]

Thus, disabling chronic pain, especially among those with SUD, often evolves and presents as multimorbidity involving varying combinations of several chronic pain conditions, psychiatric and medical comorbidities, polysubstance and medication dependencies, and a complex set of pain-related maladaptive psychopathologies influenced by all the comorbidities (see **Fig. 4**). Such patients with consequential severe disabilities and excess risk of suicide, overdose, and all-cause mortality are becoming increasingly common in physician practices, posing a great challenge to providers and health systems. Isolated focus on a single issue or limited set of issues like pain and SUD without coordinated treatment of multiple comorbidities is unlikely to lead to sustained benefit. Recently, there is growing recognition of the need for multidimensional approaches to successfully manage patients with such complex clinical conditions.[108–110]

MULTIDIMENSIONAL PHARMACOBEHAVIORAL MODEL FOR COMPLEX CHRONIC PAIN MANAGEMENT

The authors propose a multidimensional, pharmacobehavioral model for medical management of complex chronic pain with a whole person focus, rooted in the biopsychosocial framework (**Fig. 5**). This model divides the overall management of the patient into categories or steps:

1. Patient education and activation: Reexplaining pain based on modern conceptualization of the chronification of pain and shifting the locus of control to the patient
2. Dependence treatment
3. Comorbidity treatment
4. Polypharmacy reduction
5. Chronic pain treatment

Box 2
Various factors involved in chronification of pain

Demographic factors

Age

Gender

Education level

Smoking

Overweight

Disability

Receiving Workers' compensation

Higher work dissatisfaction

Higher physical work demand

Psychological pain factors

Maladaptive coping

Fear avoidance (of work, movements, activities)

Falls, fear of falls

Catastrophization (excessive negative thoughts about future in relation to pain)

Low self-efficacy

Pain hypervigilance

Overreliance on pain medications

Initial pain severity (confined to early part of chronification)

Comorbidities with psychological impact

Psychiatric
  Trauma, posttraumatic stress disorder (PTSD)
  Depression, anxiety
  Bipolar disorder
  Other severe mental illnesses
  Personality disorder

Medical
  Poor overall health
  Congestive heart failure, chronic obstructive pulmonary disease, cancer diagnosis, critical
  illness recovery
  Traumatic brain injury and concussions

Dependencies to various agents

Active substance use & recovery from SUD
  Tobacco, alcohol, opioid, cocaine, stimulants, cannabis, barbiturates, benzodiazepines, and
  other drugs

Medications
  Opioids, benzodiazepines, stimulants, anti-depressants, anti-psychotics, anticonvulsants,
  barbiturates, other psychoactive medications
  Nonsteroidal anti-inflammatory agents

Patients with disabling chronic pain and SUD/medication dependence often present in a state of personal crisis, and the initial goal of management is often achieving clinical stability. Crisis stabilization is followed by a slow transition from disease-focused,

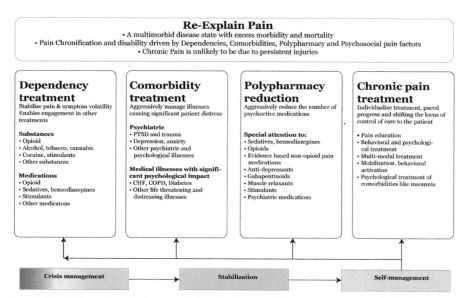

Re-Explain Pain
- A multimorbid disease state with excess morbidity and mortality
- Pain Chronification and disability driven by Dependencies, Comorbidities, Polypharmacy and Psychosocial pain factors
- Chronic Pain is unlikely to be due to persistent injuries

Dependency treatment
Stabilize pain & symptom volatility
Enables engagement in other treatments

Substances
- Opioid
- Alcohol, tobacco, cannabis
- Cocaine, stimulants
- Other substances

Medications
- Opioid
- Sedatives, benzodiazepines
- Stimulants
- Other medicatons

Comorbidity treatment
Aggressively manage illnesses causing significant patient distress

Psychiatric
- PTSD and trauma
- Depression, anxiety
- Other psychiatric and psychological illnesses

Medical illnesses with significant psychological impact
- CHF, COPD, Diabetes
- Other life threatening and distressing illnesses

Polypharmacy reduction
Aggressively reduce the number of psychotive medications

Special attention to:
- Sedatives, benzodiazepines
- Opioids
- Evidence based non-opioid pain medications
- Anti-depressants
- Gabapentinoids
- Muscle relaxants
- Stimulants
- Psychiatric medications

Chronic pain treatment
Individualize treatment, paced progress and shifting the locus of control of care to the patient

- Pain education
- Behavioral and psychological treatment
- Multi-modal treatment
- Mobilization, behavioral activation
- Psychological treatment of comorbidities like insomnia

Crisis management → Stabilization → Self-management

Fig. 5. Multidimensional pharmacobehavioral model for management of disabling pain among those with substance dependence. CHF, congestive heart failure; COPD, chronic obstructive pulmonary disease.

provider-based management to a whole person–focused paradigm with self-management of pain and comorbidities. This model could be implemented using an adequately trained single medical provider or an interdisciplinary team, both within primary care settings when feasible. A detailed discussion of each element of this complex process is beyond the scope of this review, but the authors broadly discuss each of the management categories. Although as a learning heuristic, these are described as discrete components; the management in each of these categories usually progresses simultaneously, and often one treatment intervention can impact multiple components, both positively and negatively.

Reexplaining Pain

The first and arguably most important step in treatment is developing a shared clinical conceptualization of the complex reasons for the disabling pain, or developing a more nuanced diagnosis beyond the common explanation of persistent injury, tissue damage, or disease. Such a shared conceptualization requires an initial detailed longitudinal diagnostic formulation of chronic pain as a condition caused by the persistence of perceived need to protect body tissue, driven by central nervous system neuroplasticity, under the influence of pain factors, comorbidities, dependencies, and polypharmacy (chronification of pain).

Over time, patients may acquire injury/disease-focused beliefs and cognitive narratives related to pain-driving maladaptive behaviors that sustain painful disability and suffering.[111,112] Such maladaptive beliefs and narratives are no doubt also sustained by health care systems that promote passive treatments (medications, procedures) over active self-management. Patients (and the multiple providers caring for them) are often unaware of the complex connection between pain and SUDs, and about the further contribution of multimorbidity to the chronification of pain. For example, a patient with disabling chronic back pain, failed spinal surgeries, and OUD may see the continued pain-related opioid use as a consequence of the inability to "fix" the back and may seek out additional procedures. This patient might be uninformed that persistent spine injury/disease is an unlikely explanation for disabling chronic pain, and that the comorbid SUD, PTSD, and insomnia are much more important drivers of pain chronification. This example patient may also be unaware that the polypharmacy developing from the fragmented treatment of multiple problems will also affect pain and health deleteriously. Education of patients, families, and other providers based on a nuanced longitudinal narrative enables them to integrate this new understanding into their wider pain- and function-related beliefs, attitudes, behaviors, treatment, and lifestyle choices.[113] This psychological/cognitive approach commonly known as "explaining pain" (therapeutic neuroscience or pain neuroscience education) has been shown to be an effective mode of pain treatment.[113]

Dependence Treatment

The most logical next step after the "reexplaining pain" is the treatment of significant SUD and medication dependence, which often restricts the ability of patients to engage in treatments for pain and comorbidities.

It is often difficult to control pain and other symptoms without effective treatment of SUD and medication dependencies that often drive the intensity and volatility of these symptoms. In the case of OUD or opioid medication dependence, buprenorphine treatment that can effectively manage both dependence and pain offers a viable pharmacologic treatment path.[114] Methadone is another treatment option, but can cause increasing levels of dependence with long-term use that could worsen pain and associated symptoms.[115] A more detailed description of the influence of dependence on pain and its management is beyond the scope of this review and can be found elsewhere.[4]

The influence of alcohol, tobacco, cannabis, and cocaine use in pain chronification is not often recognized; they require equal attention as other substances. Many patients often use these substances to get relief from pain. Nonopioid SUD and medication dependence are much more difficult to manage as pharmacologic treatment, like anticonvulsants, naltrexone, and antidepressants, may have limited impact on pain associated with dependence. The authors often have to judiciously use prescription opioids and/or interventional procedures to control overwhelming pain to facilitate SUD/dependence treatment engagement.

Many patients with pain often have multiple SUDs and medication dependencies, making the management even more challenging. In these situations, a nuanced individualized approach based on the longitudinal diagnostic formulation is often the way forward. The authors recommend an integrative simultaneous treatment of multiple SUDs and medication dependencies with a harm reduction approach, engaging patients at the level they are willing to engage. In addition, the authors strongly believe treaters should not deny treatment of one SUD to patients because they have another active SUD or medication dependence. It is critical not to abandon patients if their behaviors become difficult under the influence of polysubstance use. Such patients tend to be at higher risk of adverse outcomes, including overdose, suicide, and death.

Comorbidity Treatment

As noted above, psychiatric comorbidities, medical comorbidities, and pain are commonly seen as separate treatment entities with little recognition of the complex reciprocal interconnections between them. This is especially the case with medical comorbidities that often generate a sustained sense of mortality dread and anxiety (eg, congestive heart failure, coronary artery disease, chronic obstructive pulmonary disease, and cancer). Simultaneous, effective management of these comorbidities often leads to better control of pain, and effective dependence treatment often allows patients to engage in better management of comorbidities.

Polypharmacy Reduction

Patients and providers are often unaware that polypharmacy from the nonintegrated treatment of individual symptoms associated with chronic pain, SUDs, and comorbidities often worsens chronic pain and disability. Polypharmacy reduction is often an important component of chronic pain treatment. Patients are often reluctant to leave the perceived safety of taking a pill to control overwhelming symptoms. Managing patient expectation around the need for polypharmacy reduction can be extremely challenging, but is crucial to maintaining a therapeutic alliance. Patient education, psychotherapies focused on treatment of coping, insomnia, anxiety, and depression, and effective treatment of medication dependencies and SUD all can reduce medication need.

Pain Treatment

It is essential to recognize that traditional biomedically oriented treatment with a focus on pharmacotherapy and passive interventions should be abandoned as the primary treatment of chronic pain, especially among those with comorbid SUD/medication dependence. "Reexplaining pain" followed by the effective management of SUD/medication dependence, comorbidities, and polypharmacy, combined with simple behavioral activation (eg, walking 30 minutes 2 times a day at a comfortable speed), are effective for many patients. This basic approach *may* obviate evidence-based professional psychological treatments like cognitive behavioral therapy (CBT), acceptance and commitment therapy (ACT), and mindfulness,[92] which are often difficult to access currently. Also, many elements of psychological treatment of pain like motivational interviewing, goal setting, cognitive reframing, basic mindfulness, and behavioral activation are deployable in primary care clinics; models to build capacity and expand reach are under development. CBT, ACT, and mindfulness-based psychological treatment are more successful when combined with "Reexplaining pain" beyond what is offered traditionally within the respective treatment protocols.[113] Other comorbidities can create their own psychological challenges (eg, emotional volatility in SUDs, constant dread of mortality in cancer or CHF) can complicate overall treatment and may require further health psychology treatment.

Pain medications and procedural interventions to control overwhelming pain can enable engagement in the multidimensional treatment. Structured opioid therapy with close attention to patient safety can often be helpful in allaying overwhelming distress associated with pain. Structured opioid therapy, in turn, enables engagement in further treatment of multimorbidity, thus improving functionality and reducing overall risk. Although seemingly contrary to the current climate of frenzied opioid restriction, this is consistent with the whole-person approach to the treatment of SUD and chronic pain. It is also vital to recognize that surgical procedures are less likely to show sustained effectiveness in patients who have uncontrolled comorbidities, and postsurgical pain can develop into yet another chronic pain. Hence, it is important to engage in multidimensional treatment if surgical treatment of chronic pain is considered.

SUMMARY

Chronic pain combined with SUD and medication dependence often presents as a disabling multimorbid disease state with polypharmacy or polysubstance use associated with excess risk of adverse outcomes, including death. It is becoming increasingly clear that simple strategies like opioid tapering and nonpharmacologic treatment of pain are insufficient by themselves. Health systems and clinical teams must develop resources to manage this vulnerable population. Categorization of patient problems and treatment options in a multidimensional pharmacobehavioral model can help both patients and physicians to engage in more effective treatment. Acquisition of knowledge and skills spanning multiple fields of pain, addiction, psychiatry, and complex medical multimorbidity required to manage these complex conditions can be challenging, but eminently possible with effective provider education and training. Clinical and research foci in this area must shift from management of individual conditions to development of effective methods to manage multimorbidities in association with dependence.

ACKNOWLEDGMENTS

The editors wish to thank Stefan G. Kertesz, Birmingham Veterans Affairs Medical Center and University of Alabama at Birmingham, for providing a critical review of this article.

REFERENCES

1. Volkow ND, Collins FS. The role of science in addressing the opioid crisis. N Engl J Med 2017;377(4):391–4.
2. Von Korff M, Crane P, Lane M, et al. Chronic spinal pain and physical-mental comorbidity in the United States: results from the national comorbidity survey replication. Pain 2005;113(3):331–9.
3. Dowell D, Haegerich TM, Chou R. CDC guideline for prescribing opioids for chronic pain—United States, 2016. MMWR Recomm Rep 2016;65(1):1–49.
4. Manhapra A, Arias AJ, Ballantyne JC. The conundrum of opioid tapering in long-term opioid therapy for chronic pain: a commentary. Subst Abuse 2017;1–10.
5. Oliva EM, Bowe T, Tavakoli S, et al. Development and applications of the Veterans Health Administration's Stratification Tool for Opioid Risk Mitigation (STORM) to improve opioid safety and prevent overdose and suicide. Psychol Serv 2017;14(1):34–49.
6. Banta-Green CJ, Merrill JO, Doyle SR, et al. Opioid use behaviors, mental health and pain–development of a typology of chronic pain patients. Drug Alcohol Depend 2009;104(1–2):34–42.
7. Viana MC, Lim CCW, Pereira FG, et al. Previous mental disorders and subsequent onset of chronic back or neck pain: findings from 19 countries. J Pain 2017;19(1):99–110.
8. Howe CQ, Sullivan MD. The missing 'P' in pain management: how the current opioid epidemic highlights the need for psychiatric services in chronic pain care. Gen Hosp Psychiatry 2014;36(1):99–104.
9. Blanco C, Wall MM, Okuda M, et al. Pain as a predictor of opioid use disorder in a nationally representative sample. Am J Psychiatry 2016;173(12):1189–95.
10. Weiss RD, Potter JS, Griffin ML, et al. Reasons for opioid use among patients with dependence on prescription opioids: the role of chronic pain. J Subst Abuse Treat 2014;47(2):140–5.

11. Weiss RD, Rao V. The prescription opioid addiction treatment study: what have we learned. Drug Alcohol Depend 2017;173(Suppl 1):S48–54.
12. Dhingra L, Perlman DC, Masson C, et al. Longitudinal analysis of pain and illicit drug use behaviors in outpatients on methadone maintenance. Drug Alcohol Depend 2015;149:285–9.
13. Larson MJ, Paasche-Orlow M, Cheng DM, et al. Persistent pain is associated with substance use after detoxification: a prospective cohort analysis. Addiction 2007;102(5):752–60.
14. Potter JS, Chakrabarti A, Domier CP, et al. Pain and continued opioid use in individuals receiving buprenorphine-naloxone for opioid detoxification: secondary analyses from the Clinical Trials Network. J Subst Abuse Treat 2010;38(Suppl 1):S80–6.
15. Potter JS, Prather K, Weiss RD. Physical pain and associated clinical characteristics in treatment-seeking patients in four substance use disorder treatment modalities. Am J Addict 2008;17(2):121–5.
16. Rosenblum A, Joseph H, Fong C, et al. Prevalence and characteristics of chronic pain among chemically dependent patients in methadone maintenance and residential treatment facilities. JAMA 2003;289(18):2370–8.
17. Sheu R, Lussier D, Rosenblum A, et al. Prevalence and characteristics of chronic pain in patients admitted to an outpatient drug and alcohol treatment program. Pain Med 2008;9(7):911–7.
18. Caldeiro RM, Malte CA, Calsyn DA, et al. The association of persistent pain with out-patient addiction treatment outcomes and service utilization. Addiction 2008;103(12):1996–2005.
19. Barry DT, Beitel M, Joshi D, et al. Pain and substance-related pain-reduction behaviors among opioid dependent individuals seeking methadone maintenance treatment. Am J Addict 2009;18(2):117–21.
20. Barry D, Beitel M, Cutter C, et al. Allopathic, complementary, and alternative medical treatment utilization for pain among methadone-maintained patients. Am J Addict 2009;18(5):379–85.
21. Jamison RN, Kauffman J, Katz NP. Characteristics of methadone maintenance patients with chronic pain. J Pain Symptom Manage 2000;19(1):53–62.
22. Nordmann S, Vilotitch A, Lions C, et al. Pain in methadone patients: time to address undertreatment and suicide risk (ANRS-Methaville trial). PLoS One 2017;12(5):e0176288.
23. Peles E, Schreiber S, Gordon J, et al. Significantly higher methadone dose for methadone maintenance treatment (MMT) patients with chronic pain. Pain 2005;113(3):340–6.
24. Dhingra L, Masson C, Perlman DC, et al. Epidemiology of pain among outpatients in methadone maintenance treatment programs. Drug Alcohol Depend 2013;128(1–2):161–5.
25. Chakrabarti A, Woody GE, Griffin ML, et al. Predictors of buprenorphine-naloxone dosing in a 12-week treatment trial for opioid-dependent youth: secondary analyses from a NIDA Clinical Trials Network study. Drug Alcohol Depend 2010;107(2–3):253–6.
26. Fox AD, Sohler NL, Starrels JL, et al. Pain is not associated with worse office-based buprenorphine treatment outcomes. Subst Abuse 2012;33(4):361–5.
27. Griffin ML, McDermott KA, McHugh RK, et al. Longitudinal association between pain severity and subsequent opioid use in prescription opioid dependent patients with chronic pain. Drug Alcohol Depend 2016;163:216–21.

28. Han B, Compton WM, Blanco C, et al. Prescription opioid use, misuse, and use disorders in U.S. Adults: 2015 national survey on drug use and health. Ann Intern Med 2017;167(5):293–301.
29. Bohnert AS, Eisenberg A, Whiteside L, et al. Prescription opioid use among addictions treatment patients: nonmedical use for pain relief vs. other forms of nonmedical use. Addict Behav 2013;38(3):1776–81.
30. Trafton JA, Oliva EM, Horst DA, et al. Treatment needs associated with pain in substance use disorder patients: implications for concurrent treatment. Drug Alcohol Depend 2004;73(1):23–31.
31. Dahlman D, Kral AH, Wenger L, et al. Physical pain is common and associated with nonmedical prescription opioid use among people who inject drugs. Subst Abuse Treat Prev Pol 2017;12(1):29.
32. Cicero TJ, Ellis MS, Surratt HL, et al. The changing face of heroin use in the United States: a retrospective analysis of the past 50 years. JAMA Psychiatry 2014;71(7):821–6.
33. Martins SS, Sarvet A, Santaella-Tenorio J, et al. Changes in US lifetime heroin use and heroin use disorder: prevalence from the 2001-2002 to 2012-2013 National Epidemiologic Survey on alcohol and related conditions. JAMA Psychiatry 2017;74(5):445–55.
34. Cicero TJ, Ellis MS, Harney J. Shifting patterns of prescription opioid and heroin abuse in the United States. N Engl J Med 2015;373(18):1789–90.
35. Cicero TJ, Ellis MS, Kasper ZA. Increased use of heroin as an initiating opioid of abuse. Addict behaviors 2017;74:63–6.
36. Ilgen MA, Perron B, Czyz EK, et al. The timing of onset of pain and substance use disorders. Am J Addict 2010;19(5):409–15.
37. Tsui JI, Lira MC, Cheng DM, et al. Chronic pain, craving, and illicit opioid use among patients receiving opioid agonist therapy. Drug Alcohol Depend 2016; 166:26–31.
38. Alford DP, German JS, Samet JH, et al. Primary care patients with drug use report chronic pain and self-medicate with alcohol and other drugs. J Gen Intern Med 2016;31(5):486–91.
39. Brennan PL, Schutte KK, Moos RH. Pain and use of alcohol to manage pain: prevalence and 3-year outcomes among older problem and non-problem drinkers. Addiction 2005;100(6):777–86.
40. Worley MJ, Heinzerling KG, Shoptaw S, et al. Pain volatility and prescription opioid addiction treatment outcomes in patients with chronic pain. Exp Clin Psychopharmacol 2015;23(6):428–35.
41. Worley MJ, Heinzerling KG, Shoptaw S, et al. Volatility and change in chronic pain severity predict outcomes of treatment for prescription opioid addiction. Addiction 2017;112(7):1202–9.
42. Ren ZY, Shi J, Epstein DH, et al. Abnormal pain response in pain-sensitive opiate addicts after prolonged abstinence predicts increased drug craving. Psychopharmacology 2009;204(3):423–9.
43. Morasco BJ, Corson K, Turk DC, et al. Association between substance use disorder status and pain-related function following 12 months of treatment in primary care patients with musculoskeletal pain. J Pain 2011;12(3):352–9.
44. Heilig M, Egli M, Crabbe JC, et al. Acute withdrawal, protracted abstinence and negative affect in alcoholism: are they linked? Addict Biol 2010;15(2):169–84.
45. Zale EL, Maisto SA, Ditre JW. Interrelations between pain and alcohol: an integrative review. Clin Psychol Rev 2015;37:57–71.

46. Jakubczyk A, Ilgen MA, Kopera M, et al. Reductions in physical pain predict lower risk of relapse following alcohol treatment. Drug Alcohol Depend 2016; 158:167–71.
47. Riley JL 3rd, King C. Self-report of alcohol use for pain in a multi-ethnic community sample. J Pain 2009;10(9):944–52.
48. Rohilla J, Desai G, Chan P. Prevalence of chronic pain in patients with alcohol dependence syndrome in tertiary care center in India. Asian J Psychiatr 2016; 17(2):199–208.
49. Vowles KE, McEntee ML, Julnes PS, et al. Rates of opioid misuse, abuse, and addiction in chronic pain: a systematic review and data synthesis. Pain 2015; 156(4):569–76.
50. Minozzi S, Amato L, Davoli M. Development of dependence following treatment with opioid analgesics for pain relief: a systematic review. Addiction 2013; 108(4):688–98.
51. Elander J, Lusher J, Bevan D, et al. Pain management and symptoms of substance dependence among patients with sickle cell disease. Social Sci Med 2003;57(9):1683–96.
52. Ballantyne JC, Stannard C. New addiction criteria: diagnostic challenges persist in treating pain with opioids. Pain 2013;1:1–7.
53. Ballantyne JC, Sullivan MD, Kolodny A. Opioid dependence vs addiction: a distinction without a difference? Arch Intern Med 2012;172(17):1342–3.
54. Cicero TJ, Surratt HL, Kurtz S, et al. Patterns of prescription opioid abuse and comorbidity in an aging treatment population. J Subst Abuse Treat 2012; 42(1):87–94.
55. Saunders K, Merikangas K, Low NC, et al. Impact of comorbidity on headache-related disability. Neurology 2008;70(7):538–47.
56. Polatin PB, Kinney RK, Gatchel RJ, et al. Psychiatric illness and chronic low-back pain. The mind and the spine–which goes first? Spine (Phila Pa 1976) 1993;18(1):66–71.
57. Grant BF, Saha TD, Ruan WJ, et al. Epidemiology of DSM-5 drug use disorder: results from the National Epidemiologic Survey on alcohol and related conditions-III. JAMA Psychiatry 2016;73(1):39–47.
58. Fayaz A, Ayis S, Panesar SS, et al. Assessing the relationship between chronic pain and cardiovascular disease: a systematic review and meta-analysis. Scand J Pain 2016;13:76–90.
59. Heimer R, Zhan W, Grau LE. Prevalence and experience of chronic pain in suburban drug injectors. Drug Alcohol Depend 2015;151:92–100.
60. Mellbye A, Karlstad O, Skurtveit S, et al. Co-morbidity in persistent opioid users with chronic non-malignant pain in Norway. Eur J Pain 2014;18(8):1083–93.
61. Hser YI, Gelberg L, Hoffman V, et al. Health conditions among aging narcotics addicts: medical examination results. J Behav Med 2004;27(6):607–22.
62. Cicero TJ, Wong G, Tian Y, et al. Co-morbidity and utilization of medical services by pain patients receiving opioid medications: data from an insurance claims database. Pain 2009;144(1–2):20–7.
63. Morasco BJ, Duckart JP, Carr TP, et al. Clinical characteristics of veterans prescribed high doses of opioid medications for chronic non-cancer pain. Pain 2010;151(3):625–32.
64. Hudson TJ, Edlund MJ, Steffick DE, et al. Epidemiology of regular prescribed opioid use: results from a national, population-based survey. J Pain Symptom Manage 2008;36(3):280–8.

65. Parsells Kelly J, Cook SF, Kaufman DW, et al. Prevalence and characteristics of opioid use in the US adult population. Pain 2008;138(3):507–13.
66. Robinson KT, Bergeron CD, Mingo CA, et al. Factors associated with pain frequency among adults with chronic conditions. J Pain Symptom Manage 2017; 54(5):619–27.
67. Braden JB, Sullivan MD. Suicidal thoughts and behavior among adults with self-reported pain conditions in the national comorbidity survey replication. J Pain 2008;9(12):1106–15.
68. Ilgen MA, Zivin K, McCammon RJ, et al. Pain and suicidal thoughts, plans and attempts in the United States. Gen Hosp Psychiatry 2008;30(6):521–7.
69. Darke S, Ross J, Zador D, et al. Heroin-related deaths in New South Wales, Australia, 1992-1996. Drug Alcohol Depend 2000;60(2):141–50.
70. Coffin PO, Galea S, Ahern J, et al. Opiates, cocaine and alcohol combinations in accidental drug overdose deaths in New York City, 1990-98. Addiction 2003; 98(6):739–47.
71. Lyndon A, Audrey S, Wells C, et al. Risk to heroin users of polydrug use of pregabalin or gabapentin. Addiction 2017;112(9):1580–9.
72. Slavova S, Costich JF, Bunn TL, et al. Heroin and fentanyl overdoses in Kentucky: epidemiology and surveillance. Int J Drug Policy 2017;46:120–9.
73. Tomassoni AJ, Hawk KF, Jubanyik K, et al. Multiple fentanyl overdoses - New Haven, Connecticut, June 23, 2016. MMWR Morb Mortal Wkly Rep 2017; 66(4):107–11.
74. Marshall BDL, Krieger MS, Yedinak JL, et al. Epidemiology of fentanyl-involved drug overdose deaths: a geospatial retrospective study in Rhode Island, USA. Int J Drug Policy 2017;46:130–5.
75. Webb L, Oyefeso A, Schifano F, et al. Cause and manner of death in drug-related fatality: an analysis of drug-related deaths recorded by coroners in England and Wales in 2000. Drug Alcohol Depend 2003;72(1):67–74.
76. Hser YI, Evans E, Grella C, et al. Long-term course of opioid addiction. Harv Rev Psychiatry 2015;23(2):76–89.
77. Smyth B, Hoffman V, Fan J, et al. Years of potential life lost among heroin addicts 33 years after treatment. Prev Med 2007;44(4):369–74.
78. Degenhardt L, Larney S, Randall D, et al. Causes of death in a cohort treated for opioid dependence between 1985 and 2005. Addiction 2014;109(1):90–9.
79. Larney S, Bohnert AS, Ganoczy D, et al. Mortality among older adults with opioid use disorders in the Veteran's Health Administration, 2000-2011. Drug Alcohol Depend 2015;147:32–7.
80. Beynon C, McVeigh J, Hurst A, et al. Older and sicker: changing mortality of drug users in treatment in the North West of England. Int J Drug Policy 2010; 21(5):429–31.
81. Solomon DH, Rassen JA, Glynn RJ, et al. The comparative safety of analgesics in older adults with arthritis. Arch Intern Med 2010;170(22):1968–76.
82. Solomon DH, Rassen JA, Glynn RJ, et al. The comparative safety of opioids for nonmalignant pain in older adults. Arch Intern Med 2010;170(22):1979–86.
83. Gomes T, Juurlink DN, Dhalla IA, et al. Trends in opioid use and dosing among socio-economically disadvantaged patients. Open Med 2011;5(1):e13–22.
84. Eriksen J, Sjogren P, Bruera E, et al. Critical issues on opioids in chronic non-cancer pain: an epidemiological study. Pain 2006;125(1–2):172–9.
85. Ekholm O, Kurita GP, Hojsted J, et al. Chronic pain, opioid prescriptions, and mortality in Denmark: a population-based cohort study. Pain 2014;155(12): 2486–90.

86. Case A, Deaton A. Rising morbidity and mortality in midlife among white non-Hispanic Americans in the 21st century. Proc Natl Acad Sci U S A 2015; 112(49):15078–83.
87. Case A, Deaton A. Mortality and morbidity in the 21st century. Brookings Pap Econ Act 2017;397–476.
88. Apkarian AV, Baliki MN, Geha PY. Towards a theory of chronic pain. Prog Neurobiol 2009;87(2):81–97.
89. Simons LE, Elman I, Borsook D. Psychological processing in chronic pain: a neural systems approach. Neurosci Biobehav Rev 2014;39:61–78.
90. Pelletier R, Higgins J, Bourbonnais D. Is neuroplasticity in the central nervous system the missing link to our understanding of chronic musculoskeletal disorders? BMC Musculoskelet Disord 2015;16:25.
91. Chou R, Shekelle P. Will this patient develop persistent disabling low back pain? JAMA 2010;303(13):1295–302.
92. Edwards RR, Dworkin RH, Sullivan MD, et al. The role of psychosocial processes in the development and maintenance of chronic pain. J Pain 2016; 17(9 Suppl):T70–92.
93. Castillo RC, Wegener ST, Heins SE, et al. Longitudinal relationships between anxiety, depression, and pain: results from a two-year cohort study of lower extremity trauma patients. Pain 2013;154(12):2860–6.
94. Kroenke K, Outcalt S, Krebs E, et al. Association between anxiety, health-related quality of life and functional impairment in primary care patients with chronic pain. Gen Hosp Psychiatry 2013;35(4):359–65.
95. Tegethoff M, Belardi A, Stalujanis E, et al. Comorbidity of mental disorders and chronic pain: chronology of onset in adolescents of a national representative cohort. J Pain 2015;16(10):1054–64.
96. Gebhardt S, Heinzel-Gutenbrunner M, Konig U. Pain relief in depressive disorders: a meta-analysis of the effects of antidepressants. J Clin Psychopharmacol 2016;36(6):658–68.
97. Mundal I, Grawe RW, Bjorngaard JH, et al. Prevalence and long-term predictors of persistent chronic widespread pain in the general population in an 11-year prospective study: the HUNT study. BMC Musculoskelet Disord 2014;15:213.
98. van Hecke O, Torrance N, Smith BH. Chronic pain epidemiology and its clinical relevance. Br J Anaesth 2013;111(1):13–8.
99. Butchart A, Kerr EA, Heisler M, et al. Experience and management of chronic pain among patients with other complex chronic conditions. Clin J Pain 2009; 25(4):293–8.
100. Patel KV, Guralnik JM, Dansie EJ, et al. Prevalence and impact of pain among older adults in the United States: findings from the 2011 National Health and Aging Trends Study. Pain 2013;154(12):2649–57.
101. Sharpe L, McDonald S, Correia H, et al. Pain severity predicts depressive symptoms over and above individual illnesses and multimorbidity in older adults. BMC Psychiatry 2017;17(1):166.
102. Battle CE, Lovett S, Hutchings H. Chronic pain in survivors of critical illness: a retrospective analysis of incidence and risk factors. Crit Care 2013;17(3):R101.
103. Khoury S, Benavides R. Pain with traumatic brain injury and psychological disorders. Prog Neuropsychopharmacology Biol Psychiatry 2017. [Epub ahead of print].
104. Seal KH, Bertenthal D, Barnes DE, et al. Association of traumatic brain injury with chronic pain in Iraq and Afghanistan veterans: effect of comorbid mental health conditions. Arch Phys Med Rehabil 2017;98(8):1636–45.

105. Sutradhar R, Lokku A, Barbera L. Cancer survivorship and opioid prescribing rates: a population-based matched cohort study among individuals with and without a history of cancer. Cancer 2017;123(21):4286–93.
106. Hsu ES. Medication overuse in chronic pain. Curr Pain Headache Rep 2017; 21(1):2.
107. Menzies V, Thacker LR 2nd, Mayer SD, et al. Polypharmacy, opioid use, and fibromyalgia: a secondary analysis of clinical trial data. Biol Res Nurs 2016;19(1): 97–105.
108. Liu NH, Daumit GL, Dua T, et al. Excess mortality in persons with severe mental disorders: a multilevel intervention framework and priorities for clinical practice, policy and research agendas. World Psychiatry 2017;16(1):30–40.
109. Gallagher RM. Rational integration of pharmacologic, behavioral, and rehabilitation strategies in the treatment of chronic pain. Am J Phys Med Rehabil 2005; 84(3):S64–76.
110. Castillo RC, Archer KR, Newcomb AB, et al. Pain and psychological distress following orthopedic trauma: a call for collaborative models of care. Tech Orthop 2016;31(4):228–34.
111. Garland EL, Froeliger B, Zeidan F, et al. The downward spiral of chronic pain, prescription opioid misuse, and addiction: cognitive, affective, and neuropsychopharmacologic pathways. Neurosci biobehavioral Rev 2013;37(10 Pt 2): 2597–607.
112. Langer EJ. Matters of mind: mindfulness/mindlessness in perspective. Conscious Cogn 1992;1(3):289–305.
113. Moseley GL, Butler DS. Fifteen years of explaining pain: the past, present, and future. J Pain 2015;16(9):807–13.
114. Daitch D, Daitch J, Novinson D, et al. Conversion from high-dose full-opioid agonists to sublingual buprenorphine reduces pain scores and improves quality of life for chronic pain patients. Pain Med 2014;15(12):2087–94.
115. Rhodin A, Gronbladh L, Nilsson LH, et al. Methadone treatment of chronic non-malignant pain and opioid dependence–a long-term follow-up. Eur J Pain 2006; 10(3):271–8.
116. Rosenblum A, Parrino M, Schnoll SH, et al. Prescription opioid abuse among enrollees into methadone maintenance treatment. Drug Alcohol Depend 2007; 90(1):64–71.

Management of Challenging Pharmacologic Issues in Chronic Pain and Substance Abuse Disorders

Elyse M. Cornett, PhD[a],*, Rebecca Budish, MS[a],
Dustin Latimer, BS[a], Brendon Hart, DO[a],
Richard D. Urman, MD, MBA[b], Alan David Kaye, MD, PhD[c,d]

KEYWORDS

- Chronic pain • Substance abuse • Addiction • Pain management • Opioids
- Drug abuse

KEY POINTS

- Chronic pain is challenging to understand, as pain is subjective, personal, and has a vast number of causes.
- Over the past 10 years (2006–2016), the total US deaths due to drugs has doubled.
- There is a need for more psychological support in pain patients nationwide.

INTRODUCTION

Substance abuse has a major impact on health care services. These patients present challenges with regard to general management, pharmacologic treatment selections, and financial strain. According to the Substance Abuse and Mental Health Services Administration (SAMHSA), approximately 1 (8.1%) in 12 persons older than 12 had a substance use disorder (SUD) in 2014.[1] These disorders encompass both alcohol

This article originally appeared in *Anesthesiology Clinics*, Volume 36, Issue 4, December 2018. The authors have no financial disclosures and no conflicts of interest. The article has been read and approved by all the authors, the requirements for authorship have been met, and each author believes that the article represents honest work. All authors contributed equally to the article.

[a] Department of Anesthesiology, LSU Health Shreveport, 1501 Kings Highway, Shreveport, LA 71103, USA; [b] Department of Anesthesiology, Perioperative and Pain Medicine, Brigham and Women's Hospital, 75 Francis street, Boston, MA 02115, USA; [c] Department of Anesthesiology, LSU Health Science Center, Room 656, 1542 Tulane Avenue, New Orleans, LA 70112, USA; [d] Department of Pharmacology, LSU Health Science Center, Room 656, 1542 Tulane Avenue, New Orleans, LA 70112, USA
* Corresponding author. Department of Anesthesiology, LSU Health Shreveport, 1501 Kings Highway, Shreveport, LA 71103.
E-mail address: ecorne@lsuhsc.edu

and illicit drugs, including marijuana, cocaine, heroin, and nonmedical use of prescription drugs. Within that 8.1%, 0.7% had a specific pain reliever use disorder.[1] The National Center on Addiction and Substance Abuse also notes that 1 in 6 people with a substance use problem will have multiple substance disorders.[2] Although they all require treatment, only 10.9% received treatment at a specialty facility in the prior year.[3] Substance abuse costs total more than $740 billion annually in crime, health care, and lost work productivity. Further, prescription opioid misuse has contributed $78.5 billion and this number is still on the rise.

Data from the National Health Interview Survey in 2012 demonstrated 10.3% of people 18 and older report "a lot" of pain, whereas 11.2% experience chronic pain, defined as pain every day for the past 3 months.[4] Chronic pain may be challenging to understand, as pain is subjective, personal, and has a vast number of causes.[5] There are no laboratory or imaging tests to evaluate pain, thus the physician relies heavily on patient history and clinical presentation.[6] Without proper treatment, patients may experience a decline in their daily function and quality of life. Generally, it is believed that chronic pain cannot be "cured"; however, the pain can be managed through a variety of treatment approaches, including pharmacologic, surgical, and behavioral therapies.[7] In 2016, the Centers for Disease Control and Prevention (CDC) published a guideline for prescribing opioids to patients with chronic pain.[8] This guide includes recommendations for when to initiate opioid use, proper dosing, associated risks, and screening questions to evaluate a patient who may be at high risk for abuse.

When considering how many patients are prescribed chronic opioid medication, only 8% to 12% of them become addicted[9]; however, we also must consider that many people are using opioid medication for nonmedical uses. More than 67% of these people state they have obtained opioids from a friend or family member.[3] This is a concern for many reasons, the most essential being the rising rate of overdose. Over the period between 2006 and 2016, the total US deaths related to drugs doubled.[10] Natural and semisynthetic opioids were the number 1 drug type involved in overdoses, until recently, when heroin and synthetic opioid overdoses began exceeding in 2015 to 2016. Critically reviewing the statistics available, deaths by opioid overdose have continued to escalate at alarming rates, with 64,000 people dying from drug overdoses in 2016, including more than 42,000 related to opioid deaths.[11,12] These data represent a 20% increase from the 52,000 total from 2015. Overdoses related to illegally manufactured fentanyl represent the greatest contribution to the increase, accounting for 20,000 deaths in total, heroin accounted for 15,000 deaths, and prescription drugs for fewer than 15,000.

Given these current statistics, physicians must be vigilant in monitoring the trends and providing appropriate support to their patients. This review discusses the present opioid crisis, mechanisms behind chronic pain and substance abuse, and management plans for patients with these disorders.

OPIOID CRISIS

In the mid-1990s, a campaign entitled "Pain as the Fifth Vital Sign" was launched. The campaign focused on increasing both awareness and treatments of this subjective vital sign. Shortly following, the American Pain Society and the American Academy for Pain Medicine began strongly encouraging the use of opioid medication for noncancer patients with chronic pain. Since this time, the use of opioids as pain relievers has been steadily increasing. This rise was supported by an article published in 1986, stating that opioids were safe for patients with chronic pain.[13] Reasons for the increasing need for chronic pain management included aging populations, increases in the prevalence of chronic conditions, expectations from patients for complete relief of symptoms, and increasing complexity of surgical procedures.[14] The use of opioids continued to rise, and this increase was facilitated by the 1995 development of Oxycontin, an extended-release (ER) oxycodone.[15] Addiction, tolerance, and other safety concerns were diminished to promote avid prescribing.

Overdose deaths involving opioids quadrupled from 1999 to 2010, with oxycodone being the most commonly distributed during this time.[16] The number of emergency room visits increased, as an attempt to obtain additional opioid prescriptions. Opioids became a gateway to street drugs, and patients began transitioning to heroin due to its lower price and ease of obtaining. Products containing fentanyl and other analogs were becoming increasingly more common in 2013, and the death rate continued to rise over the next few years.[14] The opioid crisis was officially declared a public health emergency.

Ending this epidemic and preventing further crises is a multistep process. Public health officials suggest a primary, secondary, and tertiary prevention method. This includes preventing new-onset opioid addictions, identifying addiction earlier, and providing adequate treatments to those in need.[15] Although the focus has been on preventing new addiction through means such as pharmacist involvement[17] and modification of opioid formulations,[15] the medical community is far from achieving success. Many health care providers have been unaware of the serious risks of opioids, which include physical (ie, chronic constipation, increased pain sensitivity, respiratory depression) as well as psychological (addiction, distrust) factors. Inconsistent patient monitoring via contracts, drug screens, or state programs can create a negative environment and a fragile patient-doctor relationship if the patient senses bias or deceit.[14] Some physicians are refusing to treat patients they believe are "drug seeking," instead of uncovering the truth and guiding treatment for possible abuse. To make the problem even more challenging, Medicaid in certain states does not cover methadone as a maintenance treatment, making access to care extremely difficult for many patients.[14] Reasons for increased chronic opioid management are summarized in **Box 1**.

Many policies thus far have been focused on reducing the nonmedical use of opioids, and we have seen a mild decline in their use from 2002 to 2012.[15] However, there is a continuous rise in both overdoses and admissions to treatment centers, suggesting that even patients receiving prescription opioids for chronic pain are in danger of addiction and death.[7]

SUBSTANCE ABUSE

Substance abuse is a maladaptive pattern of drug use that leads to clinically significant impairment or distress as manifested by one or more behaviorally based criteria.[18] Substance misuse and abuse are critical to differentiate between in order

---

Box 1
Reasons for increased chronic pain management

Pain is now considered an additional vital sign

Longer life expectancy leads to continued management of chronic conditions

Patients are dissatisfied with only partial relief of pain

Failure to control initial pain

to access potential for substance addiction to develop. Substance misuse is defined as the incorrect use of medication by patients who may use a drug for a purpose other than its original intended purpose, combining medications without the instruction of physician, taking too little or too much of a drug, taking a drug too often, or taking a drug in ways the physician did not intend the patient to do.[18] Substance addiction is a primary, chronic disease of the brain involving dysfunction of reward, motivation, and memory-related circuitry. This change can be manifested in biological changes, psychological and spiritual alterations, and social shifts in a person's life. Inappropriate emotional responses and an inability to maintain lasting interpersonal relationships are often significant problems a patient suffering from addiction will face.[18] Alcohol, tobacco, marijuana, and opioids are among the most common substances associated with addiction, costing the nation more the $740 billion annually in costs related to crime, lost work productivity, and health care. Marijuana leads the nation in illicit drug use; prescription drug misuse is the second most common type of illicit drug use. Being able to understand the reasons for misuse of prescription drugs and its prevalence makes for a major economic impact.[19] Substance abuse has long been seen as a social or criminal problem. In 1935, Alcoholics Anonymous was founded in response to mainstream psychiatric and general medicine providers not attending to SUDs, and the only other option being treated in an asylum away from the rest of health care.[18] In modern times, health care systems are becoming essential in addressing substance misuse and substance addiction.[19] Physicians are key in preventing a patient's substance addiction, treating patients who suffer from addiction, and implementing a safe and combative plan to correct for their addiction.[18] See **Fig. 1** created using information from DAWN, the Drug Abuse Warning Network public health surveillance system that monitored drug-related hospital emergency room department visits to elucidate drug use patterns in patients nationwide.

Physicians take the following steps to determine the most effective plan of action for someone suffering from addiction:

- Formulate diagnosis with differentials
- Psychological assessment including risk of addictive disorder
- Informed consent
- Treatment agreement
- Preintervention and postintervention assessment of pain level and function
- Trial of opioid therapy and/or adjunctive medication
- Routinely reassess pain score and function
- Regularly assess the "4 A's" (analgesia, activity, adverse effects, aberrant behaviors)
- Periodic review of pain diagnosis and the development of comorbid conditions, including addictive disorders
- Documentation

NEUROBIOLOGY OF PAIN AND REWARD

Pain is a subjective reporting by a patient that can be broken down into psychological and biological groupings. It is an individual's experience of sensory, affective, and cognitive dimensions.[20] The classification of pain can be accomplished by determining if the pain is linked to a medical etiology (eg, pain caused by ischemia, inflammation, tissue damage) or if the pain lacks measurable biological factors. Pain can be further classified based on acute or chronic, source, pathophysiology, nociceptive quality, location, distribution, or intensity.[21]

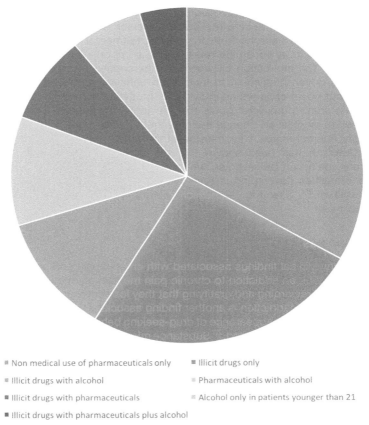

Non medical use of pharmaceuticals only   Illicit drugs only

Illicit drugs with alcohol   Pharmaceuticals with alcohol

Illicit drugs with pharmaceuticals   Alcohol only in patients younger than 21

Illicit drugs with pharmaceuticals plus alcohol

Fig. 1. Estimates of emergency department visits related to drug misuse or abuse. (*Data from* Drug abuse warning network (DAWN), Substance Abuse and Mental Health Services Administration (SAMHSA), 2008.)

The origins of pain trace back evolutionarily to elicit an amplified surge of motivation to escape or avoid the behavior that caused the pain. This allows for organisms to learn from experiences of pain and became a critical factor in future decision making.[20] The basal ganglia and associated limbic cortex became a cornerstone in the evolutionary process of vertebral brain function of selecting ideal behaviors to minimize consequences (ie, pain).[20] In modern humans, the thalamus, primary and secondary somatosensory cortex, insula, and the anterior cingulate cortex are the most commonly activated regions of the brain in response to acute pain. These regions of the brain receive direct nociceptive signaling from the spinal cord to determine the site and degree of pain to be perceived.[20] In addition to pain-receptive areas, the cortical and subcortical regions, are integrative in the reward/motivation circuit that encode for action selection and learning.[20] Scattered within the network of the subcortical region, opioid neurotransmission can be found.[21] Opioid neurotransmission activity is determined by the receptor that is activated on neurotransmission release. The μ and δ opioid receptors facilitate a dopamine release, whereas the κ receptors suppress dopamine being released.[21]

It is the dopamine neurotransmission in the nucleus accumbens of the striatum that is the main stake in reward-motivated behavior. The nucleus accumbens receives dopaminergic neurons from the ventral tegmental area, and activation of these neurons elicits a dopamine release that is important for learning and decision making.[20] The interaction between pain perceptive regions of the brain and dopaminergic-driven motivation to learn from behavior amplifies the pain-reward behavior. Acute pain engages an individual's motivational and emotional circuitry; chronic pain shifts behavioral goals toward achieving relief.[20] Chronic pain has been shown to extensively change the gray matter, alter white matter connectivity, and modify neurochemical transmission of glutamate, and opioid and dopamine transmission.[20] It has been shown that the cortical changes seen in patients with chronic pain can be reversed when pain is relieved, which it suggestive of brain abnormalities developing in response to continuous activation of the nociceptive system.[20] See **Fig. 2**, which details pain classifications, duration, and tissue type.

CLINICAL FINDINGS

There are many clinical findings associated with chronic pain and substance abuse. Patients can exhibit an addiction to chronic pain medication, meaning that they find the substance so rewarding and gratifying that they lose control despite harmful consequences.[22] Pseudoaddiction is another finding associated with chronic pain that is untreated, resulting in an appearance of drug-seeking behavior. Typically this resolves when the pain has been controlled.[23] Substance misuse and abuse are closely related. Misuse of an opioid for sleep purposes versus abuse of a medication are different in that abuse typically does not involve the physician or monitoring of the medication. Drug abuse typically gives the user a "high," whereas misuse can be accidental or intentional but the primary aim is not to have a euphoric experience.[22] Finally, dependence is broken down into tolerance and withdrawal. Many of these patients are seen in the perioperative period. Withdrawal from opioids can present with a myriad of physical and psychological symptoms. Physical symptoms include central nervous system hyperarousal responses, including diaphoresis, chills, myalgias, and diarrhea. Typically, the acute phase of withdrawal lasts 5 to 10 days, with a peak at day 2 to 3 depending on the half-life of the medication invovled.[22] Tolerance is the concept that patients require higher doses of the medication to achieve the same desired clinical effect over time. This is possibly due to the upregulation of receptors over time.[22] Other clinical symptoms from chronic opioid use are hyperalgesia and medication overuse headaches. Opioid-induced hyperalgesia is primarily mediated by N-methyl-D-aspartate and gamma-aminobutyric acid, and is defined as an increased sensitivity to an already painful stimulus, that is, surgery, in chronic opioid users. The difference between tolerance and hyperalgesia is that an increased or decreased dose of opioids will change the hyperalgesic response, whereas tolerance is gradual over time.[24] Overuse of nonsteroidal anti-inflammatory drugs (NSAIDs) in chronic pain can result in gastrointestinal, cerebrovascular, and renal adverse effects and must be monitored appropriately. Surgeons routinely prescribe opioids in the perioperative setting to help with acute pain control and, as such, can unknowingly contribute to the increasing risk of opioid abuse across the country.[25] There are a growing number of patients who receive opioids for postoperative pain control and then continue to receive them chronically thereafter. There is a risk of persistent opioid use even in opioid-naive patients who were exposed to opioids in the perioperative period.[25] Risk factors include a history of substance abuse, psychological conditions, female

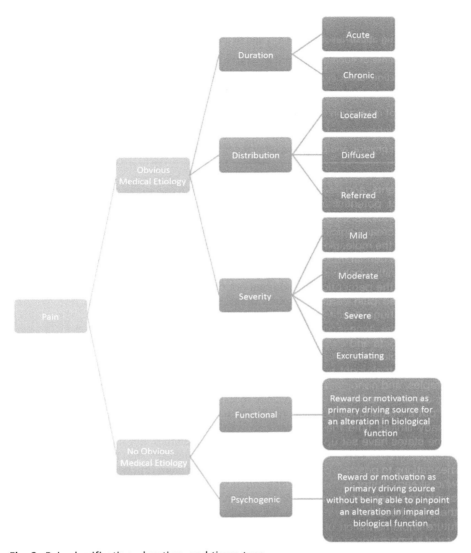

Fig. 2. Pain classification, duration, and tissue type.

sex, and low socioeconomic class.[25–27] See **Box 2** for common drug abuse–associated terms and their definitions.

TREATMENT THERAPIES

The CDC recently came out with new guidelines regarding the prescribing and use of opioid prescriptions for primary care providers. This new approach focuses on limiting opioid use in chronic pain, using the lowest effective dose possible, and ensuring close monitoring of patients who use opioids.[28] The focus has shifted to a multimodal therapy of pain control with the focus on NSAIDs, anticonvulsants, and

---

Box 2
Common drug abuse–associated terms and definitions

Addiction: sense of euphoria, reward leading to misuse or overuse of medication

Pseudoaddiction: drug-seeking behavior due to untreated pain, resolves with treatment

Misuse: use of medication for other than what it was prescribed

Abuse: use of medication without physician monitoring

Tolerance: higher levels of medication needed for same effect, happens gradually

Withdrawal: physical and psychological symptoms after abrupt discontinuation

---

antidepressants, and treating acute pain quickly with opioids to prevent the long-term chronicity of potential abuse. There are various new and promising nonopioids currently in various stages of development to target novel receptors to treat chronic pain and decrease opioid consumption. An example is the endocannabinoid system; by blocking the molecules that degrade cannabinoids endogenously, thus increasing endogenous cannabinoids.[28] Other therapies targeted and the psychosocial aspect include cognitive behavioral therapy and mindful meditation practices. Studies have shown that the perception of pain has not changed with psychological therapy, but the perceived pain control is much greater.[28] The downside is that psychological care has a huge deficit in rural areas and even in some cities, and many patients may not have access or coverage for these therapies. Using the lowest possible dose of opioids and combing with another nonopioid novel therapy can significantly decrease tolerance and dependence.[28] There are many various novel therapies currently in trials right now, including peripherally restricted opioids, other selective therapies, and nonopioid therapies, but it will be many years until any potential therapies come to market. Finally, the close monitoring of those patients on opioid therapy will put a tremendous burden on primary care physicians, which may decrease the already limited time the provider has with each patient. To alleviate this burden, some states have set up a statewide monitoring system, but this has yet to show a decrease in opioid overdose and emergency room visits.[28] The CDC has given recommendations to possibly prevent a worsening opioid crisis, but what about the patients who already suffer from opioid dependence? Current evidence supports the use of opioid replacement therapy combined with psychosocial support. As mentioned, there is a need for more psychological support in patients nationwide. One possible future implementation of this may be related to digital health technologies through use of a smartphone or the Internet to meet the psychosocial needs.[28] Another potential therapy is the use of abuse deterrent opioid formulations. These formulations aim to reduce the extraction and bioavailability of the active substance.[29] A growing body of evidence has shown that the introduction of abuse deterrents results in a decrease in potential abuse and diversion, thereby benefiting the opioid epidemic.[29] Gabapentin, Gralise, for example, gastroretentive gabapentin, and pregabalin have been incorporated into multimodal pain regimens, but are those medications addictive as well? Bonnet and Scherbaum[30] report in a review that pregabalin appears to be more addictive than gabapentin but that gabapentinoids do not have substantial addictive effects. There is no evidence to suggest that gabapentinoids increase extracellular dopamine in the mesolimbic reward center. In those with substance abuse issues, the potential to abuse gabapentin and pregabalin is elevated but low. In this regard, it is generally recommended to avoid pregabalin in those with chronic opioid use and substance abuse disorders. See **Box 3** for current therapies aimed at reducing the opioid crisis.

Box 3
Current therapies aimed at reducing the opioid crisis
Limit opioid use for chronic pain
Use lowest adequate dose
Frequent monitoring
Multimodal approach
Cognitive behavioral therapy
Mindfulness and meditation

ABUSE DETERRENTS

Prescription opioids can be abused in their current state, or manipulated to be abused in another state. Possible routes of abuse include ingestion, inhalation, or intravenous. Medications can be manipulated by grinding them into a powder, dissolving them into a solvent like alcohol, or combining with other psychoactive substances.[31] The goal of any abuse deterrent is to give effective pain relief while reducing the rate of abuse by altering the formulation. Different routes include combining agonist/antagonist formulations together, extending the release of the drug, and novel routes of admission.[31] There are currently a number of Food and Drug Administration (FDA)-approved abuse deterrent formulations that have either aversive, for example, niacin, antagonistic, for example, naloxone, or physical barrier additives, for example, polyethylene oxide.

Oxycontin is the original abuse deterrent and contains polyethylene oxide in its ER formulation. The tablet is difficult to crush and dissolve, becoming viscous, and when it came to market demonstrated an immediate reduction in overdoses in the United States.[31] This physical barrier and crush-resistant technology containing polyethylene oxide makes it hard to crush and turns into a plastic substance if dissolved.[32] Targiniq ER is a combined agonist/antagonist containing oxycodone and naloxone. The euphoric effect is blocked if attempts are made to crush the tablet. This has not yet been commercially available.[31] Embeda is a third abuse deterrent that is a combination of morphine and naloxone. The naloxone stays sequestered in the core if taken appropriately, but if crushed, then the antagonist effect blunts any euphoria from recreational use.[31] Hysingla is a fourth approved abuse deterrent and contains only hydrocodone. The formulation is difficult to crush and dissolve, making it a good abuse deterrent. It uses the same polyethylene oxide similar to Oxycontin.[32] Morphabond is a new abuse deterrent that is more resistant to crushing and cutting and becomes viscous if dissolved. This is the first morphine formulation without an antagonist serving as the deterrent.[31] Xtampza ER is another abuse deterrent and is oxycodone based. This drug is able to be opened and sprinkled on food, while still maintaining its ER potential. This makes it unattractive to drug seekers, because it maintains its ER activity even while crushed.[31] Suboxone is one of the more common agonist/antagonist formulations. It is a combination of buprenorphine and naloxone. Buprenorphine itself is a partial agonist at the mu receptor and antagonist at the kappa receptor.[33] The naloxone only takes affect if the drug is abused in ways other than sublingual absorption, for example, intravenous delivery.[32] There are other abuse deterrent drugs that are still being reviewed by the FDA. The potential to decrease opioid abuse with these formulations is great. One study even goes as far to say that it reduces overdose deaths by 87%.[34] The opioid epidemic is one that must be taken seriously in the medical community going forward. Abuse deterrents will play an increasingly important role going forward. **Box 4** lists common abuse deterrent drugs.

Box 4 Common abuse deterrents
Targiniq; oxycodone/naloxone
Embeda: morphine/naloxone
Hysingla: hydrocodone
Morphabond: morphine
Xtampza: oxycodone
Suboxone: buprenorphine/naloxone

SUMMARY

Chronic pain and opioid abuse is an ever increasing problem in the United States. It has been labeled a crisis by the federal government. This presents a number of challenges in the outpatient surgery setting for many patients with chronic pain issues and addiction because surgery typically requires the use of opioids and other pain medication. The most beneficial preoperative assessment is the establishment of realistic expectations.[35] The CDC recently came out with new guidelines regarding the prescribing and use of opioid prescriptions for primary care providers. This new approach focuses on limiting opioid use in chronic pain, using the lowest effective dose possible, and ensuring close monitoring of patients who use opioids. The CDC has also given recommendations to possibly prevent a worsening opioid crisis. However, the patients who already suffer from opioid dependence will likely need continued and longitudinal support in the form of opioid replacement therapy and psychosocial support.

REFERENCES

1. Hedden SL, Kennet J, Lipari R, et al. Behavioral health trends in the United States: results from the 2014 national survey on drug use and health.
2. Types of addiction | The National Center on Addiction and Substance Abuse.
3. Center for Behavioral Health Statistics. Results from the 2013 national survey on drug use and health: summary of national findings.
4. Nahin RL. Estimates of pain prevalence and severity in adults: United States, 2012. J Pain 2015;16(8):769–80.
5. Vadivelu N, Mitra S, Kaye AD, et al. Perioperative analgesia and challenges in the drug-addicted and drug-dependent patient. Best Pract Res Clin Anaesthesiol 2014;28(1):91–101.
6. Chronic pain: symptoms, diagnosis, & treatment | NIH MedlinePlus the Magazine.
7. Abrecht CR, Greenberg P, Song E, et al. A contemporary medicolegal analysis of implanted devices for chronic pain management. Anesth Analg 2017;124(4): 1304–10.
8. Dowell D, Haegerich TM, Chou R. CDC guideline for prescribing opioids for chronic pain—United States, 2016. MMWR Recomm Rep 2016;65(1):1–49.
9. Vowles KE, McEntee ML, Julnes PS, et al. Rates of opioid misuse, abuse, and addiction in chronic pain. Pain 2015;156(4):569–76.
10. Overdose death rates | National Institute on Drug Abuse (NIDA).
11. Dowell D, Noonan RK, Houry D. Underlying factors in drug overdose deaths. JAMA 2017;318(23):2295.

12. National Center for Health Statistics. Provisional counts of drug overdose deaths, as of 8/6/2017. 2016. Available at: https://www.cdc.gov/nchs/data/health_policy/monthly-drug-overdose-death-estimates.pdf. Accessed February 28, 2018.

13. Portenoy RK, Foley KM. Chronic use of opioid analgesics in non-malignant pain: report of 38 cases. Pain 1986;25(2):171–86.

14. Dasgupta N, Beletsky L, Ciccarone D. Opioid crisis: no easy fix to its social and economic determinants. Am J Public Health 2018;108(2):182–6.

15. Kolodny A, Courtwright DT, Hwang CS, et al. The prescription opioid and heroin crisis: a public health approach to an epidemic of addiction. Annu Rev Public Health 2015;36(1):559–74.

16. Jones CM. Trends in the distribution of selected Centers for Disease Control and Prevention.

17. Compton WM, Jones CM, Stein JB, et al. Promising roles for pharmacists in addressing the U.S. opioid crisis [published online ahead of print December 31, 2017]. Res Social Adm Pharm 2017. https://doi.org/10.1016/j.sapharm.2017.12.009.

18. Prater CD, Zylstra RG, Miller KE. Successful pain management for the recovering addicted patient. Prim Care Companion J Clin Psychiatry 2002;4(4):125–31.

19. (US). SA and MHSA (US); O of the SG. Health care systems and substance use disorders. In: Facing addiction in America: the surgeon general's report on alcohol, drugs, and health. 2016. Available at: https://addiction.surgeongeneral.gov/.

20. Navratilova E, Porreca F. Reward and motivation in pain and pain relief. Nat Neurosci 2014;17(10):1304–12.

21. Elman I, Borsook D. Common brain mechanisms of chronic pain and addiction. Neuron 2016;89(1):11–36.

22. Kahan M, Srivastava A, Wilson L, et al. Misuse of and dependence on opioids: study of chronic pain patients. Can Fam Physician 2006;52(9):1081–7.

23. Weaver M, Schnoll S. Abuse liability in opioid therapy for pain treatment in patients with an addiction history. Clin J Pain 2002;18(4 Suppl):S61–9.

24. Hsu ES. Medication overuse in chronic pain. Curr Pain Headache Rep 2017;21(1):2.

25. Demsey D, Carr NJ, Clarke H, et al. Managing opioid addiction risk in plastic surgery during the perioperative period. Plast Reconstr Surg 2017;140(4):613e–9e.

26. Kaye AD, Jones MR, Kaye AM, et al. Prescription opioid abuse in chronic pain: an updated review of opioid abuse predictors and strategies to curb opioid abuse (part 2). Pain Physician 2017;20(2S):S111–33. Available at: http://www.ncbi.nlm.nih.gov/pubmed/28226334. Accessed March 14, 2018.

27. Kaye AD, Jones MR, Kaye AM, et al. Prescription opioid abuse in chronic pain: an updated review of opioid abuse predictors and strategies to curb opioid abuse: part 1. Pain Physician 2017;20(2S):S93–109. Available at: http://www.ncbi.nlm.nih.gov/pubmed/28226333. Accessed March 14, 2018.

28. Wilson-Poe AR, Morón JA. The dynamic interaction between pain and opioid misuse. Br J Pharmacol 2018;175(14):2770–7.

29. Gasior M, Bond M, Malamut R. Routes of abuse of prescription opioid analgesics: a review and assessment of the potential impact of abuse-deterrent formulations. Postgrad Med 2016;128(1):85–96.

30. Bonnet U, Scherbaum N. How addictive are gabapentin and pregabalin? A systematic review. Eur Neuropsychopharmacol 2017;27(12):1185–215.

31. Hale ME, Moe D, Bond M, et al. Abuse-deterrent formulations of prescription opioid analgesics in the management of chronic noncancer pain. Pain Manag 2016;6(5):497–508.
32. Vadivelu N, Chang D, Lumermann L, et al. Management of patients on abuse-deterrent opioids in the ambulatory surgery setting. Curr Pain Headache Rep 2017;21(2):10.
33. Jonan AB, Kaye AD, Urman RD. Buprenorphine formulations: clinical best practice strategies recommendations for perioperative management of patients undergoing surgical or interventional pain procedures. Pain Physician 2018;21(1): E1–12. Available at: http://www.ncbi.nlm.nih.gov/pubmed/29357325. Accessed March 14, 2018.
34. Sessler NE, Downing JM, Kale H, et al. Reductions in reported deaths following the introduction of extended-release oxycodone (OxyContin) with an abuse-deterrent formulation. Pharmacoepidemiol Drug Saf 2014;23(12):1238–46.
35. Vadivelu N, Kai AM, Kodumudi V, et al. Pain management of patients with substance abuse in the ambulatory setting. Curr Pain Headache Rep 2017;21(2):9.

Medication-Assisted Treatment Considerations for Women with Opiate Addiction Disorders

Alicia A. Jacobs, MD*, Michelle Cangiano, MD

KEYWORDS

- Opioid-use disorder (OUD) • Opioid addiction • Medication-assisted therapy (MAT)
- Trauma-informed care • Buprenorphine • Hub-and-spoke model • Harm reduction

KEY POINTS

- Rates of opioid-use disorder (OUD) and its adverse outcomes are skyrocketing in women.
- Women with OUD have demographic differences that include quicker time to physical dependence, shorter duration to adverse outcomes, and higher rates of psychiatric comorbidity.
- Women have improved outcomes rates with care that is trauma-informed, gender-specific, and based in a medical home.
- Treating OUD as a chronic, relapsing, and remitting disease within the concept of a harm-reduction model vastly improves outcomes.

INTRODUCTION

Opioid-use disorder (OUD), which is used interchangeably with the term opioid addiction, has become a societal epidemic with escalating rates in women. It is a chronic illness that does not respect age or sociodemographics. To respond to this epidemic public health crisis, primary care providers need to create the access and workforce training needed to provide the highest quality care possible. Because OUD is a common, chronic disease, it is the duty of primary care providers to lean into learning and treating this condition, and supporting the patients who need assistance.

This article originally appeared in *Primary Care: Clinics in Office Practice*, Volume 45, Issue 4, December 2018.
Disclosure Statement: The authors have nothing to disclose.
Department of Family Medicine, the Larner College of Medicine at the University of Vermont, 235 Rowell, 106 Carrigan Drive, Burlington, VT 05405, USA
* Corresponding author.
E-mail address: Alicia.Jacobs@UVMHealth.org

EPIDEMIOLOGY
Risk Factors

The biggest risk factors for opioid addiction are adverse childhood events (abuse or trauma), mental health issues, family history of addiction, chronic stress, and chronic pain. In fact, almost all women who develop addiction to opioids have a history of childhood trauma. Psychological and emotional distresses are additional risk factors for women.[1] The United States consumes more than 90% of the opioid pain medications produced in the world and we are 7% of the world's population. Women are generally more likely to have chronic pain complaints. Patients who use pain medications for nonmedical reasons source them predominantly from friends and family, or receives prescription from their own medical provider.[2]

Epidemic Rates

Rates of addiction have skyrocketed in the general population, even more so in women. In 2015 alone, more than 21,500,000 Americans aged 12 years and older were reported to have a substance-use disorder (SUD). Of those, 122,000 were adolescents addicted to prescription pain relievers.[3] At younger ages, there has been full gender convergence so that girls are equally as addicted as boys. Adolescent girls report using to enhance self-esteem, decrease shyness and as a coping skill.[4] The changing burden of disease in women is outlined in **Box 1**.[5]

Complications and Outcomes

There are multiple complications and other health concerns associated with oral and intravenous opioid use, including but not limited to heart or blood stream infections, skin and muscle or bone infections, lung damage, trauma, hepatitis and human immunodeficiency virus, falls, withdrawal symptoms, and concomitant use of other drugs and alcohol. In addition, there are multiple social issues and societal costs, including job loss, family disruption, criminal activity, incarceration, social stigma, loss of housing or custody of children, and an estimated $72 billion in annual health care costs. Women have particularly high rates of multiple providers and emergency department utilization. Rates of hepatitis C more than doubled in the 4 years from 2010 to 2014.[1] Drug overdose killed 52,404 people in 2015, making it the leading cause of accidental death in the United States (**Fig. 1**).[3] Women much more frequently use concomitant benzodiazepines, which markedly increase risk of respiratory depression and death. Incarceration rates are much higher in the United States where drug abuse is predominantly addressed as a criminal behavior in the justice system.[6] Women have a much

---

Box 1
2015 opioid addiction facts and figures in opioid use disorder in women

- 48,000 died of prescription pain reliever overdose between 1999 and 2010
- Opioid death rates in women have increased by 850% between 1999 and 2015
- Heroin overdose deaths have tripled between 2010 and 2013

Data from American Society of Addiction Medicine. Opioid addiction: 2016 facts & figures. Available at: https://www.asam.org/docs/default-source/advocacy/opioid-addiction-disease-facts-figures.pdf; and Office on Women's Health. Final report: opioid use, misuse, and overdose in women. Available at: https://www.womenshealth.gov/files/documents/final-report-opioid-508.pdf. Accessed December 1, 2017.

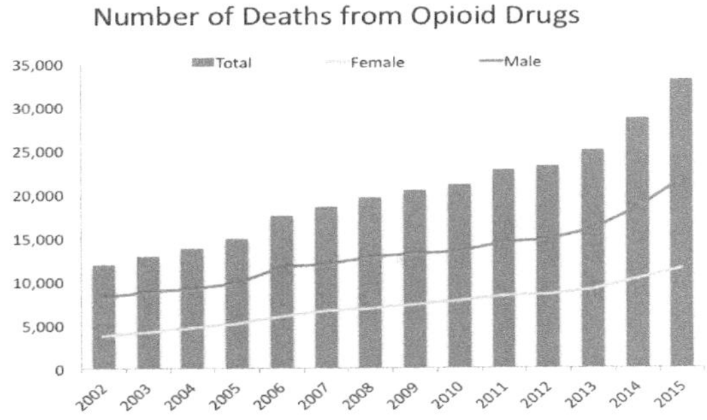

Fig. 1. National overdose deaths. (*From* National Institute on Drug Abuse. Overdose death rate. Available at: https://www.drugabuse.gov/related-topics/trends-statistics/overdose-death-rates; and *Courtesy of* National Center for Health Statistics, CDC Wonder.). Accessed December 1, 2017.

higher parenting burden and hence expose their own children to adverse childhood events of addiction, family disruption, and incarceration. This is undoubtedly a public health crisis.

NEUROBIOLOGY

Drug addiction has been defined as the pathologic seeking and using of drugs despite negative consequences.[7] The mechanism is explained by many neurobiological changes to a person's brain causing susceptibility. The most studied is the mesolimbic dopamine system. This system is centered on the nuclear accumbens in the midbrain, with the ventral tegmental area projecting neurons to the forebrain.[8] The areas of forebrain include the hippocampus, amygdala, and prefrontal cortex, which have been implicated as the reward centers of the brain (**Fig. 2**). Although drugs of abuse all are different molecules, their actions all lead to the activation of the mesolimbic dopamine system.[7] Many systems influence and mediate this process, such as gamma-aminobutyric acid (GABA), glutamate, serotonin, and so forth.[9] The stimulation leads to changes in the nerves, which cause them to respond to stimuli differently. Though the paucity of dopamine and other neurotransmitters in these regions rebound with recovery, a relative paucity often remains over time. This accounts for the continued cravings and potential relapses despite years of sobriety.

Many of the early studies on this mesolimbic pathway were conducted in male animal models. In the 1990s, the realization of the importance of the difference between the sexes sparked more research into this area. One of the main areas of study is understanding the effect of estrogen on dopamine. Studies have demonstrated that the subjective effect of cocaine varies based on the menstrual cycle. There is more of a response in the follicular phase when there are relatively high amounts of estrogen and low progesterone. There is much less of an effect in the luteal phase or when subjects have been given high doses of progesterone, indicating progesterone may attenuate the effects of drugs.[10] Estrogen likely plays a role in kappa-opiate binding and mu-opiate binding given that studies have shown increases in premenopausal women compared with men and postmenopausal women.[11] Understanding these differences may help providers in treatment decisions for their patients. For instance, buprenorphine may be a better treatment option for premenopausal women. Inversely,

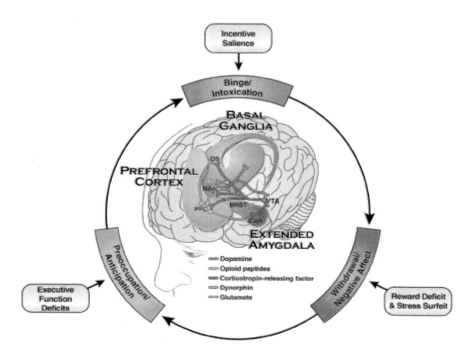

Fig. 2. Anatomy of addiction. CRAFT, car relax alone forget friends trouble. (*Adapted from* Koob GF, Everitt BJ, Robbins TW. Reward, motivation, and addiction. In: Squire LG, Berg D, Bloom FE, et al, editors. Fundamental neuroscience. 3rd edition. Amsterdam: Academic Press; 2008. p. 987–1016; with permission.)

progesterone-only contraception may be a better option for women on opioid replacement.

Women have other differences in their brains that may account for the differences in the timing of onset, severity of addiction, and the telescoping of addiction with faster progression of disease. Women have been noted to have more neurons in the ventral tegmental area. Addicting drugs increase dendritic branching of medium spiny neurons, causing more synapses to the reward centers in the forebrain. This is hypothesized to be the reason for women's more rapid progression to drug involvement and dependence.[12]

SCREENING AND DIAGNOSIS

Screening for OUD should be universal, completed with a validated tool, and integrated into standard primary care services. To minimize paperwork fatigue and optimize office workflows, patients should be given a short, evidenced-based, validated tool to assess risk of a SUD. For efficiency, screening can be tiered with a single screening question followed by a confirmatory tool. Eligibility should be based on age rather than demographics and types of visits. The authors recommend screening in the 12 years and older age group at all preventative care visits and other visits as deemed appropriate.

Ideally, questionnaires should be filled out in paper or electronic format directly by the patient because this improves sensitivity rates. In addition, when possible, the tool should be integrated into the usual workflow (integrated into both behavioral health screening and preventative care questionnaires), as well as built into electronic format when applicable.

For the cohort aged 12 to 18 years, the CRAFFT screening tool is recommended. For women 18 years and older, the Single Substance Abuse Question (SSAQ) is a validated primary screening tool recommended by both the National Institute on Drug Abuse (NIDA)[13] and the Substance Abuse and Mental Health Services Association (**Table 1**).[14] Any positive SSAQ screen should be followed with a confirmatory screen. The Drug Abuse Screening Test (DAST)-10 is recommended as an efficient and validated tool (**Table 2**).[15–17] The DAST-10 should be scored and the clinical response should be should be matched appropriately with the level of problems related to the drug use. An appropriate response for a low-level score would be brief in office counseling with shorter interval follow-up to reassess risk at a future date. Scores at the moderate to severe level require further investigation and possibly intensive biopsychosocial assessment with an addiction specialist.[18] The continuum of care starts in the primary care office and extends to drug counselor, addiction specialist, and intensive outpatient or inpatient treatment.

TREATMENT: MEDICAL

The Drug Addiction Treatment Act (DATA) was signed in 2000 in response to the increasing prevalence of opioid addiction and heroin overdoses. This effectively allowed for office-based treatment of addiction by allowing physicians to prescribe medications such as buprenorphine. In 2002, the US Food and Drug Administration (FDA) approved 2 formulations of buprenorphine. Pharmacologically, there is no difference between the film and tablet version of buprenorphine. Subjectively, patients seem to prefer the film version of the medication.[19] Buprenorphine works differently than methadone because it is a partial agonist as opposed to a full agonist. Being a partial agonist means that it activates opioid receptors but to a lesser degree than a full agonist. Therefore, people who are used to the subjectively positive effects of opioids will experience a small positive effect, which can increase compliance. It also has a strong affinity to the opioid receptors, which block the effects of full agonists. It still has the potential to be misused but the combination with naloxone minimizes this. Buprenorphine also has a ceiling effect, so increasing the dose of the medication does not produce the same effect as increasing the dose of a full agonist. Buprenorphine is metabolized by cytochrome P450 and, therefore, can have serious drug–drug interactions.[20] Therefore, many sources recommend that buprenorphine should not be used with benzodiazepines or other sedative drugs (eg, alcohol). There is some controversy about whether this is clinically significant versus theoretic risk.

For a physician to begin prescribing, a waiver from the Substance Abuse and Mental Health Service Administration (SAMHSA) must be obtained.[21] To be eligible for this waiver, they must complete an 8-hour training. It is recommended that before

Table 1			
Screening tool: Single Substance Abuse Question			
How many times in the past year have you used an illegal drug or a prescription medication for nonmedical reasons?	None = 0	Once = 1	More than once = 2

From National Institute on Drug Abuse. Resource guide: screening for drug use in general medical settings. Available at: https://www.drugabuse.gov/publications/resource-guide-screening-drug-use-in-general-medical-settings/nida-quick-screen. Accessed December 1, 2017.

Table 2
Screening tool: Drug Abuse Screening Test-10

Drug Use Questionnaire (DAST - 10)
The following questions concern information about your possible involvement with drugs not including alcoholic beverages during the past 12 mo. Carefully read each statement and decide if your answer is "Yes" or "No". Then, circle the appropriate response beside the question.
In the statements "drug abuse" refers to (1) the use of prescribed or over the counter drugs may include: cannabis (e.g. marijuana, hash), solvents, tranquillizers (e.g. Valium), barbiturates, cocaine, stimulants (e.g. speed), hallucinogens (e.g. LSD) or narcotics (e.g. heroin). Remember that the questions *do not* include alcoholic beverages.
Please answer every question. If you have difficulty with a statement, then choose the response that is mostly right.

These questions refer to the past 12 mo	Circle Your Response	
1. Have you used drugs other than those required for medical reasons?	Yes	No
2. Do you abuse more than one drug at a time?	Yes	No
3. Are you always able to stop using drugs when you want to?	Yes	No
4. Have you had "blackouts" or "flashbacks" as a result or drug use?	Yes	No
5. Do you every feel bad or guilty about your drug use?	Yes	No
6. Does your spouse (or parents) ever complain about your involvement with drugs?	Yes	No
7. Have you neglected your family because of your use of drugs?	Yes	No
8. Have you engaged in illegal activities in order to obtain drugs?	Yes	No
9. Have you ever experienced withdrawal symptoms (felt sick) when you stopped taking drugs?	Yes	No
10. Have you had medical problems as a result of your drug use (e.g. memory loss, hepatitis, convulsions, bleeding, etc.)?	Yes	No

beginning to provide office-based addiction treatment services, practices have trained physicians and support staff, as well as connections to mental health resources. In fact, DATA 2000 stipulates that when physicians submit notification to SAMHSA to obtain the required waiver, they must attest to their ability to refer patients for appropriate counseling and other nonpharmacologic therapy. During the first year, a physician may not treat more than 30 patients. After that time, physicians may request a limit increase to treat no more than 100 patients. Further information on requirements and to find a DATA-approved buprenorphine 8-hour training session can be found on the SAMHSA website. Advanced Practices Providers can also obtain waivers with a 24-hour training.

There are 3 phases to medication-assisted therapy (MAT): induction, stabilization, and maintenance. Induction is the process of switching from the drug of abuse to buprenorphine. The goal is to find the minimum dose at which the patient stops opioid use, has no withdrawal symptoms, has no side effects, and has no cravings. It is recommended that the induction dose or doses be observed, and the patient be followed very closely (1–2 times/week). Stabilization occurs when these criteria have been met. Dosage adjustments may be necessary during early stabilization; however, when the patient reaches maintenance further dose adjustments are not necessary. Frequent contact during stabilization increases likelihood of compliance. It is recommended the patient be seen at least weekly for the first 4 to 5 weeks. The maintenance phase occurs after stabilization and may be indefinite. The visits are spaced out; however, urine drug screening should occur monthly. Because addiction is a relapsing and remitting disease and causes alterations in brain chemistry, patients may need maintenance lifetime treatment. Physicians should be knowledgeable about brief interventions in case of relapse and should give care in a nonjudgmental way. During the maintenance phase, the focus is on psychosocial issues that have been identified during treatment that may contribute to the person's addiction. Many women with SUDs also have a history of trauma. It is important to provide trauma-informed care to these women to reduce the risk of retraumatization and help improve the efficacy of treatment.[22]

TREATMENT: CHRONIC DISEASE, HARM REDUCTION, AND SYSTEMS OF CARE

There has been significant change in the understanding of SUDs over the past few decades. OUD is truly a chronic disease with a relapsing, remitting pattern that includes treatment lapses with nonadherence to recommended treatment, and significant morbidity and mortality. In the past, opioid addiction had been primarily addressed within an abstinence model of care in which treatment was predominantly provided in treatment centers and aimed at complete abstinence from any psychoactive substance use. Any relapse was deemed a failure of treatment.

Understanding the concept of opioid addiction as a chronic disease can help alleviate any perception of treating provider or patient failure. Indeed, when a woman with opioid addiction has a relapse, she is relapsing at a rate comparable to patients with other chronic diseases such as uncontrolled diabetes, hypertension, or asthma (**Fig. 3**).[23] Despite understanding opioid addiction as a chronic disease, many patients and providers still see relapse as a moral failing and shared failure, which can lead to either shame and/or judgment in either party. Relapse in chronic opioid addiction can additionally have more societal impacts due to theft and other crimes. However, the appropriate response to relapse is more targeted wrap-around services rather than discontinuing the doctor and patient relationship.

Understanding opioid addiction as a chronic disease leads to the best outcomes; access to treatment understandably improves outcomes (**Fig. 4**). Using a harm-reduction model of care, access to MAT is ideally made universally available to even further improve outcomes in this epidemic. It is recognized that integrating MAT into the routine, normalized chronic disease management of primary care offices is the ideal mechanism for creating adequate access to care.[24]

Though there could be many models, Vermont uses the hub-and-spoke model, which creates a dynamic movement of patients to and from centralized treatment to decentralized primary care offices, depending on their chronic disease state of remission. The hub is the traditional methadone clinic and there are many spokes where patients receive care in ambulatory and other settings. The ideal spoke is the revolutionary, normalized MAT chronic care in the medical home (**Fig. 5**).

Women, in particular, fair less well in the treatment center model of care due to higher rates of parenting responsibilities, more psychiatric comorbidities, and high rates of previous trauma and shame. This centralized model tends to have more associated stigma. In addition, participants can be exposed to supply in the small subset of relapsing patients in this centralized locations. In a primary care office, appointments can be scheduled around child care, the care is normalized, and psychiatric or other medical concerns can be integrated.

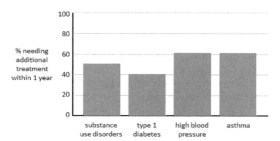

Fig. 3. Relapse rates in chronic medical conditions. (*Data from* McLellan A, Lewis D, O'Brien CP, et al. Drug dependence, a chronic medical illness: implications for treatment, insurance and outcomes evaluation. JAMA 2000;284(13):1689–95.)

WHOLE PERSON CARE

Working with this high-risk, vulnerable population of women with chronic OUD is a unique opportunity to give whole person care with unconditional regard and a potentially healing relationship. Too often, nonaddiction care is neglected when a patient attends a specialty treatment center. Any of those other health problems, including psychiatric symptoms and untreated medical issues, can affect stress, relapse rates, and overall outcomes. When MAT is provided in a primary care office, it provides a venue of regularly scheduled visits in which other medical and psychiatric care can be provided.

In addition, these more frequent visits provide an opportunity for deeply meaningful connection, which can create an opportunity to provide universal compassion and, therefore, potentially healing relationships. Many of these women have not experienced an unconditional regard to their being and struggles. Validating their struggles, ongoing symptoms of trauma, and right to dignified care is therapeutic for the patient and hence rewarding for the provider to give.

Indeed, in a qualitative study of the Vermont hub-and-spoke model of care, 70% of the participants receiving MAT in the primary care spoke cited the relationship with the doctor as the most important aspect of the location of their care. They also cited access to concomitant medical care, being treated with respect, and being treated without shaming; that is, as a person, not an addict. (Rawson R: Vermont hub-and-

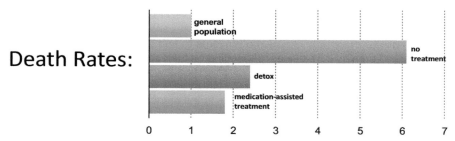

Fig. 4. Outcomes in OUD. (*Data from* Evans E, Li L, Min J, et al. Mortality among individuals accessing pharmacological treatment for opioid dependence in California, 2006-2010. Addiction 2015;110:996–1005; and Mohlman MK, Tanzman B, Finison K, et al. Impact of medication-assisted treatment for opioid addiction on Medicaid expenditures and health services utilization rates in Vermont. J Subst Abuse Treat 2016;67:9–14.)

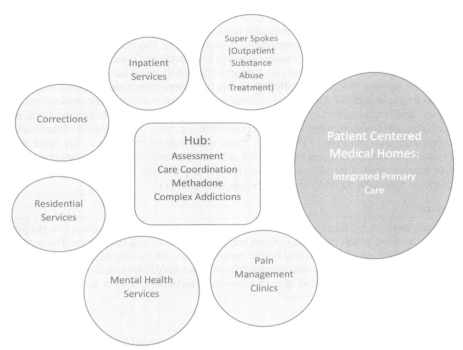

Fig. 5. Hub-and-spoke model of care. (*Used with Permission* of the Vermont Department of Health © 2018.)

spoke model of care for opioid use disorders: An Evaluation. Submitted for publication.) None of the patients receiving care in the centralized hub noted these connections in their treatment center–based care.

SPECIAL CIRCUMSTANCES
Maternity Care

The treatment of drug addiction in pregnancy is a major consideration due to the epidemiology of dependence in women. One-third of all women are in their childbearing years.[25] Both methadone and buprenorphine are approved to treat opioid addiction in nonpregnant patients but both are classified as FDA pregnancy category C medications due to insufficient data regarding their use during pregnancy. It is known that all opioids cross the placental barrier. Prolonged use of any opioids during pregnancy is associated with adverse obstetric outcomes, as well as fetal adverse effects.[26] Neonatal symptoms can include respiratory depression and physical dependence in the neonate and neonatal abstinence syndrome (NAS) shortly after birth. Symptoms of NAS include irritability, hyperactivity, abnormal sleep patterns, failure to gain weight, poor feeding, tremors, vomiting, diarrhea, and high-pitched cry. This condition may become life-threatening without early recognition and treatment.[27] Outcomes in babies are much improved with medically supervised buprenorphine treatment of the gravid mother during pregnancy due to early recognition of NAS symptoms.

Despite the risk of opioid exposure in pregnancy, maternal treatment of OUD during pregnancy is strongly recommended for overall harm reduction. There have been numerous small studies comparing buprenorphine and methadone. One double-blind randomized control study by Jones and colleagues[28] showed no significant difference in the incidence of maternal or neonatal adverse effects. The group treated with buprenorphine had decreased morphine needed to treat NAS and decreased hospital stays. In recent years, buprenorphine has become the standard of care in the treatment of pregnant women.[29] More recently naltrexone has been compared with both buprenorphine and methadone. One study compared naltrexone with buprenorphine, methadone, and nonexposed controls. Results showed that both buprenorphine and naltrexone did not have higher rates of neonatal mortality or congenital abnormalities compared with controls.[30] Based on these early results, providers now have more choice in treatment options for pregnant women. Because buprenorphine monoagent has more potential for abuse and diversion, many centers are now using buprenorphine or naloxone for MAT therapy in pregnant women.

Dental

Any person on long-term opioids is at higher risk for dental caries, periodontal disease, and tooth loss, which can lead to taste impairment and eating difficulties. The reasons behind this increased risk of oral health problems may be multifactorial, including poor oral hygiene, chronic pain, and xerostomia from salivary hypofunction (from the medications). All patients on MAT should have an assessment of their oral health and be connected with a dental home.[31]

Tobacco

Tobacco use is 4 times higher in patients with opioid abuse history than the general population. Tobacco abuse is a high-prevalence preventable cause of morbidity and mortality in the United States. In fact, the prevalence of smoking in patients with SUDs exceeds 70%.[18] Although nicotine triggers the same pleasure pathways in the brain as opioids, medications used to treat opioid dependence do not seem to have a significant effect on smoking cessation.[32] These patients also tend to minimize the importance of cigarette smoking in their overall health.[33] Due to frequency of visits for MAT, there is ample opportunity to address tobacco use in this population. Likewise, because smoking can cause serious complications in pregnancy, this is an important time to address smoking cessation.

Other Comorbidities

More than 60% of patients with SUD have coexisting psychiatric illness, including mood, anxiety, psychotic, attention-deficit hyperactivity, and antisocial personality disorders. In addition, other drug use, posttraumatic stress disorder, unwanted pregnancies, eating disorders, and premenstrual dysphoric disorder occur at higher rates.

Lapses in Care

Of note, many patients experience lapses in insurance coverage and hence coverage of their care that puts them at increased risk for relapse. Inversely, relapse can put these patients at increased risk for neglect of maintaining their insurance coverage.

SUMMARY

Societally, the deadly epidemic of OUD is skyrocketing in women, causing increasing disease burden and fatalities. Primary care clinicians must consider the top reasons to provide integrated management of opioid addiction in women in the primary care office:

1. Opioid addiction is epidemic and rates are rising even faster in women.
2. Treating the addiction with MAT vastly improves outcomes, particularly in women who have disproportionate parenting responsibilities.
3. Providing MAT in primary care normalizes the care and reduces shame.
4. Providing MAT in primary care creates the opportunity for whole person care, including every psychiatric and medical problem.
5. Women with OUD are a vulnerable population and each person needs a champion.
6. Providing this type of integrated care creates the opportunity for primary care practice to be inspired, inspirational, and unconditional.

ACKNOWLEDGMENTS

Many thanks to Drs Patricia Fisher and Sanchit Maruti for their expert input into this article, and to Dr Michael Goedde for statistics and figures.

REFERENCES

1. Final Report: Opioid use, Misues and Overdose in Women. 2017. Available at: https://www.womenshealth.gov/files/documents/final-report-opioid-508.pdf. Accessed December 1, 2017.
2. Jones C, Paulozzi L, Mack K. Sources of Prescription opioid pain relievers by frequency of past year non-medical use: United States, 2008-2011. JAMA 2014; 174(5):802–3.
3. A. S. o. A. Medicine. 2016. Available at: http://www.asam.org/docs/default-source/advocacy/opioid-addiction-disease-facts-figures.pdf. Accessed December 1, 2017.
4. Zilberman M. Substance abuse across the lifespan in women, in Women & Addiction. The Guilford Press; 2009. p. 3–13.
5. Opioid Addiction Facts & Figures 2016, American Society of Addiction Medicine. Available: https://www.asam.org/docs/default-source/advocacy/opioid-addiction-disease-facts-figures.pdf. Accessed December 1, 2017.
6. Hser Y, Evans E, Grella C, et al. Long-term course of opioid addiction. Harv Rev Psychiatry 2014;23(2):76–89.
7. Hyman SE. Addiction: a disease of learning and memory. Am J Psychiatry 2005; 162:1414–22.
8. Nestler EJ. Cellular basis of memory for addiction. Dialogues Clin Neurosci 2013; 15:431–43.
9. Nestler EJ. Molecular basis of long-term plasticity underlying addiction. Nat Rev Neurosci 2001;2:119–28.
10. Evans SM, Foltin RW. Exogenous progesterone attenuates the subjective effects of smoked cocaine in women, but not in men. Neuropsychopharmacology 2006; 31:659–74.
11. Zubieta J-K, Dannals RF, Frost J. Gender and age influences on human brain mu-opioid receptor binding measured by PET. Am J Psychiatry 1999;156:842–8.
12. Bobzean S, DeNorbrega A, Perrotti L. Sex differences in the neurobiology of drug addiction. Exp Neurol 2014;259:64–74.
13. National Institute on Drug Abuse. Available at: https://www.drugabuse.gov/publications/resource-guide-screening-drug-use-in-general-medical-settings/nida-quick-screen. Accessed December 1, 2017.
14. Substance Abuse and Mental Health Services Association. Available at: https://www.samhsa.gov/. Accessed December 1, 2017.

15. Yudko E, Lozhkina O, Fouts A. A comprehensive review of the psychometric properties of the Drug Abuse Screening Test. J Subst Abuse Treat 2007;32: 189–98.
16. Gavin D, Ross H, Skinner H. Diagnostic validity of the Drug Abuse Screening Test in the assessment of DSM-III drug disorders. Br J Addict 1989;84(3):301–7.
17. Skinner HA. The Drug Abuse Screening Test. Addict Behav 1982;7(4):363–71.
18. LaPaglia D. Substance use disorders and systems of care. In: Yale textbook of public psychiatry. Oxford University Press; 2016. p. 81–96.
19. Soyka M. Buprenorphine-naloxone buccal soluble film for the treatment of opioid dependence: current update. Expert Opin Drug Deliv 2015;12(2):339–47.
20. Johnson R, Strain E, Amass L. Buprenorphine: how to use it right. Drug Alcohol Depend 2003;70:59–77.
21. Samhsa, Samhsa. 2016. Available at: https://www.samhsa.gov/medication-assisted-treatment/buprenorphine-waiver-management/. Accessed November 30, 2017.
22. Brown V, Harris M, Fallot R. Moving toward trauma-informed practice in addiction treatment: a collaborative model of agency assessment. J Psychoactive Drugs 2013;45(5):386–93.
23. McLellan AT, Lewis DC, O'Brien CP, et al. Drug dependence, a chronic medical illness: implications for treatment, insurance, and outcomes evaluation. JAMA 2000;284:1689–95.
24. Brooklyn J, Sigmon S. Vermont hub-and-spoke model of care for opioid use disorder: development, implementation, and impact. J Addict Med 2017;11:286–92.
25. Unger A, Jung E, Winklbaur B, et al. Gender issues in the pharmacotherapy of opioid-addicted women: buprenorphine. J Addict Dis 2010;29:217–30.
26. Ludlow JP, Evans SF, Hulse G. Obstetric and perinatal outcomes in pregnancies associated with illicit substance abuse. Aust N Z J Obstet Gynaecol 2004;44: 302–6.
27. Oei J, Lui K. Managment of the newborn infant affected by maternal opiates and other drugs of dependency. J Paediatr Child Health 2007;43:9–18.
28. Jones HE, Kaltenbach K, Heil SH, et al. Neonatal abstinence syndrome after methadone or buprenorphine exposure. N Engl J Med 2010;363:2320–31.
29. Soyka M. Buprenorphine use in pregnant opioid users: a critical review. CNS Drugs 2013;27(8):653–62.
30. Kelty E, Hulse G. A retrospective cohort study of obstetric outcomes in opioid-dependent women treated with implant naltrexone, oral methadone or sublingual buprenorphine, and non-dependent controls. Drugs 2017;77:1199–210.
31. Shekarchizadeh H, Khami MR, Mohebbi SZ. Oral health of drug abusers: a review of health effects and care. Iran J Public Health 2013;42(9):929–40.
32. David SP, Lancaster T, Stead L, et al. Opioid antagonists for smoking cessation. Cochrane Database Syst Rev 2013;(6):CD003086.
33. Mandal P, Jain R, Jhanjee S, et al. Psychological barriers to tobacco cessation in Indian buprenorphine-naloxone maintained patients: a pilot study. Indian J Psychol Med 2015;37:299–304.

Analgesia, Opioids, and Other Drug Use During Pregnancy and Neonatal Abstinence Syndrome

Hendrée E. Jones, PhD[a,b,c,]*, Walter K. Kraft, MD[d]

KEYWORDS

- Neonatal abstinence syndrome • NAS • Neonatal opioid withdrawal • NOWS
- Neonatal • Addiction • Opioid use disorder • Prenatal

KEY POINTS

- A life course perspective helps patients stop substance use. Pregnancy is a critical time for behavior change. Healing opioid use disorder requires an individualized multifactorial approach.
- Buprenorphine formulations (alone and those with naloxone) and methadone show relative safety and efficacy for the fetus, mother, and child. Medications works best with comprehensive physical, psychological, and case management.
- Infants with significant in utero opioid exposure need observation for neonatal abstinence syndrome (NAS). At least half of infants with NAS can be managed solely with nonpharmacologic approaches.
- Future genetic factor research may yield (1) infant risk stratification to minimize NAS intensity and duration and (2) optimizing NAS treatments based on drug disposition and effect differences.

This article originally appeared in *Clinics in Perinatology*, Volume 46, Issue 2, June 2019.
Disclosure Statement: H.E. Jones has no relationship with a commercial company that has a direct financial interest in subject matter or materials discussed in article or with a company making a competing product. W.K. Kraft has received research funding from Chiesi.
a Department of Obstetrics and Gynecology, University of North Carolina at Chapel Hill, UNC Horizons, 410 North Greensboro Street, Chapel Hill, NC, USA; b Department of Psychiatry and Behavioral Sciences, School of Medicine, Johns Hopkins University, Baltimore, MD, USA; c Department of Obstetrics and Gynecology, School of Medicine, Johns Hopkins University, Baltimore, MD, USA; d Clinical Research Unit, Department of Pharmacology and Experimental Therapeutics, Thomas Jefferson University, 1170 Main Building, 132 South 10th Street, Philadelphia, PA 19107-5244, USA
* Corresponding author. Department of Obstetrics and Gynecology, UNC Horizons, University of North Carolina at Chapel Hill, 410 North Greensboro Street, Chapel Hill, NC 27510.
E-mail address: Hendree_Jones@med.unc.edu

OPIOID USE CONTINUES TO RISE AMONG THE GENERAL POPULATION: PREGNANT WOMAN ARE NOT SPARED

The opioid crisis was a recognized threat to public health in the United States since 2009 when annual deaths due to opioid overdose surpassed motor vehicle accidents.[1] Nationally,630,000 people died from a drug overdose between 1999 and 2016 with opioid deaths 5 times higher in 2016 compared with 1999.[2] Although more men than women report illicit (eg, heroin) and nonmedical (eg, prescription opioids) opioid use, it is a concerning problem for women.[3] For heroin, women tend to use smaller amounts, for less time, and are less likely to inject it compared with men.[4–7] For prescription opioids, women report using them (eg, oxycodone, hydrocodone, fentanyl) to relieve pain (physical and psychological), reduce weight, reduce stress, and reduce exhaustion.[8] Although fewer women than men died from opioid overdoses in 2016 (ie, 7109 women and 9978 men), from 1999 to 2016, prescription opioid overdose deaths rose more rapidly for women (sevenfold) than for men (fourfold). Thus, gender-responsive interventions need development to reduce overdose deaths.

OPIOID USE OCCURS ON A CONTINUUM: IDENTIFICATION AND TREATMENT IS NEEDED FOR OPIOID USE DISORDERS DURING PREGNANCY

All substance use, including opioids, occurs on a continuum that encompasses no, occasional, and regular use. Substance use occurring despite adverse consequences leads to a diagnosis of opioid use disorder (OUD) that is graded as mild, moderate, or severe. For women who continue to use opioids after pregnancy awareness, the Diagnostic and Statistical Manual, Fifth Edition (DSM-5) criteria indicates that they have at least a mild OUD that merits intervention. Consistent with the general population, the prevalence of OUD during pregnancy, measured at delivery, has greatly increased from 1999 to 2014 (from 1.5 per 1000 to 6.5 per 1000 delivery hospitalizations; $P<.05$).[9] Likewise, the diagnosis of neonatal abstinence syndrome (NAS) (see the section "Defining neonatal abstinence syndrome" for definition) has increased from 1.2 per 1000 hospital births in 2000 to 8.0 per 1000 in 2014.[10] This almost sevenfold increase in NAS nationally suggests that approximately every 15 minutes an infant is born with a NAS diagnosis.[11,12]

Before women can be treated for OUD during pregnancy, they must be identified. Opioid and/or other substance use is most commonly initiated before pregnancy. Thus, all women of childbearing age deserve regular screening for substance use problems to prevent and respond to substance-exposed pregnancies. The American College of Obstetrics and Gynecology (ACOG) recommends repeated substance use disorder screening across prenatal visits.[13] Of note, substance use screening (via instrument/questionnaire) differs from drug testing (via *confirmed* biologic samples, such as urine via gas chromatography–mass spectrometry). A positive urine drug screen is not a diagnosis of a substance use disorder; such results indicate only the presence or absence of the parent drug and/or its metabolites indicating recent substance use.[14] Universal *voluntary* screening using a validated instrument must be conducted with a nonpunitive, supportive treatment approach.

A life course perspective is needed to help patients stop harmful substance use. For women, the pregnancy life event can be a critical time for behavior change. Ending substance use, including opioids, requires an individualized multifactorial approach. Factors associated with the risk of substance use disorders are genetic (eg, ~50% of substance use disorder vulnerability),[15] as well as environmental issues specific to women (eg, 40%–70% of women in treatment have been the victim of physical or sexual abuse).[16,17] Thus, treatment first requires access to appropriate care and a personalized approach. Access to the appropriate level of care is the first step of treatment initiation, engagement, and retention. For women with OUD who become pregnant, prenatal care and OUD treatment ideally require integration or at least coordination of providers.[18] Appropriate perinatal care also includes identifying and responding to multiple life domain needs such as physical health, concurrent substance use (eg, tobacco, alcohol, and marijuana), dental health, psychological health, interpersonal, economic, housing, parenting, and family. Such comprehensive treatment must be continued based on the patient's needs, often encompassing at least a year after pregnancy ends.

BUPRENORPHINE AND METHADONE: PART OF A COMPLETE TREATMENT APPROACH

An important, but not only, part of care of women with OUD includes the use of opioid agonist medication (buprenorphine or methadone). Recommendations to use methadone pharmacotherapy over medically assisted withdrawal (also known commonly as detoxification) resulted from reports of medically assisted withdrawal leading to maternal opioid relapse and fetal demise.[19,20] Although data to date do not support an association between medically assisted withdrawal and fetal demise, they also do not support either equivalence or benefit of such an approach relative to maternal opioid agonist pharmacotherapy.[20,21] In fact, medically assisted withdrawal can increase the risk of maternal relapse (up to 100%), reduce treatment engagement (treatment completion rates as low as 9%),[21] and fail to prevent NAS. Given these issues, medically assisted withdrawal is not considered a first-line approach and needs more systematic investigation to determine its role, if any, as a treatment approach to OUD during the perinatal period. In contrast to medically assisted withdrawal, medication treatment using either buprenorphine or methadone is endorsed by the ACOG,[22] American Society for Addiction Medicine,[23] United Nations,[24] World Health Organization,[25] and other government agencies[26] as the optimal approach for treating OUD during pregnancy.

Buprenorphine or methadone, if taken in adequate doses, can stabilize the OUD of the pregnant woman and prevent relapse.[27,28] Methadone treatment, compared with untreated use of heroin, improves maternal medical outcomes (eg, less human immunodeficiency virus [HIV] infection due to reduced drug risk, decreased preeclampsia risk, and more obstetric visits completed).[29] For the fetus, methadone versus untreated OUD has been associated with less fetal death, less fetal exposure to cycles of heroin-induced intoxication and withdrawal,[30] and improved fetal growth.[27] Buprenorphine is approved by the Food and Drug Administration (FDA) to treat OUD and has been investigated in pregnant patients.[31] The MOTHER study[32] assessed buprenorphine compared with methadone in a randomized trial that focused on pregnant women with OUD throughout pregnancy and their neonates. Both buprenorphine and methadone had similar maternal and delivery outcomes. Relative to methadone, among patients retained in the study, in utero buprenorphine-exposed neonates required 89% less morphine to treat NAS, spent 58% less time in the hospital being medicated for NAS, and spent 43% less time in the hospital. A systematic review of research regarding buprenorphine to treat OUD during pregnancy concludes the following: (1) buprenorphine and methadone have comparable maternal outcomes; (2) buprenorphine produces less fetal heart rate and movement suppression; (3) buprenorphine produces less severe NAS; (4) both drugs are compatible with breastfeeding; and (5) deleterious effects of buprenorphine on subsequent infant development are not apparent.[33]

The FDA approved products containing both buprenorphine and naloxone (an opioid antagonist added to deter buprenorphine product injecting the medication) to treat adult OUD. All labels include pregnancy, neonatal, and lactation information and note the accepted use of the medication during the perinatal period if the benefits outweigh the risks. Although the product insert contains updated information, national and international guidance documents are slow to catch up with science to support the use of combination products. Buprenorphine + naloxone during pregnancy shows no obvious adverse maternal or neonatal outcomes, a reduced incidence of NAS, lower peak NAS scores, and shorter overall mean length of hospitalization than neonates with in utero methadone exposure.[34–36] Prospective large-sample results would benefit future practice.

Every national and international guideline on the treatment of OUD endorses buprenorphine and methadone as the first-line approach for pregnant women. In addition, federal regulations require priority access to opioid treatment programs for pregnant women (eg, no need to fully meet DSM-5 criteria for OUD to initiate medication). However, only a third of pregnant women who qualify actually receive opioid agonist pharmacotherapy in the United States.[37] Thus, although treatment programs have increased capacity to treat more pregnant women with OUD, focusing on certain risk groups and increasing utilization of opioid medication should be emphasized (eg, young, unemployed, uninsured have less access).[38] Further, increasing the numbers of active medical buprenorphine prescribers is needed to expand access for all pregnant patients.

WOMEN RECEIVING BUPRENORPHINE OR METHADONE DURING PREGNANCY: PAIN MANAGEMENT: LABOR, DELIVERY, AND POSTPARTUM

Delivery universally produces acute pain with a clearly defined onset and resolution.[39] Women with OUD require assessment for appropriate analgesia and anesthesia options, with adequate pain management provided at delivery. Regardless of treatment status, women with OUD may by hyperanalgesic, have opioid tolerance, and need greater amounts of opioid for relief of pain compared with patients without OUD.[40] Pain medication must be provided regardless of current or past OUD. For women treated with buprenorphine or methadone, the medication should not be withheld or altered in terms of quantity or frequency of dosing during labor and delivery or the immediate postpartum period. Women treated with buprenorphine or methadone for OUD can experience adequate pain control postpartum with the use of other opioids in combination with acetaminophen and a nonsteroidal anti-inflammatory drugs.[41] Women receiving methadone during pregnancy were found to have similar analgesic requirements and response during labor but required more opioid analgesic after cesarean delivery when compared with women not on methadone maintenance.[39] Of great importance, women who use heroin or prescription opioids and/or are prescribed chronic opioids (including methadone or buprenorphine) should *not* receive opioid agonist/antagonist pain medications (eg, butorphanol, nalbuphine, and pentazocine) for acute pain because these medications may cause an acute opioid withdrawal syndrome.[42]

BREASTFEEDING IS COMPATIBLE AND ENCOURAGED: BUPRENORPHINE OR METHADONE

Breastfeeding helps to build a strong mother-infant bond and provides optimal nutrition and passive immunization for the child. Women with OUD may struggle with using their breasts for food (eg, due to sexual abuse and trauma). They may also struggle with the responsibilities of motherhood (eg, no parenting role models due to being raised in foster care, loss of custody of other children, their own adverse childhood experiences). Successful establishment of breastfeeding can be quite empowering for some women. Women should not be forced to breastfeed. Women receiving buprenorphine or methadone should be encouraged to breastfeed if they are HIV negative.[43] Women with hepatitis B or C may also breastfeed as long as the nipple and surrounding areola are not cracked and/or bleeding to avoid direct contact with maternal blood.[44] If this does occur, women should be encouraged to pump and discard breast milk and to resume nursing when the skin has healed. Because negligible amounts of methadone are excreted in human milk across the dose range, there is no contraindication to nursing while prescribed methadone.[45] Although little buprenorphine or methadone is transferred in breast milk, the act of breastfeeding may ease neonatal withdrawal from opioids.[46] Similarly, little buprenorphine is excreted in breast milk, and its low oral bioavailability is not thought to impact NAS or infant behavior.[47] Given that some women use other substances while taking buprenorphine or methadone, such substances deserve discussion. Neonatal exposure to nicotine may cause irritability, poor feeding, and sleep disruption.[48] Infants can have irritability, gastrointestinal disruptions, and sleep issues with cocaine exposure.[49] Breastfeeding during maternal use of benzodiazepines should be discouraged. ACOG discourages any use of cannabis during preconception, pregnancy, and lactation.[50] Finally, alcohol use and breastfeeding are not compatible.

The need for treatment continues postpartum. A review of methadone discontinuation in pregnant and postpartum women concluded that methadone discontinuation at or up to 6 months postpartum was 56%.[51] Although the discontinuation reasons are elusive, program policies that withdraw medication from women after delivery and loss of Medicaid coverage may be contributing issues. Opioid-related overdoses contribute to pregnancy-associated deaths in many states (11%–20% of cases).[52,53] At 12 months postpartum, treatment retention negatively correlated with illicit drug use during the third trimester.[54] Expanding coverage of OUD treatment for pregnant and postpartum women is critical to maternal and neonatal health.[55]

DEFINING NEONATAL ABSTINENCE SYNDROME

In utero transfer of opioids is associated with a withdrawal syndrome in the neonate after the umbilical cord is cut. The pathobiology of opioid withdrawal prompts a similar set of physical signs in the neonate as in the adult, although the manifestations and medical implications differ. As in adults, the neonate with significant symptoms will have difficulty with gastrointestinal function with loose stools and vomiting, autonomic dysfunction with temperature dysregulation and sneezing, and neurologic signs of irritability and tremors. Unlike the adult, the neonate differs in a developmental arc of growth and development. Severe withdrawal impairs the ability of the neonate to feed properly, which can lead to poor weight gain and development. Irritability also impairs maternal-infant bonding. The mechanistic basis for the clinical presentation is not fully defined; however, tolerance to opioids is primarily medicated by receptor downregulation coupled with upregulation in the cyclic adenosine monophosphate pathway.[56] Although NAS is a nonspecific term, it has traditionally referred to signs due to primarily opioid withdrawal and its defining manifestations are those associated with opioid withdrawal. To more clearly link the etiology of the discrete syndrome to an in utero exposure, federal agencies have suggested the more specific term neonatal opioid withdrawal syndrome (NOWS).[57]

Although not causing a withdrawal syndrome severe enough requiring individualized treatment on their own, many medications and exposures along with in utero opioid exposure can worsen the severity of neonatal withdrawal symptoms (eg, tobacco or medications such as antidepressants, benzodiazepines, and gabapentin).[58–63] Other factors that impact the need for pharmacologic treatment include concurrent use of alcohol, tobacco, and other drugs.[63] Maternal methadone dose as a potential modifiable covariate of NAS severity has been extensively investigated, with varied methodological quality of studies. Although meta-analysis did not identify a statistically significant difference in outcomes between high-dose and low-dose methadone, there is a trend suggestive of a modest maternal dose–NAS severity relationship.[64] This dose relationship, if it exists, is at best loosely tied to the severity of withdrawal signs and not relevant in terms of choosing a maternal dose or differential NAS treatment approaches. Lower maternal methadone doses have been associated with higher rates of illicit drug use. ACOG and others suggest that maternal doses of methadone should not be reduced solely to reduce NAS severity.[52]

NEONATAL ABSTINENCE SYNDROME TREATMENT APPROACHES

Infants with documented or suspected in utero opioid exposure need monitoring with a standard assessment instrument. Although a number of scoring systems have been developed,[65–68] the Finnegan[69] remains the de facto standard for clinical care. A score of greater than 8 is highly correlated with in utero opioid exposure, even in the absence of declared use during pregnancy.[70] When informed by at least moderate pretest probability, performance in defining a high degree of symptoms is excellent. Elements that make up the score have drifted over time, with individual sites modifying the instrument over the years. These changes reflect practice changes (eg, removal of seizures only seen in the early NAS practice history). Thus, the terms "Finnegan" or "modified Finnegan" generally describe scoring systems that vary in minor ways across sites. Regardless of the NAS scoring instrument used, key elements are ensuring uniformity in scoring through a process of continuous training and quality assessment of nursing staff. In-service sessions paired with observed assessment by a site-level gold standard assessor comprises quality NAS assessment.

Attempts to simplify NAS assessment approaches (Jones and colleagues,[71,72] Isemann and colleagues[73]) include quick screening instruments with a goal of predicting those infants most likely to need pharmacologic treatment. Others have focused on shortening the Finnegan while retaining the instrument's discrimination for both identifying the neonates who need pharmacologic treatment and informing treatment decisions following medication initiation. Maguire and colleagues[74] and Gomez-Pomar and colleagues[75] used quantitative methods comparing Finnegan as the gold standard with the explicit goal to remove less informative scoring elements to reduce nursing burden. Most recently, the scoring elements have focused on the infant's ability to eat, sleep, and be consoled (sometimes identified by the acronym ESC). This approach was 1 of 8 elements comprising a quality improvement project.[76,77] The ESC approach has not been compared with the Finnegan and the test characteristics of sensitivity, specificity, and receiver operator curves have not been published. Comprehensive approaches to NAS treatment that include ESC as one of many elements have demonstrated decreased resource utilization. However, which specific interventions are responsible for less resource utilization is unknown. The benefits in reduction of nursing time with the use of ESC score have not been quantitated. In addition, NAS is a condition with heterogeneous expression of symptoms covering multiple organ systems. Systematic evaluation of ESC compared with the Finnegan scoring systems would be welcomed to assess if simplification of the score to 3 domains results in missing signs of concern in certain neonates, or if it provides a similar result to current standard assessment tools.

NONPHARMACOLOGIC TREATMENT OF NEONATAL ABSTINENCE SYNDROME

All neonates, regardless of initial manifestations, should first be treated with nonpharmacologic approaches. Nonpharmacologic approaches should not be considered an alternative to medication therapy, but instead the baseline for all patients. Nonpharmacologic approaches are effective in reducing the number of infants treated with pharmacologic treatments.[76,78] No standard set of interventions constitute a definitive "nonpharmacologic treatment bundle." Some sites have embarked on large-scale changes to NAS care. These approaches often yield an impressive reduction in length of stay. Such interventions involve many changes at once and it is difficult to identify which specific intervention is associated with the greatest impact. Interventions, such a use of small, frequent formula feedings for those not breastfeeding, have not been (and likely will never be) individually examined but are considered safe and widely practiced. A few key interventions have been examined more closely. Those with the most evidence to support are breastfeeding, rooming in, swaddling, and skin-to-skin contact.[79] Breastfeeding is associated with clear improvements in NAS outcomes of need for treatment, duration of hospitalization, and length of pharmacologic treatment.[80,81] In retrospective studies, rooming in has been associated with significant improvement in outcomes.[82–84] These interventions select out a very specific group of mothers who are able to be integrated into the neonatal care plan. In addition to these specific interventions, parallel attention to trust building with mothers is a key element in fostering the health of infants with NAS. Above all, successful outcomes are more likely when the parents trust the caregiver's and clinician's approach interactions with an understanding of the stages of addiction recovery and a lack of preconceived notions of how an individual parent is anticipated to act. Ideally, the flow of information from the newborn nursery to the mother occurs before the baby is born. This includes a discussion of scoring, treatment approaches, and empowering mothers to aid in activities that have been shown to reduce the need for pharmacologic treatment.

PHARMACOLOGIC TREATMENT OF NEONATAL ABSTINENCE SYNDROME

Pharmacologic treatment is used in neonates with severe NAS (**Fig. 1**). End points in clinical trials of pharmacologic therapy are length of treatment and duration of

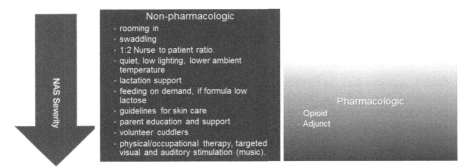

Fig. 1. Approach to infants with in utero opioid exposure. All infants should be provided a base of nonpharmacologic therapies. Specific measures will vary with the ability of the local site to provide. Some potential approaches are listed. Pharmacologic therapy is added only in those for whom symptoms are not controlled with nonpharmacologic means.

hospitalization. However, these measures assume that the other goals of treatment (relief of discomfort, appropriate growth and development, and maximizing parental bonding) are being met. Some of these goals are less easily quantified. It is possible for example, that low doses of control medications and aggressive weaning schedules could reduce length of stay but at the cost of accepting a higher degree of infant discomfort. Weight and some measure of symptom scores could capture this difference, but mother-infant bonding is more difficult to assess. Thus, despite the primacy of length of treatment in clinical trials, secondary measures of neonatal well-being should be considered when judging various treatments.

The foundation of pharmacologic treatment for opioid NAS is replacement with an opioid. Compared with other classes of agents, the opioids are consistently superior in clinical trials and retrospective examinations. This is consistent with observations in the treatment of adult opioid withdrawal.[85,86] Continued elevated symptom scores and clinical signs of severe NAS trigger the use of pharmacologic treatment. Doses are titrated up until signs/symptoms are controlled, or a second medication is added. After a period of clinical stability, doses are gradually weaned to a target dose and then discontinued. Regardless of the specific drugs or regimens used, standardization of treatment is a key element in optimizing therapy. Published examples in which improvement programs stressing uniform use of institutional treatment protocol have resulted in 15% to 50% reduction in length of treatment and duration of hospitalization.[87–91]

There are significant differences in treatment regimens between institutions. Eighty percent of US sites use morphine as the primary opioid, with the remainder using methadone.[91] A small but growing number of sites are using buprenorphine as the primary opioid. In the inpatient setting, all 3 opioids have excellent safety records. Comparing morphine and methadone efficacy, the randomized controlled data suggest an advantage of methadone (**Table 1**). The largest multicenter study of 117 neonates with mixed in utero exposure (~60% methadone and 30% buprenorphine) demonstrated a 14% shorter mean length of treatment with methadone than morphine.[92] Real-world data from the Pediatrix Clinical Data Warehouse of 7667 infants showed a 22% reduction in length of hospitalization for neonates treated with methadone compared with morphine.[93] Sublingual buprenorphine was compared with oral morphine in the BBORN, a blinded controlled study in 63 neonates almost all who were exposed to methadone in utero.[94] Buprenorphine had a 42% shorter

Table 1					
Methadone versus morphine: median length of treatment					
Author	Design	n	Morphine (Number of Days)	Methadone (Number of Days)	P
Lainwala et al,[112] 2005	Retrospective	46	36	40	NS
Hall et al,[88] 2014	Retrospective	383	16[a]	16[a]	NS
Young et al,[113] 2015	Retrospective	26	7[a]	38[a]	.001
Brown et al,[114] 2015	Blinded RCT	31	21	14	.008
Davis et al,[92] 2018	Blinded RCT	183	15	11.5	.02
Tolia et al,[93] 2018	Retrospective	7667	23[b]	18[b]	<.001

Abbreviations: NS, not significant; RCT, randomized controlled trial.
[a] Mean.
[b] Length of stay.

length of stay compared with a weight-based morphine comparison. Hall and colleagues[95,96] reported retrospective cohort data from southern Ohio of 212 neonates treated with buprenorphine compared with 349 treated with morphine and morphine as a comparison cohort. Buprenorphine use was associated with a 29% reduction in length of treatment. Compared with the BBORN controlled trial, the buprenorphine and morphine treatment regimens differed, and the Ohio cohort had more heterogeneous exposures in utero. The similarity of effect size using different study designs, populations, and drug regimens suggests an advantage for buprenorphine. The preparation used in all published reports contains 30% ethanol. The safety profile of ethanol in infants has not been established, but serum concentrations after buprenorphine administration generally fall within regulatory guidelines.[97]

Ultimately, the answer to "what is the best opioid for NAS?" is not straightforward. We have the results of randomized controlled trials, but the better question is "what is the best opioid treatment regimen for which neonate?" A treatment protocol identifies not only the specific opioid, but defines starting dose, rate of up-titration, maximum dose, weaning rate, and a cessation dose. Other differences are the severity score cut points used to initiate and intensify pharmacologic treatment, as well as the choice and dose of other pharmacologic adjunct therapy. Up to this point, the endpoint used to gauge success of a regimen has been the drug dose, and not the drug concentration within the neonate. Pharmacometric modeling is a quantitative approach that has particular value in the neonatal population. The strengths include an ability to (1) use a small number of blood draws per patient, (2) define the variability in pharmacokinetics between individuals, (3) identify covariates associated with the variation, (4) incorporate developmental changes with maturation of hepatic and renal function, and (5) establish a relationship between drug exposure and pharmacodynamic response. A number of investigators have begun to use pharmacometrics to describe drug behavior in NAS[98–101] and to generate dosing regiments.[102]

NONOPIOID ADJUNCT THERAPY

Phenobarbital and clonidine are nonopioid drugs that can be used in conjunction with an opioid. These adjunctive therapies aim to synergize treatment. Several small studies compared an adjunct medication with an opioid to treat NAS. Commonly, an adjunct is given only when symptoms are not controlled and then weaned before cessation of the opioid. Other centers will wean the opioid first and discontinue the adjunct later as an inpatient or outpatient. This approach is much more common for phenobarbital than clonidine. The third approach is that of parallel opioid and clonidine therapy, with a goal of reducing opioid exposure, as well as length of treatment. Neither the optimal adjunctive drug nor treatment regimen have been clearly defined for specific populations.

TREATMENT LOCATION

NAS treatment has increasingly moved out of the intensive care unit to areas of the hospital with less stimulation. Alternatively, specialized areas have been designated that are optimized not only in environment control, but also in staff support. There are treatment protocols in which pharmacologic treatment is transitioned to the outpatient management with methadone. Another approach is to discharge with phenobarbital as the primary pharmacologic therapy after inpatient opioid weaning. Inpatient pharmacologic treatment is consistently reported as being associated with longer lengths of hospitalization compared with outpatient weaning, but shorter total duration of treatment.[103] The best documented experience is a population-based retrospective cohort study of 532 neonates primarily treated with phenobarbital.[104] Consistent with prior studies, the median (interquartile range) length of pharmacologic therapy was significantly shorter in inpatients compared with outpatients. However, neonates treated as outpatients had an increased number of emergency room visits within 6 months of discharge when compared with those treated as inpatients alone. Although not statistically significant, the point estimate odds ratio for an emergency visit at 6 weeks, or any hospitalization at 6 or 24 weeks was approximately 1.5 for outpatient compared with inpatient treatment. This suggests that caution is indicated when transitioning a neonate to outpatient treatment, which should be considered only when there is a comprehensive support structure in place and pediatricians are familiar and comfortable with weaning a neonate as an outpatient.

GENETICS

OUD heritability in adults, derived from an examination of twins, is high and accounts for approximately 50% of the risk being genetic.[15] Similar data are lacking for neonates, but a small investigation of in utero opioid exposure revealed high concordance of NAS scores and need for treatment in 5 of 7 mostly dizygotic twin sets.[105] Primarily single-nucleotide polymorphism (SNP) approaches in adults have identified variants in the mu-opioid receptor (OPRM1), delta-opioid receptor (OPRD1), the dopamine D2 receptor (DRD2), and brain-derived neurotrophic factor.[106] Initial studies in neonates with in utero opioid exposure suggested OPRRM1 118A > G AG/GG and COMT 158A > G AG/GG genotype were associated with improved outcomes in NAS.[107] A microarray replication identified pointwise, but not experiment-wise significance of these 2 SNPs as well as OPRK1 rs702764 C allele and PNOC rs732636 A allele.[108] Genes in the inflammatory pathway have also been implicated,[109] as well as epigenetic factors.[110,111] In aggregate, early signals suggest that with larger sample sizes, more definitive causal relationships can be established and may lead to a better understanding of NAS biology. Several factors should be noted in comparing adult and neonatal genetic investigations of opioid withdrawal. First, the phenotypic endpoints in neonates are small and generally well established. However, there is drift in standard of care with a greater emphasis on nonpharmacologic care, so a metric such as the need for pharmacologic therapy may differ between older and more recent cohorts. Endpoints of length of stay will vary between institutions, depending on a specific pharmacologic regimen used. The use of morphine equivalents between different opioids widely used in adults and lacks validation in neonates, so comparisons between institutions with different drug regimens are problematic. Alternatively, there is increasing standardization of regimens. All neonates are at least initially treated in the hospital, and the electronic health record provides the ability to generate accurate data with more ease than in adults. The pathology is somewhat simpler in that NAS is withdrawal and not addiction. Future directions will generate larger and more comprehensive data sets with standard data elements. The long-term goal would be to have more solidly associated genetic factors that would allow for the generation of a risk score that would allow for (1) risk stratification of neonates to optimize intensity and duration of monitoring of symptoms and (2) optimizing pharmacologic treatments based on differences in drug disposition and effect. Personalized models will not be based on a single SNP, but polygenic and include nongenetic covariates associated with severity, such as gestational age and other maternal substance use. Such models are aspirational and genetics remains a research tool at the current time.

Best Practices

What is the current practice for

The treatment of women who have substance use disorders, including OUD during the pregnancy period and how their infants cared for.

Best Practice/Guidelines/Care Path Objective

What changes in current practice are likely to improve outcomes?
- All maternal and child health care providers need to be trained to engage all women in a short conversation (universal screening), to provide nonjudgmental feedback/advice about substance use, as needed, and have the knowledge to refer patients to appropriate treatment options. Such actions can improve maternal and infant outcomes.
- For pregnant and postpartum women with an OUD, national and international guidelines recommend the use of methadone and buprenorphine as medications over medically supervised withdrawal given that withdrawal yields high relapse rates and untreated addiction can lead to worse outcomes. However, only a third of pregnant women who qualify, actually receive opioid agonist pharmacotherapy in the United States. Thus, increasing the numbers of active medical buprenorphine prescribers is needed to expand access for all perinatal patients.
- Although national and international guidance recommends encouraging breastfeeding in women receiving methadone or buprenorphine who are not using illicit drugs, and who have no other contraindications (eg, HIV infection), not all providers follow this practice. Thus, more providers need education and support to help women.
- Women who have an opioid use during pregnancy are at high risk of postpartum mortality, and need access to adequate postpartum psychosocial support services, including substance use disorder treatment, relapse prevention programs, case management, and parenting support.
- Approaching NAS treatment from a dyad perspective may improve outcomes. NAS treatment has increasingly moved out of the intensive care unit to areas of the hospital with less stimulation. Alternatively, specialized areas have been designated that are optimized not only in environment control, but also in staff support When the mother or other caregiver is part of the NAS care approach, fewer resources may be needed.

Major Recommendations

- Taking a life course perspective and dyadic approach to the care and treatment of mothers for substance use disorders (including OUD) and their prenatally substance-exposed child will promote healthy outcomes.

- Treatment access to methadone and buprenorphine for pregnant and postpartum women is needed.

- Treatment cannot end at the postpartum period, the mother-child dyad continues to need support and resources are needed to provide adequate comprehensive care to them.

- Newer NAS approaches need to be evaluated in a rigorously scientific manner.

Summary Statement

Healing women who have substance use disorders, including OUD, requires an individualized multifactorial approach. Methadone and buprenorphine are important parts of treatment and work best with comprehensive physical, psychological, and case management. Infants with significant in utero opioid exposure need observation for NAS. At least half of infants with NAS can be managed solely with nonpharmacologic approaches. A dyadic approach to care is an important key to improving outcomes for the mother and child.

Data from The American College of Obstetricians and Gynecologists. Opioid use and opioid use disorder in pregnancy. Committee Opinion No. 711. American College of Obstetricians and Gynecologists. Obstet Gynecol 2017;130:e81–94; and Substance Abuse and Mental Health Services Administration. Clinical guidance for treating pregnant and parenting women with opioid use disorder and their infants. 2018 SMA18-5054. Available at: https://store.samhsa.gov/product/Clinical-Guidance-for-Treating-Pregnant-and-Parenting-Women-With-Opioid-Use-Disorder-and-Their-Infants/SMA18-5054. Accessed March 13, 2019.

REFERENCES

1. Waite T. American security today. DEA: fentanyl-related overdose deaths rising at an alarming rate 2016. Available at: https://americansecuritytoday.com/dea-fentanyl-related-overdose-deaths-rising-alarming-rate/. Accessed September 15, 2018.
2. Centers for disease control and prevention (CDC). Drug overdose death data 2017. Available at: https://www.cdc.gov/drugoverdose/index.html. Accessed September 15, 2018.
3. Center for behavioral health statistics and quality. Results from the 2016 national survey on drug use and health: detailed tables. Rockville (MD): Substance Abuse and Mental Health Services Administration; 2017. Available at: https://www.samhsa.gov/data/sites/default/files/NSDUH-DetTabs-2016/NSDUH-DetTabs-2016.pdf. Accessed September 15, 2018.
4. Powis B, Griffiths P, Gossop M, et al. The differences between male and female drug users: community samples of heroin and cocaine users compared. Subst Use Misuse 1996;31(5):529–43.
5. Bryant J, Brener L, Hull P, et al. Needle sharing in regular sexual relationships: an examination of serodiscordance, drug using practices, and the gendered character of injecting. Drug Alcohol Depend 2010;107(2–3):182–7.
6. Lum PJ, Sears C, Guydish J. Injection risk behavior among women syringe exchangers in San Francisco. Subst Use Misuse 2005;40(11):1681–96.
7. Dwyer R, Richardson D, Ross MW, et al. A comparison of HIV risk between women and men who inject drugs. AIDS Educ Prev 1994;6(5):379–89.
8. McHugh RK, Devito EE, Dodd D, et al. Gender differences in a clinical trial for prescription opioid dependence. J Subst Abuse Treat 2013;45(1):38–43.
9. Haight SC, Ko JY, Tong VT, et al. Opioid use disorder documented at delivery hospitalization - United States, 1999-2014. MMWR Morb Mortal Wkly Rep 2018;67(31):845–9.
10. Winkelman TNA, Villapiano N, Kozhimannil KB, et al. Incidence and costs of neonatal abstinence syndrome among infants with Medicaid: 2004-2014. Pediatrics 2018;141(4). https://doi.org/10.1542/peds.2017-3520.
11. Patrick SW, Schumacher RE, Benneyworth BD, et al. Neonatal abstinence syndrome and associated health care expenditures: United States, 2000-2009. JAMA 2012;307(18):1934–40.
12. Ko JY, Patrick SW, Tong VT, et al. Incidence of neonatal abstinence syndrome - 28 states, 1999-2013. MMWR Morb Mortal Wkly Rep 2016;65(31):799–802.
13. American College of Obstetricians and Gynecologists, Committee on Health Care for Undeserved Women. ACOG committee opinion no. 343: psychosocial risk factors: perinatal screening and intervention. Obstet Gynecol 2006;108(2):469–77.
14. Terplan M, Minkoff H. Neonatal abstinence syndrome and ethical approaches to the identification of pregnant women who use drugs. Obstet Gynecol 2017;129(1):164–7.
15. Berrettini W. A brief review of the genetics and pharmacogenetics of opioid use disorders. Dialogues Clin Neurosci 2017;19(3):229–36.
16. Martin SL, English KT, Clark KA, et al. Violence and substance use among North Carolina pregnant women. Am J Public Health 1996;86(7):991–8.
17. Okuda M, Olfson M, Hasin D, et al. Mental health of victims of intimate partner violence: results from a national epidemiologic survey. Psychiatr Serv 2011;62(8):959–62.

18. Murphy J, Goodman D, Johnson MC, et al. The comprehensive addiction and recovery act: opioid use disorder and midwifery practice. Obstet Gynecol 2018;131(3):542–4.
19. Center for Substance Abuse Treatment. 1993. Available at: http://adaiclearinghouse.org/downloads/TIP-2-Pregnant-Substance-Using-Women-83.pdf. Accessed March 18, 2019.
20. Jones HE, Terplan M, Meyer M. Medically assisted withdrawal (detoxification): considering the mother-infant dyad. J Addict Med 2017;11(2):90–2.
21. Terplan M, Laird HJ, Hand DJ, et al. Opioid detoxification during pregnancy: a systematic review. Obstet Gynecol 2018;131(5):803–14.
22. ACOG Committee on Health Care for Underserved Women, American Society of Addiction Medicine. ACOG committee opinion no. 524: opioid abuse, dependence, and addiction in pregnancy. Obstet Gynecol 2012;119(5):1070–6.
23. Kampman K, Jarvis M. American Society of Addiction Medicine (ASAM) national practice guideline for the use of medications in the treatment of addiction involving opioid use. J Addict Med 2015;9(5):358–67.
24. United Nations. International standards for the treatment of drug use disorders. Vienna (Austria): United Nations; 2016. Commission on Narcotic Drugs Fifty-Ninth Session.
25. World Health Organization. Guidelines for the identification and management of substance use and substance use disorders in pregnancy. Geneva (Switzerland): World Health Organization; 2014.
26. Substance Abuse and Mental Health Services Administration. Federal guidelines for opioid treatment programs. HS publication no. (SMA)PEP 15-FEDGUI-DEOTP. Rockville (MD): Substance Abuse and Mental Health Services Administration; 2015.
27. Kaltenbach K, Berghella V, Finnegan L. Opioid dependence during pregnancy. Effects and management. Obstet Gynecol Clin North Am 1998;25(1):139–51.
28. Center for substance abuse treatment. Medication-assisted treatment for opioid addiction in opioid treatment programs inservice training. HHS publication no. (SMA) 09-4341. Rockville (MD): Substance Abuse and Mental Health Services Administration; 2008. Available at: https://Store.samhsa.gov/shin/content/SMA09-4341/SMA09-4341.pdf.
29. Jones HE. Specialty treatment for women. In: Strain EC, Stitzer ML, editors. Methadone treatment for opioid dependence. Baltimore (MD): Johns Hopkins University Press; 2006. p. 455–84.
30. Kandall SR, Albin S, Gartner LM, et al. The narcotic-dependent mother: fetal and neonatal consequences. Early Hum Dev 1977;1(2):159–69.
31. Jones HE, Heil SH, Baewert A, et al. Buprenorphine treatment of opioid-dependent pregnant women: a comprehensive review. Addiction 2012;107(Suppl 1):5–27.
32. Jones HE, Kaltenbach K, Heil SH, et al. Neonatal abstinence syndrome after methadone or buprenorphine exposure. N Engl J Med 2010;363(24):2320–31.
33. Zedler BK, Mann AL, Kim MM, et al. Buprenorphine compared with methadone to treat pregnant women with opioid use disorder: a systematic review and meta-analysis of safety in the mother, fetus and child. Addiction 2016;111(12):2115–28.
34. Debelak K, Morrone WR, O'Grady KE, et al. Buprenorphine + naloxone in the treatment of opioid dependence during pregnancy-initial patient care and outcome data. Am J Addict 2013;22(3):252–4.

35. Lund IO, Fischer G, Welle-Strand GK, et al. A comparison of buprenorphine + naloxone to buprenorphine and methadone in the treatment of opioid dependence during pregnancy: maternal and neonatal outcomes. Subst Abuse 2013;7:61–74.
36. Jumah NA, Edwards C, Balfour-Boehm J, et al. Observational study of the safety of buprenorphine+naloxone in pregnancy in a rural and remote population. BMJ Open 2016;6(10):e011774.
37. Martin CE, Longinaker N, Terplan M. Recent trends in treatment admissions for prescription opioid abuse during pregnancy. J Subst Abuse Treat 2015;48(1):37–42.
38. Krans EE, Bogen D, Richardson G, et al. Factors associated with buprenorphine versus methadone use in pregnancy. Subst Abus 2016;37(4):550–7.
39. Meyer M, Wagner K, Benvenuto A, et al. Intrapartum and postpartum analgesia for women maintained on methadone during pregnancy. Obstet Gynecol 2007;110(2 Pt 1):261–6.
40. Weaver M, Schnoll S. Abuse liability in opioid therapy for pain treatment in patients with an addiction history. Clin J Pain 2002;18(4 Suppl):S61–9.
41. Jones HE, O'Grady K, Dahne J, et al. Management of acute postpartum pain in patients maintained on methadone or buprenorphine during pregnancy. Am J Drug Alcohol Abuse 2009;35(3):151–6.
42. Strain EC, Preston KL, Liebson IA, et al. Precipitated withdrawal by pentazocine in methadone-maintained volunteers. J Pharmacol Exp Ther 1993;267(2):624–34.
43. McCarthy JJ, Posey BL. Methadone levels in human milk. J Hum Lact 2000;16(2):115–20.
44. Section on Breastfeeding. Breastfeeding and the use of human milk. Pediatrics 2012;129(3):e827–41.
45. Jansson LM, Velez M, Harrow C. Methadone maintenance and lactation: a review of the literature and current management guidelines. J Hum Lact 2004;20(1):62–71.
46. Abdel-Latif ME, Pinner J, Clews S, et al. Effects of breast milk on the severity and outcome of neonatal abstinence syndrome among infants of drug-dependent mothers. Pediatrics 2006;117(6):e1163–9.
47. Marquet P, Chevrel J, Lavignasse P, et al. Buprenorphine withdrawal syndrome in a newborn. Clin Pharmacol Ther 1997;62(5):569–71.
48. Pichini S, Puig C, Zuccaro P, et al. Assessment of exposure to opiates and cocaine during pregnancy in a Mediterranean city: preliminary results of the "meconium project.". Forensic Sci Int 2005;153(1):59–65.
49. Jones W. Cocaine use and the breastfeeding mother. Pract Midwife 2015;18(1):19–22.
50. American College of Obstetricians and Gynecologists Committee on Obstetric Practice. Committee opinion no. 637: marijuana use during pregnancy and lactation. Obstet Gynecol 2015;126(1):234–8.
51. Wilder C, Lewis D, Winhusen T. Medication assisted treatment discontinuation in pregnant and postpartum women with opioid use disorder. Drug Alcohol Depend 2015;149:225–31.
52. Committee on Obstetric Practice. Committee opinion no. 711: opioid use and opioid use disorder in pregnancy. Obstet Gynecol 2017;130(2):e81–94.
53. Metz TD, Rovner P, Hoffman MC, et al. Maternal deaths from suicide and overdose in Colorado, 2004-2012. Obstet Gynecol 2016;128(6):1233–40.

54. O'Connor AB, Uhler B, O'Brien LM, et al. Predictors of treatment retention in postpartum women prescribed buprenorphine during pregnancy. J Subst Abuse Treat 2018;86:26–9.

55. Schiff DM, Patrick SW, Terplan M. Maternal health in the United States. N Engl J Med 2018;378(6):587.

56. Anand KJ, Willson DF, Berger J, et al. Tolerance and withdrawal from prolonged opioid use in critically ill children. Pediatrics 2010;125(5):e1208–25.

57. FDA. Neonatal Opioid withdrawal syndrome and medication-assisted treatment with methadone and buprenorphine 2016. Available at: https://www.fda.gov/Drugs/DrugSafety/ucm503630.htm. Accessed August 8, 2017.

58. Law KL, Stroud LR, LaGasse LL, et al. Smoking during pregnancy and newborn neurobehavior. Pediatrics 2003;111(6 Pt 1):1318–23.

59. Food and Drug Administration. FDA drug safety communication: antipsychotic drug labels updated on use during pregnancy and risk of abnormal muscle movements and withdrawal symptoms in newborns. Silver Spring, MD: U.S. Food and Drug Administration Location; 2011.

60. Koren G, Matsui D, Einarson A, et al. Is maternal use of selective serotonin re-uptake inhibitors in the third trimester of pregnancy harmful to neonates? CMAJ 2005;172(11):1457–9.

61. Huybrechts KF, Bateman BT, Desai RJ, et al. Risk of neonatal drug withdrawal after intrauterine co-exposure to opioids and psychotropic medications: cohort study. BMJ 2017;358:j3326.

62. Jones HE, Heil SH, Tuten M, et al. Cigarette smoking in opioid-dependent pregnant women: neonatal and maternal outcomes. Drug Alcohol Depend 2013; 131(3):271–7.

63. Desai RJ, Huybrechts KF, Hernandez-Diaz S, et al. Exposure to prescription opioid analgesics in utero and risk of neonatal abstinence syndrome: population based cohort study. BMJ 2015;350:h2102.

64. Cleary BJ, Donnelly J, Strawbridge J, et al. Methadone dose and neonatal abstinence syndrome-systematic review and meta-analysis. Addiction 2010;105(12): 2071–84.

65. Zahorodny W, Rom C, Whitney W, et al. The neonatal withdrawal inventory: a simplified score of newborn withdrawal. J Dev Behav Pediatr 1998;19(2):89–93.

66. Lipsitz PJ. A proposed narcotic withdrawal score for use with newborn infants. A pragmatic evaluation of its efficacy. Clin Pediatr (phila) 1975;14(6):592–4.

67. Ostrea E. Infants of drug-dependent mothers. In: Burg F, Ingelfinger J, Wald R, editors. Current pediatric therapy. 14th edition. Philadelphia: WB Saunders; 1993. p. 800–1.

68. Green M, Suffet F. The neonatal narcotic withdrawal index: a device for the improvement of care in the abstinence syndrome. Am J Drug Alcohol Abuse 1981;8(2):203–13.

69. Finnegan LP, Connaughton JF Jr, Kron RE, et al. Neonatal abstinence syndrome: assessment and management. Addict Dis 1975;2(1–2):141–58.

70. Zimmermann-Baer U, Notzli U, Rentsch K, et al. Finnegan neonatal abstinence scoring system: normal values for first 3 days and weeks 5-6 in non-addicted infants. Addiction 2010;105(3):524–8.

71. Jones HE, Harrow C, O'Grady KE, et al. Neonatal abstinence scores in opioid-exposed and nonexposed neonates: a blinded comparison. J Opioid Manag 2010;6(6):409–13.

72. Jones HE, Seashore C, Johnson E, et al. Measurement of neonatal abstinence syndrome: evaluation of short forms. J Opioid Manag 2016;12(1):19–23.

73. Isemann BT, Stoeckle EC, Taleghani AA, et al. Early prediction tool to identify the need for pharmacotherapy in infants at risk of neonatal abstinence syndrome. Pharmacotherapy 2017;37(7):840–8.
74. Maguire D, Cline GJ, Parnell L, et al. Validation of the Finnegan neonatal abstinence syndrome tool-short form. Adv Neonatal Care 2013;13(6):430–7.
75. Gomez Pomar E, Finnegan LP, Devlin L, et al. Simplification of the Finnegan neonatal abstinence scoring system: retrospective study of two institutions in the USA. BMJ Open 2017;7(9):e016176.
76. Wachman EM, Grossman M, Schiff DM, et al. Quality improvement initiative to improve inpatient outcomes for neonatal abstinence syndrome. J Perinatol 2018;38(8):1114–22.
77. Grossman MR, Berkwitt AK, Osborn RR, et al. An initiative to improve the quality of care of infants with neonatal abstinence syndrome. Pediatrics 2017;139(6). https://doi.org/10.1542/peds.2016-3360.
78. Holmes AV, Atwood EC, Whalen B, et al. Rooming-in to treat neonatal abstinence syndrome: improved family-centered care at lower cost. Pediatrics 2016;137(6). https://doi.org/10.1542/peds.2015-2929.
79. Ryan G, Dooley J, Gerber Finn L, et al. Nonpharmacological management of neonatal abstinence syndrome: a review of the literature. J Matern Fetal Neonatal Med 2019;32(10):1735–40.
80. Tsai LC, Doan TJ. Breastfeeding among mothers on opioid maintenance treatment: a literature review. J Hum Lact 2016;32(3):521–9.
81. Short VL, Gannon M, Abatemarco DJ. The association between breastfeeding and length of hospital stay among infants diagnosed with neonatal abstinence syndrome: a population-based study of in-hospital births. Breastfeed Med 2016;11:343–9.
82. Newman A, Davies GA, Dow K, et al. Rooming-in care for infants of opioid-dependent mothers: implementation and evaluation at a tertiary care hospital. Can Fam Physician 2015;61(12):e555–61.
83. Abrahams RR, Kelly SA, Payne S, et al. Rooming-in compared with standard care for newborns of mothers using methadone or heroin. Can Fam Physician 2007;53(10):1722–30.
84. McKnight S, Coo H, Davies G, et al. Rooming-in for infants at risk of neonatal abstinence syndrome. Am J Perinatol 2016;33(5):495–501.
85. Gowing L, Ali R, White JM, et al. Buprenorphine for managing opioid withdrawal. Cochrane Database Syst Rev 2017;(2):CD002025.
86. Gowing L, Farrell M, Ali R, et al. Alpha(2)-adrenergic agonists for the management of opioid withdrawal. Cochrane Database Syst Rev 2016;(5):CD002024.
87. Burnette T, Chernicky L, Towers CV. The effect of standardizing treatment when managing neonatal abstinence syndrome. J Matern Fetal Neonatal Med 2018;1–5. https://doi.org/10.1080/14767058.2018.1465038.
88. Hall ES, Wexelblatt SL, Crowley M, et al. A multicenter cohort study of treatments and hospital outcomes in neonatal abstinence syndrome. Pediatrics 2014;134(2):e527–34.
89. Hall ES, Wexelblatt SL, Crowley M, et al. Implementation of a neonatal abstinence syndrome weaning protocol: a multicenter cohort study. Pediatrics 2015;136(4):e803–10.
90. Asti L, Magers JS, Keels E, et al. A quality improvement project to reduce length of stay for neonatal abstinence syndrome. Pediatrics 2015;135(6):e1494–500.

91. Patrick SW, Schumacher RE, Horbar JD, et al. Improving care for neonatal abstinence syndrome. Pediatrics 2016;137(5). https://doi.org/10.1542/peds.2015-3835.
92. Davis JM, Shenberger J, Terrin N, et al. Comparison of safety and efficacy of methadone vs morphine for treatment of neonatal abstinence syndrome: a randomized clinical trial. JAMA Pediatr 2018;172(8):741–8.
93. Tolia VN, Murthy K, Bennett MM, et al. Morphine vs methadone treatment for infants with neonatal abstinence syndrome. J Pediatr 2018;203:185–9.
94. Kraft WK, Adeniyi-Jones SC, Chervoneva I, et al. Buprenorphine for the treatment of the neonatal abstinence syndrome. N Engl J Med 2017;376(24):2341–8.
95. Hall ES, Isemann BT, Wexelblatt SL, et al. A cohort comparison of buprenorphine versus methadone treatment for neonatal abstinence syndrome. J Pediatr 2016;170:39–44.e1.
96. Hall ES, Rice WR, Folger AT, et al. Comparison of neonatal abstinence syndrome treatment with sublingual buprenorphine versus conventional opioids. Am J Perinatol 2018;35(4):405–12.
97. Kraft WK, Adeniyi-Jones SC, Ehrlich ME. Buprenorphine for the neonatal abstinence syndrome. N Engl J Med 2017;377(10):997–8.
98. Liu T, Lewis T, Gauda E, et al. Mechanistic population pharmacokinetics of morphine in neonates with abstinence syndrome after oral administration of diluted tincture of opium. J Clin Pharmacol 2016;56(8):1009–18.
99. Moore JN, Healy JR, Thoma BN, et al. A population pharmacokinetic model for vancomycin in adult patients receiving extracorporeal membrane oxygenation therapy. CPT Pharmacometrics Syst Pharmacol 2016;5(9):495–502. Available at: http://www.ncbi.nlm.nih.gov/pmc/articles/PMC5036424/.
100. Wiles JR, Isemann B, Mizuno T, et al. Pharmacokinetics of oral methadone in the treatment of neonatal abstinence syndrome: a pilot study. J Pediatr 2015;167(6):1214–20.e3.
101. Xie HG, Cao YJ, Gauda EB, et al. Clonidine clearance matures rapidly during the early postnatal period: a population pharmacokinetic analysis in newborns with neonatal abstinence syndrome. J Clin Pharmacol 2011;51(4):502–11.
102. Hall ES, Meinzen-Derr J, Wexelblatt SL. Cohort analysis of a pharmacokinetic-modeled methadone weaning optimization for neonatal abstinence syndrome. J Pediatr 2015;167(6):1221–5.e1.
103. Murphy-Oikonen J, McQueen K. Outpatient pharmacologic weaning for neonatal abstinence syndrome: a systematic review. Prim Health Care Res Dev 2018;1–9. https://doi.org/10.1017/S1463423618000270.
104. Maalouf FI, Cooper WO, Slaughter JC, et al. Outpatient pharmacotherapy for neonatal abstinence syndrome. J Pediatr 2018;199:151–7.e1.
105. Pandey R, Pandey Sapkota N, Kumar D. Neonatal abstinence syndrome: twins case series. Front Pediatr 2017;5:242.
106. Crist RC, Reiner BC, Berrettini WH. A review of opioid addiction genetics. Curr Opin Psychol 2018;27:31–5.
107. Wachman EM, Hayes MJ, Brown MS, et al. Association of OPRM1 and COMT single-nucleotide polymorphisms with hospital length of stay and treatment of neonatal abstinence syndrome. JAMA 2013;309(17):1821–7.
108. Wachman EM, Hayes MJ, Sherva R, et al. Variations in opioid receptor genes in neonatal abstinence syndrome. Drug Alcohol Depend 2015;155:253–9.
109. Fielder A, Coller J, Hutchinson M, et al. Neonatal abstinence syndrome in methadone exposed infants: role of genetic variability. Drug Alcohol Depend 2015;146:e202–84.

110. Wachman EM, Hayes MJ, Shrestha H, et al. Epigenetic variation in OPRM1 gene in opioid-exposed mother-infant dyads. Genes Brain Behav 2018;17(7):e12476.
111. Wachman EM, Hayes MJ, Lester BM, et al. Epigenetic variation in the mu-opioid receptor gene in infants with neonatal abstinence syndrome. J Pediatr 2014; 165(3):472–8.
112. Lainwala S, Brown ER, Weinschenk NP, et al. A retrospective study of length of hospital stay in infants treated for neonatal abstinence syndrome with methadone versus oral morphine preparations. Adv Neonatal Care 2005;5(5):265–72.
113. Young ME, Hager SJ, Spurlock D Jr. Retrospective chart review comparing morphine and methadone in neonates treated for neonatal abstinence syndrome. Am J Health Syst Pharm 2015;72(23 Suppl 3):S162–7.
114. Brown MS, Hayes MJ, Thornton LM. Methadone versus morphine for treatment of neonatal abstinence syndrome: a prospective randomized clinical trial. J Perinatol 2015;35(4):278–83.

Safety of Psychotropic Medications During Pregnancy

Edwin R. Raffi, MD, MPH*, Ruta Nonacs, MD, PhD, Lee S. Cohen, MD

KEYWORDS

- Perinatal reproductive psychiatry • Women's mental health • Pregnancy
- Psychopharmacology • Perinatal addiction

KEY POINTS

- Common psychiatric disorders during pregnancy and risks of no treatment in patients with moderate and severe disorder, including substance use disorders are reviewed.
- Selecting the best medications during pregnancy and the reproductive safety of psychotropic medications is discussed.
- Management of substance use disorders in pregnancy using medication-assisted treatments is explored.

INTRODUCTION

The objective of this article is to discuss the safety and efficacy of psychotropic medications during pregnancy. The common disorders and the risks of not receiving treatment of certain psychiatric conditions, including substance use disorders (SUDs), also are discussed.

Pregnancy is a time of stress. Stressing the nervous system—whether positive stress (eg, weddings and graduations) or negative stress, also referred to as distress (eg, loss of a loved one)—can precipitate psychiatric symptoms, especially in a mental

This article originally appeared in *Clinics in Perinatology*, Volume 46, Issue 2, June 2019.
Disclosure Statement: Dr E.R. Raffi has no disclosure for any relationship with a commercial company that has a direct financial interest in subject matter or materials discussed in article or with a company making a competing product. Dr R. Nonacs: Simon & Schuster. Dr L.S. Cohen: Research support for the National Pregnancy Registry for Atypical Antipsychotics (tAlkermes Biopharmaceuticals; Forest/Actavis Pharmaceuticals; Otsuka Pharmaceuticals; Sunovion Pharmaceuticals, Inc.; and Teva Pharmaceutical Industries). Other research support: Brain & Behavior Research Foundation; JayMac Pharmaceuticals; National Institute on Aging; National Institutes of Health; and SAGE Therapeutics. Advisory/Consulting: Alkermes Biopharmaceuticals (through MGH Clinical Trials Network Initiative).
Perinatal and Reproductive Psychiatry Program, Massachusetts General Hospital Center for Women's Mental Health, Harvard Medical School, Simches Research Building, 185 Cambridge Street, Suite 2200, Boston, MA 02114, USA
* Corresponding author.
E-mail address: eraffi@mgh.harvard.edu

Clinics Collections 9 (2020) 99–118
https://doi.org/10.1016/j.ccol.2020.07.028

health–vulnerable individual. Data show that pregnancy does not protect against relapse of symptoms in disorders, such as depression.[1]

Treatment recommendations for patients often are individualized. When developing a management plan, the provider should consider the patient's detailed psychiatric history: diagnostic work-up, previous treatment regimens that have failed, treatment modalities that have resulted in achieving euthymia (including past and current medication responses), current presentation, history of mental health during previous pregnancies, family history, social history, substance use history, and the timeline during which the course of treatment is proposed (whether or not the patient currently is pregnant or planning a pregnancy and so forth).

We will first start by reviewing common psychiatric disorders during pregnancy and risk of no treatment followed by a discussion of psychotropic medications in 6 drug categories as follows:

1. Considering psychopharmacology during pregnancy: common psychiatric disorders and risk of no treatment
2. Antidepressant medications, including selective serotonin reuptake inhibitors (SSRIs), serotonin-norepinephrine uptake inhibitors (SNRIs), bupropion, and other antidepressants
3. Mood-stabilizing medications, including lithium, lamotrigine, valproic acid, other antiepileptic mood stabilizers, and antipsychotics as mood stabilizers
4. Antipsychotic medications, both typical antipsychotics and atypical antipsychotics
5. Anxiolytic/sedative hypnotic medications, including benzodiazepines, gabapentin, and other anxiolytics
6. Stimulants in pregnancy
7. Medication-assisted treatment (MAT) of SUDs, including opioid use disorders (OUDs), alcohol use disorder, smoking cessation, and cocaine/stimulant use disorder

If patient and provider decide to use pharmacologic treatment during pregnancy, efforts should be made to

- Select medications that have a well-studied reproductive safety profile. Ideally, all women of reproductive age should be continued on medication regimens that are safe in case of an unplanned pregnancy.
- Make modifications to medication regimens prior to pregnancy when possible, to confirm a stable and euthymic state on the new regimen prior to conception
- Limit the number of medication exposures to the fetus during pregnancy by maximizing 1 medication at effective doses instead of using multiple medications at lower doses.

In December 2014, the Food and Drug Administration (FDA) published the Content and Format of Labeling for Human Prescription Drug and Biological Products; Requirements for Pregnancy and Lactation Labeling, referred to as the Pregnancy and Lactation Labeling Rule.[2] This new system removes the previous letter categories— A, B, C, D, and X—as a means of determining medication safety for treatment of pregnant and lactating mothers. It requires a change to the content of the prescription drug labeling, which would now have to include up-to-date data to allow providers and mothers to make educated decisions.[2] As such, the following information aims to help providers guide patients in their decision-making process within the new and improved FDA guidelines.

Considering Psychopharmacology During Pregnancy: Common Psychiatric Disorders and Risk of No Treatment

When making considerations for treatment, variables to consider are severity of underlying disorder (during current episode and in the past), history of response to treatment, and patient preference and attitude toward treatment. The effect of maternal psychiatric illness (eg, depression) on fetal and neonatal well-being must be taken into account in the risk-benefit decision-making process with respect to use or choice to defer use of medication (ie, no treatment).[3–7]

Discontinuation of medication can be considered for people with a history of mild psychiatric illness. This change ideally should be done in conjunction with continuation or addition of nonpharmacologic treatments modalities.[8] In treatment of depression, for example, such modalities can include supportive therapy, cognitive-behavior therapy, or interpersonal therapy.[9–12]

Many women with history of depression who discontinue antidepressant medications during pregnancy may experience recurrent symptoms.[13] In a prospective study of 201 women, Cohen and colleagues[1] showed that patients who discontinued their antidepressants were 5 times more likely to relapse (rate of relapse of 68%) compared with women who maintained their antidepressants across pregnancy. This study also showed that 26% of women who continue antidepressants had a relapse of major depressive disorder during pregnancy.

Bipolar illness in pregnant patients carries a high risk of poor prenatal outcomes,[14,15] including but not limited to risk of self-harm, substance use, and poor compliance with prenatal care. Relapse rates in women with bipolar disorder are high in women who discontinue mood stabilizers proximate to conception (71% according to 1 study[15]).

Emergence of psychosis during pregnancy is an obstetric and psychiatric emergency. Psychosis could pose a risk to the mother and her infant. It can also hinder a patient's capability to participate in prenatal care or cooperate with care during delivery.[16,17]

More than 10% of women experience clinically significant symptoms of anxiety during pregnancy,[18] particularly during the first trimester. Pathologic anxiety has been correlated with a variety of poor obstetric outcomes, including increased rates of premature labor, low Apgar scores, and placental abruption.[19]

Many women with polysubstance use disorder are likely to attempt to abstain from using during pregnancy.[20] Continued use or relapse of SUD during pregnancy, however, can have devastating results.

Illicit opioid use is most prominent in the under-25 age group, which includes women of reproductive age. Withdrawal from opioids is known to cause premature labor, miscarriages, and fetal distress. There also is an increased risk for relapse, overdose, and death by patients who go through withdrawals.[21] In addition to OUD, alcohol use disorder (leading to fetal alcohol syndrome), cocaine/stimulant use disorder, nicotine use disorder, and other substances pose a danger to the health of young women of reproductive age and their fetuses during pregnancy.

Early screening, diagnosis, and intervention prior to and/or during pregnancy often reduce morbidity and mortality of mental health disorders for mothers and infants.

Pharmacologic treatment is usually recommended when nonpharmacologic strategies have not been efficacious and/or the risks of being psychiatrically ill during pregnancy might outweigh the benefits of nontreatment or the risks of fetal exposure to the medication.

Clinicians should attempt to make modifications to medication regimens prior to pregnancy to confirm a stable and euthymic state on the new regimen prior to conception. The goal also should be to limit the number of medications exposures to infant during pregnancy. Maximizing 1 medication at affective doses is preferred to using more medications at lower doses.

Regardless of whether or not medication is used, vulnerable patients should be monitored closely because they are at a high risk for relapse during pregnancy and in the postpartum period.

ANTIDEPRESSANT MEDICATIONS
Risks Associated with Fetal Exposure to Antidepressant Medications

Most studies related to fetal risks associated with antidepressant use during pregnancy have been on SSRIs and tricyclic antidepressants (TCAs.) These studies have provided reassurance that SSRI medications, as a group, are not considered teratogenic[5,22,23]; however, research on the complete safety profile of these medications remains ongoing.

Although the relative safety of this class of medication with respect to fetal exposure has been reported,[24–26] other reports have described adverse perinatal outcomes, such as decreased gestational age, poor neonatal adaptation, and low birthweight. These studies are controversial, however, because other investigators have not observed the same associations.[27–29] Side effects, such as neurocognitive sequelae, are controversial at best, and further investigations are needed to determine if these are a direct result of antidepressants or of other confounders, such as parental ailment.[30–32]

A majority of reports studying the potential adverse outcomes of peripartum exposure to SSRI medications have been limited by nonsystematic assessment of infant outcomes, nonblinded raters, and small sample sizes. Most of such studies fail to assess the impact of other confounders, especially maternal depression or other psychiatric comorbidities, which by themselves can be associated with compromised perinatal outcomes.[33]

Neonatal adaptation is of some concern with antidepressant medications.[34] Symptoms include jitteriness, tachypnea, tremulousness, which usually are mild, are transient, and resolve without much medical intervention within the first few days of birth. It is important for pediatricians to be aware of infants' exposure and monitor them for supportive therapy.

Some studies have associated SSRI use in late pregnancy with persistent pulmonary hypertension of the newborn (PPHN), a serious and rare developmental lung condition. Chambers and colleagues[35] reported the risk of PPHN with exposure to SSRIs after 20 weeks at approximately 1%. Multiple large studies, however, have shown there is much lower risk of PPHN or no association at all between SSRI use and PPHN.[36,37] A large Medicaid database studied 3.8 million pregnancy outcomes and demonstrated that the risk of PPHN was 0.3% for women who were treated with SSRIs versus 0.2% among the nonexposed.[37] PPHN is correlated with multiple other risk factors that are not associated with SSRI use, such as cesarean delivery, race, and body mass index.[38]

There are fewer reports and sparse research conducted on the long-term sequelae of prenatal antidepressant exposure. In children (followed through early childhood), exposure to fluoxetine, venlafaxine, TCAs, or no medication has shown no differences in behavioral or cognitive development. These measures include IQ, language, temperament, behavior, reactivity, mood, distractibility, and activity level.[39,40] At least 1 study has shown no difference between children exposed to fluoxetine or TCAs during pregnancy and those not exposed in relation to the neurocognitive measures discussed preivously.[28,39]

Although some studies have reported that autism spectrum disorders, anxiety, and attention-deficit disorder (ADD) are more common in antidepressant-exposed children,[41] these studies do not account for many confounders, perhaps the most important of which is maternal psychiatric illness as a major contributing confounder.[42,43] The intuitive notion that the higher prevalence of these disorders is likely due to genetics or maternal illness is supported by studies that have controlled for variables, such as maternal psychiatric diagnosis and exposure to other medications.[44-47]

The data suggest that the risk of postpartum hemorrhage seems slightly increased in women taking serotonin reuptake inhibitors near the time of delivery.[48-50] Given the inconsistencies across findings on this topic and the small increase in risk observed in studies on this issue, there is no compelling evidence to change prescribing practices during pregnancy. Obstetricians, however, should be alert to the possibility of an increased risk of postpartum hemorrhage in this population, so that hemorrhage, should it occur, may be managed aggressively, with the goal of minimizing maternal morbidity.

Selective Serotonin Reuptake Inhibitor Medications: Sertraline, Fluoxetine, Citalopram, Escitalopram, Paroxetine, and Fluvoxamine

A large Medicaid data study (n = 949,504) by Huybrechts and colleagues[51] and another by Furu and colleagues[52] have concluded that SSRI (fluoxetine, citalopram, paroxetine, sertraline, fluvoxamine, or escitalopram) exposure was not associated with an increased risk of any specific congenital malformations. This has also been shown in various other meta-analyses, which has been reassuring.[16]

Paroxetine is the 1 antidepressant, however, with previously concerning yet still controversial risks for fetal malformations. Reports have suggested that first-trimester exposure to paroxetine is correlated with an increased risk of cardiac malformations, such as atrial and ventricular septal defects.[53,54] Again, other peer-reviewed studies, including 2 independent, comprehensive meta-analysis studies, have not demonstrated the same increased risks of teratogenicity with first-trimester exposure to paroxetine.[55-58] Thus, although some still avoid paroxetine as first-line medication for an antidepressant-naive woman of reproductive age, this medication should surely be considered as a treatment option during pregnancy, given the previously noted reassuring data.

It has generally been assumed that the reproductive safety of escitalopram would be similar to that of the parent drug citalopram, because "S"-citalopram is 1 component of this racemic mixture. An observational multicenter prospective cohort study showed escitalopram does not seem associated with an increased risk for major malformations.[59] As seen in other studies of antidepressants, escitalopram was associated with higher rates of low birthweight (<2500 g). As is often seen in such studies, without a comparison group of women diagnosed with depression who are not taking an antidepressant, it is difficult to determine whether this adverse effect is due to the depression itself or exposure to the drug. This is particularly relevant given the multiple studies that have associated low birthweight with untreated depression and anxiety.

Fluvoxamine, a newer SSRI antidepressant, is FDA approved specifically for treatment of obsessive-compulsive disorder (OCD). Some patients who might not have responded to first-line antidepressant for the obsessive qualities of their anxiety may respond to this medication. Two large studies have shown no major congenital malformations in infants exposed to fluvoxamine compared with the unexposed infants.[52,60] The current data on fluvoxamine, however, is not as expansive of that of other antidepressants, simply due to the fact that it is not as widely prescribed.

Serotonin-Norepinephrine Uptake Inhibitor Medications: Duloxetine and Venlafaxine

Although there are fewer data on SNRI medications than on SSRI medications, so far these medications seem comparable in safety profile. A 2015 article, pooling data from 8 large cohort studies (3186 exposed to venlafaxine and 668 exposed to duloxetine), provides reassuring information regarding the reproductive safety of both venlafaxine and duloxetine after first-trimester exposure, concluding no association between exposure and increased risk of major congenital malformations.[61]

Currently, there are more data about the general safety of venlafaxine[52,62] compared with duloxetine. There is mounting evidence, however, for general safety of the latter during pregnancy. Despite some studies discussing possible association between duloxetine and increased risk of spontaneous abortion and poor neonatal adaptation syndrome,[63,64] causation is difficult and complicated to determine because it seems that having depression itself may have an impact on the risk of miscarriage.[65] Two prospective observational studies of safety of duloxetine can be combined to show that in 439 pregnancies, there were a total of 9 malformations (approximately 2.1%), which is comparable to the rate seen in the general population.

Gestational hypertension has been found significantly associated with the use of SNRI medications; thus, women on these medications should be monitored for hypertension. In a study of 686 women, gestational hypertension was significantly associated with the use of psychostimulants (odds ratio [OR] 6.11; 95% CI, 1.79–20.9) and SNRIs (OR 2.57; 95% CI, 1.34–4.93) after 20 weeks of gestation. Use of serotonin reuptake inhibitors was not associated with increased risk for hypertension. In women taking the SNRI venlafaxine or amphetamine stimulants, risk for gestational hypertension was seen more commonly at higher medication doses.[66]

Bupropion

There are data supporting the use of bupropion during pregnancy.[67–69] The Bupropion Pregnancy Registry concludes no major congenital malformation in association with this exposure in early pregnancy (n = 806).[67]

Although this information regarding the overall risk of malformation is reassuring, earlier reports had concerns of cardiac malformations in bupropion-exposed infants. To more carefully quantify this, a large insurance claims–based study was conducted. This retrospective cohort study, including more than 1200 infants exposed to bupropion during the first trimester, did not demonstrate an increased risk for cardiovascular malformations.[69]

Bupropion can be especially useful for patients with comorbid nicotine use disorder who are motivated to quit smoking and/or those with ADD (discussed later). Further studies are required to assess the risk of neonatal symptoms in bupropion-exposed infants and to better evaluate the long-term neurobehavioral effects of bupropion exposure.

Other Antidepressant Medications: Tricyclic Antidepressants, Mirtazapine, and Trazodone

TCAs, as a class, are not contraindicated for use during pregnancy. This class of medication, however, is not considered first line for treatment of mood and anxiety disorders due to generally increased and unwanted side effects (sedation, anticholinergic side effects, and so forth).[5,70,71] Desipramine and nortriptyline are preferred TCAs due to their less anticholinergic profile and less likely to exacerbate orthostatic hypotension during pregnancy.[72,73]

Data on the safety profile of mirtazapine for infants exposed in utero are considered limited (although reassuring)[6,74,75] and thus this medication should not be used as first-line treatment of mood or anxiety. Unlike typical SSRI medications, mirtazapine seems to have antiemetic properties[74] and has been used in case reports for treatment of hyperemesis gravidarum.[76] Given that hyperemesis gravidarum often is associated with significant anxiety, this medication may be a promising intervention for women with these comorbidities in the future.

The same is true for trazodone (often used as a sleep aid). Despite minimal reassuring data,[77] this medication should not use as first line for treatment of insomnia during pregnancy.

MOOD-STABILIZING MEDICATIONS

The 2 mood stabilizers most commonly considered during pregnancy are lithium and lamotrigine. Antipsychotic medications also play a major role in treatment of patients with manic-depressive disorder.

Lithium

The risk of prenatal exposure to lithium is notoriously coupled with fears of cardiovascular malformations (eg, Ebstein anomaly).[78] Previous reports have indicated that, although a signal for an increased risk of this cardiovascular malformation might be present, this risk is rare. In comparison to the general population, in which Ebstein anomaly occurs in 1/20,000 live births, lithium exposure in the first trimester was estimated to change this risk to at most 1/1000.[79] Despite approximately 50 years of data on this medication, new studies on the reproductive safety of this medication still continue.

A large retrospective cohort study of 1,325,563 pregnant women studied in utero exposure to lithium and risks of cardiovascular malformations.[80] This study, which included 663 women who used lithium during the first trimester of pregnancy, is the largest study of prenatal lithium exposure to date. Two comparison groups were women with no lithium exposure and women with bipolar disorder who used lamotrigine as a mood stabilizer. The findings of this study indicate a modest increase in the risk of cardiac malformations in infants with prenatal exposure to lithium. Compared with women with no known exposures, the relative risk of cardiac malformations calculated here was 1.65. Translating this into absolute risk, this means that if the risk of cardiovascular malformations is 1.15% in women with no exposure, the risk rises to approximately 1.90% in infants exposed to lithium. In this study, the risk of right ventricular outflow tract obstruction defects was 0.60 per 100 live births among infants exposed to lithium and 0.18 per 100 among unexposed infants.[80] The researchers also observed the increase in relative risk to be dose related. Such analysis, however, should be considered premature, considering lack of causation and possibility of other confounders.

Although the absolute risk discussed is not dramatic, this study confirms that lithium carries some teratogenic risk. Although the authors try to avoid prescribing teratogens during pregnancy, with lithium, at times, the benefits outweigh the risks.

Prenatal screening with fetal echocardiography and high-resolution ultrasound is recommended in patients who take lithium during pregnancy (approximately 16–18 weeks of gestation).[16]

Lamotrigine

Lamotrigine is another mood stabilizer used for treatment of bipolar disorder in pregnancy. This medication might not be as effective, however, as lithium in protecting against manic symptoms and is usually used for patients with a history of bipolar traits or hypomania (ie, bipolar II disorder).

Earlier reports warned of possible increased risk of increased risk of cleft palate or cleft lip deformity in infants exposed to lamotrigine during the first trimester.[81] Multiple large studies have indicated that this risk is either nonexistent or very low.[82–84] In 1 study, researchers analyzed a total of 21 studies describing pregnancy outcomes and rates of congenital malformations. Compared with disease-matched controls (n = 1412) and healthy controls (n = 774,571), in utero exposure to lamotrigine monotherapy was not associated with an increased risk of major malformations. Rates of miscarriages, stillbirths, preterm deliveries, and small-for-gestational age neonates were similar in lamotrigine-exposed pregnancies compared with the general population.[85]

In short, lamotrigine is believed to be a relatively safe mood stabilizer for use during pregnancy.

Valproic Acid

Prenatal exposure to valproic acid is strongly associated with neural tube defects, such as spina bifida, and many other anomalies, including midface hypoplasia, congenital heart disease, cleft lip and/or cleft palate, growth retardation, and microcephaly, have been observed.[16,86]

In utero valproic acid has also exposure been associated other developmental neurocognitive deficiencies, including lower IQ and impaired cognition across several domains,[87] and increased risks of autism and ADDs later in childhood.[88,89]

As a general rule, women of reproductive age should not be prescribed valproic acid. If this agent is prescribed, patients should be fully educated on the risks profile of this medication, and robust contraceptive measures should be put in place. This medication ideally should be discontinued at least 6 months prior to planning for conception of any new pregnancy. This would allow for ample time to taper off the valproate, start a new medication, and ensure euthymia and mood stabilization on the new regimen.

Other Antiepileptic Mood-Stabilizing Medications

Information about the reproductive safety of other anticonvulsants, such as oxcarbazepine and topiramate is limited. These medications generally are not first line for the treatment of bipolar disorder, and therefore, ideally should be avoided during pregnancy. The same is true for carbamazepine, especially because prenatal exposure to this substance also has been associated with neural tube defects.[90] Teratogenicity is believed to increase with high maternal serum levels of anticonvulsant and exposure to more than 1 anticonvulsant.[16]

For patients exposed to anticonvulsants during pregnancy, neural tube defects should be evaluated with ultrasonography and maternal serum α-fetoprotein. Increase of folic acid supplementation (4 mg a day) prior to conception and during the first trimester is often recommended,[16] although the general efficacy of this intervention is not clear.

Antipsychotic Medications as Mood Stabilizers

Atypical antipsychotic drugs are commonly used in treatment of bipolar affective disorder (discussed later). Judicial use of adjunctive antipsychotic medication, or at times monotherapy, is common in patients with bipolar disorder. As-needed dosing of these medications (such as olanzapine or quetiapine) can be helpful in managing issues related to insomnia, anxiety, agitation, or irritability related to bipolar disorder.

ANTIPSYCHOTIC MEDICATIONS
Typical (First-Generation) Antipsychotics

Due to the long history of use of typical antipsychotics, there are considerable data available on the reproductive safety of these medications. There is no definitive association between typical antipsychotic exposure during pregnancy and risk of congenital malformations.[91,92] When using a typical antipsychotic, a high-potency neuroleptic (eg, haloperidol) should be used. Although lower-potency typical antipsychotics are not contraindicated, some historical data do exist for their increased risk of congenital malformations associated with prenatal exposure.[93]

Haloperidol, which has much historical data, is a good medication for use in medical settings, such as in florid psychosis during labor and delivery. This is especially true because this medication can be used intravenously, intramuscularly, and orally. The wide range of dosing of this drug also can facilitate improvement of symptoms and cooperation with care, improving safety of patient, safety of care providers, and delivery outcomes.[94]

Atypical (Second-Generation) Antipsychotics

The atypical (second-generation) antipsychotics medications currently serve multiple purposes in the treatment of mental health conditions. They also are used more frequently because they are associated with fewer side effects. In addition to treating psychotic disorders, such as schizophrenia, many are approved for treatment of bipolar disorder, and anxiety disorders. For this reason, this class of medication is perhaps the most multifunctional class of medication at the disposal of care providers.

The versatile use of these medications is important in pregnancy, because prescribers should try to minimize a fetus's exposure to multiple medications. Thus, a medication that could serve multiple purposes is of great value (eg, Seroquel for treatment of anxiety, insomnia, and psychosis.)

Although there are fewer data available on the reproductive safety of this class of medication, multiple large studies have shown that, as a class, they do not seem to have an association with any congenital malformations.[91,95–98]

One study concludes that prenatal exposure to quetiapine, aripiprazole, olanzapine, and ziprasidone does not increase the risk for congenital malformation or cardiac malformations. The possible exception noted is risperidone.[92] The data regarding the safety profile of risperidone are not easy to interpret. Another similar study on risperidone notes that data "should be interpreted with caution because no apparent biological mechanism can readily explain this outcome, and the possibility of a chance finding cannot be ruled out."[99] That said, even if we assume an increased risk is associated with the use of risperidone exists, the risk appears to be small.

Newer antipsychotics, such as lurasidone, iloperidone, and brexpiprazole, are under-represented in most large-scale studies, and more studies need to be done on their perinatal safety profile.

Pregnant patients on second-generation antipsychotics should be closely monitored and screened for gestational diabetes mellitus. Polypharmacy should be avoided to the extent possible to minimize the exposure to the fetus.

ANXIOLYTIC/SEDATIVE HYPNOTIC MEDICATIONS
Benzodiazepines

According to 1 study, 3.9% of American women with private insurance use a benzodiazepine during pregnancy.[100] First-trimester exposure to benzodiazepines has been reported to increase the risk for oral cleft formation for infants (estimated increase of 0.6%).[101] Other studies (including studies with pooled data analysis),[102–104] however, have not supported this association. Although some patients might avoid first-trimester exposure to benzodiazepines, this class of medication can be useful during the second and third trimesters, especially on an as-needed basis.

A 2018 prospective study compared 144 pregnancies exposed to benzodiazepines to a group of 650 unexposed. Infants exposed to benzodiazepines in utero were more likely to be admitted to a neonatal ICU (OR 2.02; 95% CI, 1.11–3.66) and to have a small head circumference (OR 3.89; 95% CI, 1.25–12.03) compared with unexposed infants. Other adverse effects, such as low birthweight, preterm birth, respiratory distress, and muscular symptoms, including hypotonia, were not observed.[105] This study did not find a significant increase in respiratory difficulties, as observed by Yonkers and colleagues.[106] There are reports of peripartum sedation, decreased muscle tone (floppiness), and breathing problems in some infants exposed to benzodiazepines.[107,108] In general, these symptoms appear infrequently and likely are more common in women who take high dosages of these medications.

The results of most benzodiazepine studies are challenging to analyze because in most cases of benzodiazepine exposure, women were also treated with other psychotropic medications. Some providers recommend tapering and discontinuing benzodiazepines around the time of parturition. This rationale is not fully supported, however, given the risk of puerperal worsening of anxiety disorders in women with a history of panic disorder and OCD.[109,110] In a case series, clonazepam-only use during pregnancy and labor did not cause any maternal or fetal compromise.[111]

For patients who conceive on benzodiazepines and do not wish to continue to take these medications over the course of their pregnancy, a gradual taper of these medications is required to prevent rebound anxiety, panic, insomnia, and serious withdrawal side effects, such as seizures. The slower the taper, the better it is tolerated.

Gabapentin

Gabapentin is used in a wide variety of clinical settings (epilepsy, pain management, restless leg syndrome, anxiety, and sleep disturbance); however, there is small amount of information available in regard to the reproductive safety of this medication,[112] and a greater number of exposed infants are required to definitively quantify the reproductive risk profile of this medication. One report reviews the accumulated data regarding the reproductive safety of gabapentin. Pooling all of the available data estimated the risk of malformation in gabapentin only–exposed infants to be less than that of the congenital malformations observed in the general population.[113]

Other Anxiolytics: Antipsychotics, Hydroxyzine, and Buspirone

Antipsychotic medications, such as Seroquel and olanzapine, can be used for as-needed treatment of anxiety (discussed previously). Hydroxyzine has limited but reassuring reproductive safety data.[114] Currently, no systematic data are available on the reproductive safety of buspirone.

STIMULANT MEDICATIONS AND PREGNANCY

Psychostimulants may be used for treatment of variety of reasons, including ADD, management of side effects (such as fatigue and cognitive deficits), enhancement of antidepressant medications, and treatment of narcolepsy.

A 2017 study has shown that infants exposed during pregnancy had increased risk for neonatal ICU admission, were more likely to have central nervous system–related disorders and were more often moderately preterm than nonexposed infants. There was no increased risk for congenital malformations or perinatal death.[115] These findings are consistent with previous studies. What makes this study more useful and clinically relevant, however, is that it focuses on exposure to stimulants prescribed in standard doses as opposed to previous studies, which studied outcomes primarily in women who were abusing or misusing stimulants in combination with other substances.

Most of the studies that have focused on risk for major malformations have not demonstrated any increase in risk of major malformations with first-trimester exposure to methylphenidate. There are fewer available data on dextroamphetamine and amphetamine but still no evidence of teratogenesis.

Gestational hypertension also has been found significantly associated with the use of psychostimulants and seems dose-dependent.[66] Some studies of stimulants, including in women who abuse stimulants, have suggested higher rates of preterm birth, lower birthweight, and other adverse outcomes in infants exposed to stimulants during pregnancy.

The recommendations for use of these medications during pregnancy should be to try to taper off the medications, if feasible, or alternatively decrease the medication to the lowest possible dose and take it at the least number of times possible, on an as-needed basis. There are exceptions to this approach for patients who have challenged functionality if these medications are discontinued. Some examples include severe cases of attention-deficit/hyperactivity disorder (ADHD), leading to accidental injuries, such as car accidents, or cases of treating narcolepsy.

In some cases, bupropion, can be a consideration for replacement of stimulants during pregnancy. This can especially be useful for patients with comorbid depression and/or nicotine use disorder (discussed previously). Bupropion is also used by some providers (off table) for treatment of Attention Deficit Disorder.

MEDICATION-ASSISTED TREATMENT FOR SUBSTANCE USE DISORDERS
Opioid Maintenance Therapy: Methadone Versus Buprenorphine

Treatment with methadone had been considered the gold standard of care for patients requiring opioid maintenance therapy during pregnancy.[116,117] There is a growing body of evidence, however, that indicates buprenorphine should be considered equally efficacious or even as first-line therapy, especially due to its potential advantages for neonatal outcomes.[118,119] Often the decision to choose between these 2 agents is guided by patient history of use and treatment, preference, history of relapse, and need for closer monitoring.

The Maternal Opioid Treatment: Human Experimental Research (MOTHER) project, an 8-site randomized, double blind, double-dummy, flexible-dosing, parallel-group clinical trial compared treatment with methadone to that of buprenorphine. The study showed that neonates exposed to buprenorphine required shorter hospital stays, lower morphine requirements, and an average of 4.1 days of treatment of neonatal adaptation syndrome compared with 9.9 days for the methadone group ($P<.01$).[119]

SUD is a disorder plagued by risk of relapse, which is a main concern of treatment with buprenorphine (a partial agonist) versus methadone (a full opioid agonist). Full agonists might leave patients with less cravings and lower risk of concomitant opioid use.[120] In the MOTHER study, 33% of women on buprenorphine therapy stopped treatment compared with 18% of the methadone group ($P = .02$).[119] In this study, however, women in both groups had to present to a clinic daily. Buprenorphine in the outpatient setting can be prescribed on a monthly basis for patients in long-standing sustained remission, whereas most patients on methadone maintenance need to present to a specialized methadone clinic daily. As such, retention and compliance between the 2 can differ in the outpatient setting.

Special attention should be paid to the risk of polypharmacy with MAT for OUD for patients and their infants. When opiates were coadministered with psychotropic medications, the risk for neonatal drug withdrawal increased.[121] There also are increased risks for accidents, injuries, and respiratory depression for patients who use both opioids and benzodiazepines.[122,123]

Other Medication-Assisted Treatments for Opioid Use Disorder and Alcohol Use Disorder

Naltrexone is not a first-line treatment during pregnancy, especially for patients who are not on this medication prior to their pregnancy. For women who become pregnant while on treatment with naltrexone, this medication should be discontinued if the risk of relapse is low. In cases of high concern about relapse, risks, benefits, and alternatives should be discussed, including treatment with methadone or buprenorphine. Unfortunately, data on the safety profile of this medication are limited.[124]

Naltrexone is also used for treatment of alcohol use disorder. Other medications used for MAT for alcohol use disorder, including disulfiram and acamprosate, likely should be discontinued during pregnancy. The use of naloxone during pregnancy should be limited to cases of maternal overdose only to save a mother's life.

Medication-Assisted Treatments for Smoking Cessation in Pregnancy

The 3 MATs for nicotine use disorder for the general public are nicotine replacement therapy, bupropion, and varenicline. Data regarding the reproductive safety of nicotine replacement therapy are limited and controversial.[125] According to the American College of Obstetricians and Gynecologists recommendations, nicotine replacement therapy should be undertaken "only with close supervision and after careful consideration of the known risks of continued smoking versus the possible risks of nicotine replacement therapy."[126]

At this point, there is no information regarding the reproductive safety of varenicline; thus, it is generally not used in pregnancy.

In contrast, there are data to support the use of bupropion in pregnancy (discussed previously). This medication would be especially efficacious for patients with comorbid depression or ADHD requiring treatment with medications during pregnancy.

Cocaine/Stimulant Use Disorder In Pregnancy

Patients with a history of cocaine or stimulant dependence are at an increased risk for relapse of primary mood and anxiety disorders in addition to substance-induced mood disorder. Medications aimed at curbing cravings (such as topiramate and naltrexone) have been discussed. Patients with a history of cocaine dependence (with no current use) have an increased risk of hypertension. Thus, caution should be taken when prescribing SNRI medications to patients with current or remote history of cocaine use disorder with close observation for possible gestational hypertension.[66]

Best practices

What is the current best practice?

Psychopharmacology and pregnancy
- Screen, diagnose, and treat common mental health conditions prior to pregnancy when possible and/or otherwise during pregnancy
- Understand risks, benefits, alternatives, and appropriateness of psychopharmacologic treatment, including risk of no treatment
- Select medications that have a well-studied reproductive safety profile
- When possible, make modifications to medication regimens prior to pregnancy to confirm a stable and euthymic state on the new regimen prior to conception.
- Limit the number of medication exposures to infant during pregnancy.

What changes in current practice are likely to improve outcomes?

- Appropriate planning prior to pregnancy
- Early intervention prior to or during pregnancy or postpartum
- Continuous and close monitoring of symptoms
- Further research on safety and efficacy of medications during pregnancy

Major recommendations

- Screen all women of reproductive age for common mental health conditions, including, but not limited to, mood and anxiety disorders, OCD posttraumatic stress disorder (history of trauma past and present), ADHD, psychotic disorders (a medical emergency during pregnancy or postpartum), and SUDs.
- Treat women of reproductive age in need of psychiatric medications with medication that have a known favorable perinatal safety profile.
- Engage patients in conversations about family planning, including contraception, and adjust psychiatric medications before conception.
- Monitor patients during pregnancy and in the postpartum period for recurrence of symptoms, regardless of use of psychotropic medications.

Summary statement

Risks, benefits, alternatives, and appropriateness of psychotropic medications, including risks of no treatment, are discussed. Early screening, diagnosis, and intervention prior to and/or during pregnancy often reduce morbidity and mortality of mental health disorders.

REFERENCES

1. Cohen LS, Altshuler LL, Harlow BL, et al. Relapse of major depression during pregnancy in women who maintain or discontinue antidepressant treatment. JAMA 2006;295:499–507.
2. Research C for DE and. Labeling - pregnancy and lactation labeling (Drugs) final rule. Available at: https://www.fda.gov/drugs/developmentapprovalprocess/developmentresources/labeling/ucm093307.htm. Accessed August 6, 2018.
3. Altshuler LL, Cohen LS, Moline ML, et al. The expert consensus guideline series. Treatment of depression in women. Postgrad Med 2001;(Spec No):1–107.
4. Margulis AV, Abou-Ali A, Strazzeri MM, et al. Use of selective serotonin reuptake inhibitors in pregnancy and cardiac malformations: a propensity-score matched cohort in CPRD. Pharmacoepidemiol Drug Saf 2013;22:942–51.
5. Altshuler LL, Cohen L, Szuba MP, et al. Pharmacologic management of psychiatric illness during pregnancy: dilemmas and guidelines. Am J Psychiatry 1996;153:592–606.

6. Djulus J, Koren G, Einarson T, et al. Exposure to mirtazapine during pregnancy: a prospective comparative study of birth outcomes. J Clin Psychiatry 2006;67: 1280–4.

7. Bonari L, Pinto N, Ahn E, et al. Perinatal risks of untreated depression during pregnancy. Can J Psychiatry 2004;49:726–35.

8. Yonkers KA, Wisner KL, Stewart DE, et al. The management of depression during pregnancy: a report from the American Psychiatric Association and the American College of Obstetricians and Gynecologists. Obstet Gynecol 2009; 114:703–13.

9. Freeman MP, Davis M, Sinha P, et al. Omega-3 fatty acids and supportive psychotherapy for perinatal depression: a randomized placebo-controlled study. J Affect Disord 2008;110:1420148.

10. King R. Cognitive therapy of depression. Aaon Beck, John Rush, Brian Shaw, Gary Emery. New York: Guilford, 1979. Aust N Z J Psychiatry 2002;36:272–5.

11. Spinelli MG. Interpersonal psychotherapy for depressed antepartum women: a pilot study. Am J Psychiatry 1997;154:1028–30.

12. Weissman MM, Kleramna GL. Interpersonal psychotherapy for depression. Chase (MD): International Psychotherapy Institute; 2015. Available at: https://www.israpsych.org/books/wp-content/uploads/2015/06/interpersonal_psychotherapy_for_depression_-_myrna_m__weissman_phd.pdf.   Accessed August 11, 2018.

13. Cohen LS, Altshuler LL, Stowe ZN, et al. Reintroduction of antidepressant therapy across pregnancy in women who previously discontinued treatment. Psychother Psychosom 2004;73:255–8.

14. Bodén R, Lundgren M, Brandt L, et al. Risks of adverse pregnancy and birth outcomes in women treated or not treated with mood stabilisers for bipolar disorder: population based cohort study. BMJ 2012;345:e7085.

15. Viguera AC, Whitfield T, Baldessarini RJ, et al. Risk of recurrence in women with bipolar disorder during pregnancy: prospective study of mood stabilizer discontinuation. Am J Psychiatry 2007;164:1817–24.

16. Hogan C, Wang B, Freeman M, et al. Psychiatric illness during pregnancy and the postpartum period. In: Stern T, Freudenreich O, Smith F, et al, editors. Massachusetts general hospital handbook of general hospital psychiatry. 7th edition. Philadelphia: Elsevier Inc.; 2018. Available at: https://phstwlp2.partners.org:2093/#!/content/book/3-s2.0-B9780323484114000497. Accessed August 11, 2018.

17. Spielvogel A, Wile J. Treatment and outcomes of psychotic patients during pregnancy and childbirth. Birth 1992;19:131–7.

18. Buist A, Gotman N, Yonkers KA. Generalized anxiety disorder: course and risk factors in pregnancy. J Affect Disord 2011;131:277–83.

19. Cohen LS, Rosenbaum JF, Heller VL. Panic attack-associated placental abruption: a case report. J Clin Psychiatry 1989;50:266–7.

20. Ebrahim SH, Gfroerer J. Pregnancy-related substance use in the United States during 1996-1998. Obstet Gynecol 2003;101:374–9.

21. Tran TH, Griffin BL, Stone RH, et al. Methadone, buprenorphine, and naltrexone for the treatment of opioid use disorder in pregnant women. Pharmacotherapy 2017;37:824–39.

22. Wisner KL, Gelenberg AJ, Leonard H, et al. Pharmacologic treatment of depression during pregnancy. JAMA 1999;282:1264–9.

23. Ornoy A, Koren G. Selective serotonin reuptake inhibitors in human pregnancy: on the way to resolving the controversy. Semin Fetal Neonatal Med 2014;19: 188–94.
24. Chambers CD, Johnson KA, Dick LM, et al. Birth outcomes in pregnant women taking fluoxetine. N Engl J Med 1996;335:1010–5.
25. Zeskind PS, Stephens LE. Maternal selective serotonin reuptake inhibitor use during pregnancy and newborn neurobehavior. Pediatrics 2004;113:368–75.
26. Simon GE, Cunningham ML, Davis RL. Outcomes of prenatal antidepressant exposure. Am J Psychiatry 2002;159:2055–61.
27. Pastuszak A, Schick-Boschetto B, Zuber C, et al. Pregnancy outcome following first-trimester exposure to fluoxetine (Prozac). JAMA 1993;269:2246–8.
28. Nulman I, Rovet J, Stewart DE, et al. Child development following exposure to tricyclic antidepressants or fluoxetine throughout fetal life: a prospective, controlled study. Am J Psychiatry 2002;159:1889–95.
29. Suri R, Altshuler L, Hendrick V, et al. The impact of depression and fluoxetine treatment on obstetrical outcome. Arch Womens Ment Health 2004;7:193–200.
30. Lupattelli A, Wood M, Ystrom E, et al. New research: effect of time-dependent selective serotonin reuptake inhibitor antidepressants during pregnancy on behavioral, emotional, and social development in preschool-aged children. J Am Acad Child Adolesc Psychiatry 2018;57:200–8.
31. Lattimore KA, Donn SM, Kaciroti N, et al. Selective serotonin reuptake inhibitor (SSRI) use during pregnancy and effects on the fetus and newborn: a meta-analysis. J Perinatol 2005;25:595–604.
32. Cohen LS, Nonacs R. Neurodevelopmental implications of fetal exposure to selective serotonin reuptake inhibitors and untreated maternal depression: weighing relative risks. JAMA Psychiatry 2016;73:1170–2.
33. Steer RA, Scholl TO, Hediger ML, et al. Self-reported depression and negative pregnancy outcomes. J Clin Epidemiol 1992;45:1093–9.
34. Levinson-Castiel R, Merlob P, Linder N, et al. Neonatal abstinence syndrome after in utero exposure to selective serotonin reuptake inhibitors in term infants. Arch Pediatr Adolesc Med 2006;160:173–6.
35. Chambers CD, Hernandez-Diaz S, Van Marter LJ, et al. Selective serotonin-reuptake inhibitors and risk of persistent pulmonary hypertension of the newborn. N Engl J Med 2006;354:579–87.
36. Andrade SE, McPhillips H, Loren D, et al. Antidepressant medication use and risk of persistent pulmonary hypertension of the newborn. Pharmacoepidemiol Drug Saf 2009;18:246–52.
37. Huybrechts KF, Bateman BT, Palmsten K, et al. Antidepressant use late in pregnancy and risk of persistent pulmonary hypertension of the newborn. JAMA 2015;313:2142–51.
38. Hernández-Díaz S, Marter LJV, Werler MM, et al. Risk factors for persistent pulmonary hypertension of the newborn. Pediatrics 2007;120:e272–82.
39. Nulman I, Rovet J, Stewart DE, et al. Neurodevelopment of children exposed in utero to antidepressant drugs. N Engl J Med 1997;336:258–62.
40. Nulman I, Koren G, Rovet J, et al. Neurodevelopment of children following prenatal exposure to venlafaxine, selective serotonin reuptake inhibitors, or untreated maternal depression. Am J Psychiatry 2012;169:1165–74.
41. Boukhris T, Sheehy O, Mottron L, et al. Antidepressant use during pregnancy and the risk of autism spectrum disorder in children. JAMA Pediatr 2016;170: 117–24.

42. Malm H, Brown AS, Gissler M, et al. Gestational exposure to selective serotonin reuptake inhibitors and offspring psychiatric disorders: a national register-based study. J Am Acad Child Adolesc Psychiatry 2016;55:359–66.
43. Figueroa R. Use of antidepressants during pregnancy and risk of attention-deficit/hyperactivity disorder in the offspring. J Dev Behav Pediatr 2010;31: 641–8.
44. Hviid A, Melbye M, Pasternak B. Use of selective serotonin reuptake inhibitors during pregnancy and risk of autism. N Engl J Med 2013;369:2406–15.
45. Sørensen MJ, Grønborg TK, Christensen J, et al. Antidepressant exposure in pregnancy and risk of autism spectrum disorders. Clin Epidemiol 2013;5: 449–59.
46. Andrade C. Antidepressant exposure during pregnancy and risk of autism in the offspring: do the new studies add anything new? J Clin Psychiatry 2017;78: e1052–6.
47. Mezzacappa A, Lasica P-A, Gianfagna F, et al. Risk for autism spectrum disorders according to period of prenatal antidepressant exposure: a systematic review and meta-analysis. JAMA Pediatr 2017;171:555–63.
48. Heller HM, Ravelli ACJ, Bruning AHL, et al. Increased postpartum haemorrhage, the possible relation with serotonergic and other psychopharmacological drugs: a matched cohort study. BMC Pregnancy Childbirth 2017;17:166.
49. Hanley GE, Smolina K, Mintzes B, et al. Postpartum hemorrhage and use of serotonin reuptake inhibitor antidepressants in pregnancy. Obstet Gynecol 2016; 127:553–61.
50. Palmsten K, Hernández-Díaz S, Huybrechts KF, et al. Use of antidepressants near delivery and risk of postpartum hemorrhage: cohort study of low income women in the United States. BMJ 2013;347:f4877.
51. Huybrechts KF, Palmsten K, Avorn J, et al. Antidepressant use in pregnancy and the risk of cardiac defects. N Engl J Med 2014;370:2397–407.
52. Furu K, Kieler H, Haglund B, et al. Selective serotonin reuptake inhibitors and venlafaxine in early pregnancy and risk of birth defects: population based cohort study and sibling design. BMJ 2015;350:h1798.
53. Wogelius P, Nørgaard M, Gislum M, et al. Maternal use of selective serotonin reuptake inhibitors and risk of congenital malformations. Epidemiology 2006;17: 701–4.
54. Paroxetine and pregnancy | GSK. Available at: https://www.gsk.com/en-gb/media/resource-centre/paroxetine-information/paroxetine-and-pregnancy/. Accessed August 22, 2018.
55. Alwan S, Reefhuis J, Rasmussen SA, et al, National Birth Defects Prevention Study. Use of selective serotonin-reuptake inhibitors in pregnancy and the risk of birth defects. N Engl J Med 2007;356:2684–92.
56. Louik C, Lin AE, Werler MM, et al. First-trimester use of selective serotonin-reuptake inhibitors and the risk of birth defects. N Engl J Med 2007;356: 2675–83.
57. Gentile S. Pregnancy Exposure to serotonin reuptake inhibitors and the risk of spontaneous abortions. CNS Spectr 2008;13:960–6.
58. Einarson A, Pistelli A, DeSantis M, et al. Evaluation of the risk of congenital cardiovascular defects associated with use of paroxetine during pregnancy. Am J Psychiatry 2008;165:749–52.
59. Klieger-Grossmann C, Weitzner B, Panchaud A, et al. Pregnancy outcomes following use of escitalopram: a prospective comparative cohort study. J Clin Pharmacol 2012;52:766–70.

60. Malm H, Artama M, Gissler M, et al. Selective serotonin reuptake inhibitors and risk for major congenital anomalies. Obstet Gynecol 2011;118:111–20.

61. Lassen D, Ennis ZN, Damkier P. First-trimester pregnancy exposure to venlafaxine or duloxetine and risk of major congenital malformations: a systematic review. Basic Clin Pharmacol Toxicol 2016;118:32–6.

62. Einarson A, Fatoye B, Sarkar M, et al. Pregnancy outcome following gestational exposure to venlafaxine: a multicenter prospective controlled study. Am J Psychiatry 2001;158:1728–30.

63. Andrade C. The safety of duloxetine during pregnancy and lactation. J Clin Psychiatry 2014;75:e1423–7.

64. Hoog SL, Cheng Y, Elpers J, et al. Duloxetine and pregnancy outcomes: safety surveillance findings. Int J Med Sci 2013;10:413–9.

65. Kjaersgaard MIS, Parner ET, Vestergaard M, et al. Prenatal antidepressant exposure and risk of spontaneous abortion - a population-based study. PLoS One 2013;8:e72095.

66. Newport DJ, Hostetter AL, Juul SH, et al. Prenatal psychostimulant and antidepressant exposure and risk of hypertensive disorders of pregnancy. J Clin Psychiatry 2016;77:1538–45.

67. GalxoSmithKline. GSK pregnancy registry for Bupropioin. Available at: http://pregnancyregistry.gsk.com/documents/bup_report_final_2008.pdf. Accessed August 11, 2018.

68. Chun-Fai-Chan B, Koren G, Fayez I, et al. Pregnancy outcome of women exposed to bupropion during pregnancy: a prospective comparative study. Am J Obstet Gynecol 2005;192:932–6.

69. Cole JA, Modell JG, Haight BR, et al. Bupropion in pregnancy and the prevalence of congenital malformations. Pharmacoepidemiol Drug Saf 2007;16:474–84.

70. Emslie G, Judge R. Tricyclic antidepressants and selective serotonin reuptake inhibitors: use during pregnancy, in children/adolescents and in the elderly. Acta Psychiatr Scand 2000;101:26–34.

71. Pariante CM, Seneviratne G, Howard L. Should we stop using tricyclic antidepressants in pregnancy? Psychol Med 2011;41:15–7.

72. Suri R, Altshuler LL. No decision is without risk. J Clin Psychiatry 2009;70:1319–20.

73. Cohen LS, Wang B, Nonacs R, et al. Treatment of mood disorders during pregnancy and postpartum. Psychiatr Clin North Am 2010;33:273–93.

74. Alam A, Voronovich Z, Carley JA. A review of therapeutic uses of mirtazapine in psychiatric and medical conditions. Prim Care Companion CNS Disord 2013;15 [pii:PCC.13r01525].

75. Smit M, Dolman KM, Honig A. Mirtazapine in pregnancy and lactation - a systematic review. Eur Neuropsychopharmacol 2016;26:126–35.

76. Uguz F, Turgut K, Aydin A, et al. Low-dose mirtazapine in major depression developed after hyperemesis gravidarum: a case series. Am J Ther 2018. https://doi.org/10.1097/MJT.0000000000000698.

77. Einarson A, Bonari L, Voyer-Lavigne S, et al. A multicentre prospective controlled study to determine the safety of trazodone and nefazodone use during pregnancy. Can J Psychiatry 2003;48:106–10.

78. Weinstein MR, Goldfield M. Cardiovascular malformations with lithium use during pregnancy. Am J Psychiatry 1975;132:529–31.

79. Newport DJ, Viguera AC, Beach AJ, et al. Lithium placental passage and obstetrical outcome: implications for clinical management during late pregnancy. Am J Psychiatry 2005;162:2162-70.
80. Patorno E, Huybrechts KF, Bateman BT, et al. Lithium use in pregnancy and the risk of cardiac malformations. N Engl J Med 2017;376:2245-54.
81. Holmes LB, Baldwin EJ, Smith CR, et al. Increased frequency of isolated cleft palate in infants exposed to lamotrigine during pregnancy. Neurology 2008; 70:2152-8.
82. Cunnington MC, Weil JG, Messenheimer JA, et al. Final results from 18 years of the International lamotrigine pregnancy registry. Neurology 2011;76:1817-23.
83. Dolk H, Wang H, Loane M, et al. Lamotrigine use in pregnancy and risk of orofacial cleft and other congenital anomalies. Neurology 2016;86:1716-25.
84. Hernández-Díaz S, Smith CR, Shen A, et al. Comparative safety of antiepileptic drugs during pregnancy. Neurology 2012;78:1692-9.
85. Pariente G, Leibson T, Shulman T, et al. Pregnancy outcomes following in utero exposure to lamotrigine: a systematic review and meta-Analysis. CNS Drugs 2017;31:439-50.
86. Wyszynski DF, Nambisan M, Surve T, et al. Increased rate of major malformations in offspring exposed to valproate during pregnancy. Neurology 2005;64: 961-5.
87. Meador KJ, Baker GA, Browning N, et al. Fetal antiepileptic drug exposure and cognitive outcomes at age 6 years (NEAD study): a prospective observational study. Lancet Neurol 2013;12:244-52.
88. Cohen MJ, Meador KJ, Browning N, et al. Fetal antiepileptic drug exposure: adaptive and emotional/behavioral functioning at age 6 years. Epilepsy Behav 2013;29:308-15.
89. Christensen J, Grønborg TK, Sørensen MJ, et al. Prenatal valproate exposure and risk of autism spectrum disorders and childhood autism. JAMA 2013;309: 1696-703.
90. Rosa FW. Spina bifida in infants of women treated with carbamazepine during pregnancy. N Engl J Med 1991;324:674-7.
91. Einarson A, Boskovic R. Use and safety of antipsychotic drugs during pregnancy. J Psychiatr Pract 2009;15:183-92.
92. Huybrechts KF, Hernández-Díaz S, Patorno E, et al. Antipsychotic use in pregnancy and the risk for congenital malformations. JAMA Psychiatry 2016;73: 938-46.
93. Rumeau-Rouquette C, Goujard J, Huel G. Possible teratogenic effect of phenothiazines in human beings. Teratology 1977;15:57-64.
94. Tesar GE, Stern TA. Evaluation and treatment of agitation in the intensive care unit. J Intensive Care Med 1986;1:137-48.
95. McKenna K, Koren G, Tetelbaum M, et al. Pregnancy outcome of women using atypical antipsychotic drugs: a prospective comparative study. J Clin Psychiatry 2005;66:444-9.
96. Habermann F, Fritzsche J, Fuhlbrück F, et al. Atypical antipsychotic drugs and pregnancy outcome: a prospective, cohort study. J Clin Psychopharmacol 2013;33:453-62.
97. Cohen LS, Viguera AC, McInerney KA, et al. Reproductive safety of second-generation antipsychotics: current data from the Massachusetts general hospital national pregnancy registry for atypical antipsychotics. Am J Psychiatr 2015; 173:263-70.

98. Petersen I, Sammon CJ, McCrea RL, et al. Risks associated with antipsychotic treatment in pregnancy: comparative cohort studies based on electronic health records. Schizophr Res 2016;176:349–56.
99. Ennis ZN, Damkier P. Pregnancy exposure to olanzapine, quetiapine, risperidone, aripiprazole and risk of congenital malformations. A systematic review. Basic Clin Pharmacol Toxicol 2015;116:315–20.
100. Hanley GE, Mintzes B. Patterns of psychotropic medicine use in pregnancy in the United States from 2006 to 2011 among women with private insurance. BMC Pregnancy Childbirth 2014;14:242.
101. Safra MJ, Oakley GP. Association between cleft lip with or without cleft palate and prenatal exposure to diazepam. Lancet 1975;2:478–80.
102. Ban L, West J, Gibson JE, et al. First trimester exposure to anxiolytic and hypnotic drugs and the risks of major congenital anomalies: a United Kingdom population-based cohort study. PLoS One 2014;9:e100996.
103. Bellantuono C, Tofani S, Di Sciascio G, et al. Benzodiazepine exposure in pregnancy and risk of major malformations: a critical overview. Gen Hosp Psychiatry 2013;35:3–8.
104. Enato E, Moretti M, Koren G. The fetal safety of benzodiazepines: an updated meta-analysis. J Obstet Gynaecol Can 2011;33:46–8.
105. Freeman MP, Góez-Mogollón L, McInerney KA, et al. Obstetrical and neonatal outcomes after benzodiazepine exposure during pregnancy: results from a prospective registry of women with psychiatric disorders. Gen Hosp Psychiatry 2018;53:73–9.
106. Yonkers KA, Gilstad-Hayden K, Forray A, et al. Association of panic disorder, generalized anxiety disorder, and benzodiazepine treatment during pregnancy with risk of adverse birth outcomes. JAMA Psychiatry 2017;74:1145–52.
107. Fisher JB, Edgren BE, Mammel MC, et al. Neonatal apnea associated with maternal clonazepam therapy: a case report. Obstet Gynecol 1985;66:34S–5S.
108. Whitelaw AG, Cummings AJ, McFadyen IR. Effect of maternal lorazepam on the neonate. Br Med J 1981;282:1106–8.
109. Cohen LS, Sichel DA, Dimmock JA, et al. Postpartum course in women with pre-existing panic disorder. J Clin Psychiatry 1994;55:289–92.
110. Sichel DA, Cohen LS, Dimmock JA, et al. Postpartum obsessive compulsive disorder: a case series. J Clin Psychiatry 1993;54:156–9.
111. Weinstock L, Cohen LS, Bailey JW, et al. Obstetrical and neonatal outcome following clonazepam use during pregnancy: a case series. Psychother Psychosom 2001;70:158–62.
112. Fujii H, Goel A, Bernard N, et al. Pregnancy outcomes following gabapentin use: results of a prospective comparative cohort study. Neurology 2013;80:1565–70.
113. Guttuso T, Shaman M, Thornburg LL. Potential maternal symptomatic benefit of gabapentin and review of its safety in pregnancy. Eur J Obstet Gynecol Reprod Biol 2014;181:280–3.
114. Einarson A, Bailey B, Jung G, et al. Prospective controlled study of hydroxyzine and cetirizine in pregnancy. Ann Allergy Asthma Immunol 1997;78:183–6.
115. Nörby U, Winbladh B, Källén K. Perinatal outcomes after treatment with ADHD medication during pregnancy. Pediatrics 2017;140 [pii:20170747].
116. Krans EE, Cochran G, Bogen DL. Caring for opioid-dependent pregnant women: prenatal and postpartum care considerations. Clin Obstet Gynecol 2015;58:370–9.
117. Winhusen T, Wilder C, Wexelblatt SL, et al. Design considerations for point-of-care clinical trials comparing methadone and buprenorphine treatment for

opioid dependence in pregnancy and for neonatal abstinence syndrome. Contemp Clin Trials 2014;39:158–65.

118. American College of Obsetrics and Gynecology. ACOG committee opinion no. 524: opioid abuse, dependence, and addiction in pregnancy. Obstet Gynecol 2012;119:1070–6.

119. Jones HE, Kaltenbach K, Heil SH, et al. Neonatal abstinence syndrome after methadone or buprenorphine exposure. N Engl J Med 2010;363:2320–31.

120. Fischer G, Ortner R, Rohrmeister K, et al. Methadone versus buprenorphine in pregnant addicts: a double-blind, double-dummy comparison study. Addiction 2006;101:275–81.

121. Huybrechts KF, Bateman BT, Desai RJ, et al. Risk of neonatal drug withdrawal after intrauterine co-exposure to opioids and psychotropic medications: cohort study. BMJ 2017;358:j3326.

122. Hirschtritt ME, Delucchi KL, Olfson M. Outpatient, combined use of opioid and benzodiazepine medications in the United States, 1993-2014. Prev Med Rep 2018;9:49–54.

123. Schuman-Olivier Z, Hoeppner BB, Weiss RD, et al. Benzodiazepine use during buprenorphine treatment for opioid dependence: clinical and safety outcomes. Drug Alcohol Depend 2013;132:580–6.

124. National practice guideline. Available at: https://www.asam.org/resources/guidelines-and-consensus-documents/npg. Accessed August 22, 2018.

125. Forinash AB, Pitlick JM, Clark K, et al. Nicotine replacement therapy effect on pregnancy outcomes. Ann Pharmacother 2010;44:1817–21.

126. American College of Obsetrics and Gynecology. ACOG committee opinion no. 721. Smoking cessation during pregnancy. Obstet Gynecol 2017;130:e200–4.

Opioid Use Disorders and Pregnancy

Amanda J. Johnson, MD[a], Cresta W. Jones, MD[b],*

KEYWORDS

- Opioid use disorder • Methadone • Buprenorphine • Pregnancy
- Neonatal abstinence syndrome

KEY POINTS

- Opioid use disorder is associated with an increased risk of pregnancy complications.
- Recommended treatment of opioid use disorder in pregnancy includes medication-assisted therapy using methadone or buprenorphine.
- Medically assisted withdrawal may be considered for women for whom medication-assisted therapy is not a current treatment option, but has a higher risk of maternal relapse.
- Both opioid use disorder and medication assisted therapy are associated with neonatal withdrawal, or neonatal abstinence syndrome.
- A comprehensive care approach is recommended for optimal outcomes with opioid use disorder in pregnancy.

INTRODUCTION

Over the last several decades, the United States has suffered from an increasing epidemic of opioid misuse and dependence, with opioid related overdoses among US adults increasing by 200%.[1] This crisis spans across demographics, including women of childbearing age and who are pregnant.[2,3] As the crisis has intensified, so have the costs of opioid use disorder (OUD) and its sequelae increased. The care of pregnant women affected by opioid use is associated with a substantial

This article originally appeared in *Obstetrics and Gynecology Clinics*, Volume 45, Issue 2, June 2018.

Disclosure Statement: Neither author has any relationship with a commercial company that has a direct financial interest in subject matter or materials discussed in article or with a company making a competing product.

[a] Department of Obstetrics and Gynecology, Division of Maternal-Fetal Medicine, Medical College of Wisconsin, 9200 West Wisconsin Avenue, Milwaukee, WI 53226, USA; [b] Department of Obstetrics, Gynecology and Women's Health, Division of Maternal-Fetal Medicine, University of Minnesota Medical School, 606 24th Avenue S, Suite 400, Minneapolis, MN 55455, USA

* Corresponding author.

E-mail address: jonesc@umn.edu

economic burden to the health care system, with mean hospital charges for infants affected by opioid withdrawal, or neonatal abstinence syndrome (NAS), at approximately 19 times the costs of non-NAS infants.[4,5] This article provides an overview of significant issues associated with OUDs that are of importance to providers of obstetric care.

Defining Opioid Use Disorder

An OUD is currently defined as the repeated occurrence, over a 1-year time period, of 2 or more specific criteria related to opioid use. These criteria include giving up important life events to use more opioids, excessive time spent obtaining and using opioids, and withdrawal when opioid use is stopped abruptly.[6] It is important to note that women on chronic opioids for medically indicated treatment may have opioid withdrawal when medications are abruptly stopped, but withdrawal alone does not identify a patient as suffering from an OUD.

ISSUES IN PREGNANCY
Screening

The identification of opioid misuse and dependence is key to optimizing patient outcomes. Because the misuse of opioids crosses societal boundaries, and risk factor-based screening may lead to missed cases,[7] it is essential that substance use screening be universal.[8] Screening for substance use should, therefore, be considered a routine component of initial prenatal care.[9] Multiple screening tools for substance use and abuse are available, although few have been validated for opioid misuse in pregnancy.[10] Most tools can be administered in written or verbal fashion during the history component of a clinical visit, by any trained health care provider. Urine drug testing as a primary screening tool cannot be recommended at this time, owing to ongoing concerns about the ability to accurately identify patients with substance use disorders. Urine drug screening only assesses recent use, it may miss many substances of abuse, and it is associated with a high false-positive rate.[8,11,12] The Screening, Brief Intervention, and Referral for Treatment technique is recommended for use in pregnancy as a helpful tool for identifying patients with substance use disorders and for providing the first steps to initiating treatment.[13] Because of societal stereotypes and stigmas associated with substance use disorders, health care providers should screen patients in a caring and nonjudgmental manner, and should assure patients that screening is undertaken to allow for optimal maternal care and outcomes during pregnancy and beyond. It is important for all providers to educate themselves on state and federal laws surrounding substance use screening and reporting, before implementing any universal screening protocols, owing to the potential for mandatory reporting of use in some states.

Complications of Opioid Use Disorder

Untreated OUD has been associated with significant complications during pregnancy for the mother, fetus, and neonate (**Table 1**).[14,15] Women experiencing OUD in pregnancy without treatment often have limited prenatal care and are exposed to at-risk behaviors, which increases the risk of sexually transmitted infections, violence, and adverse legal consequences, as well as to a significant risk of overdose and death. The fetus is at an increased risk of intrauterine growth restriction, placental abruption, preterm birth, and fetal death. Many of these complications are significantly reduced or improved with maternal treatment,[16,17] although some complications may persist, such as suboptimal fetal growth and risk of neonatal opioid withdrawal syndrome

Table 1
Complications of untreated opioid use disorder in pregnancy

Maternal	• Limited prenatal care • Infectious exposure • Miscarriage • Preterm labor and delivery • Opioid overdose and death
Fetal	• Intrauterine growth restriction • Preterm birth • Congenital anomalies (uncertain)
Neonatal	• Small for gestational age • Neonatal abstinence syndrome • Long-term developmental effects (uncertain)

(also known as NAS). NAS is characterized by disturbances in the gastrointestinal, autonomic, and central nervous systems, and can be associated with extended newborn hospitalizations to treat withdrawal symptoms. Infants exposed to chronic opioids in utero are typically observed for a minimum of 4 to 7 days for signs or symptoms of NAS. If NAS is identified, it is often treated with oral morphine or methadone at a dose that alleviates the signs and symptoms of withdrawal, with the dose weaned over days to weeks.[12]

Although NAS is the most common term used to represent the pattern of findings typically associated with opioid withdrawal in the newborn, it is important to note that the US Food and Drug Administration now embraces the term "neonatal opioid withdrawal syndrome," which more accurately identifies the constellation of symptoms specifically associated with prenatal exposure to opioids.[18]

NAS was described initially in infants of mothers with illicit opioid use, but its development can be associated with any chronic maternal opioid use in pregnancy, including for treatment of OUD as well as of chronic pain. Rates of development of NAS have varied widely, from 30% to 80%,[12,19] and the incidence cannot be predicted by the amount of opioids used by the mother before delivery.[20,21] The incidence of NAS in the United States has increased approximately 400% in recent years.[4] In addition, NAS risk seems to be doubled in infants of mothers with coexposure to antidepressants, benzodiazepines, and gabapentin.[22] Patient should be counseled to limit exposure to these medications if not medically indicated.

Treatment

Although not approved for use in pregnancy by the US Food and Drug Administration, several therapies are currently considered standard of care for maternal treatment, and several others require additional data on outcomes before recommendations can be made (**Table 2**).[12,15]

Table 2
Treatment options for opioid use disorder in pregnancy

Preferred treatment	• Methadone • Buprenorphine
Treatment reported, not preferred	• Buprenorphine/naloxone combination therapy • Medically supervised withdrawal
Limited data in pregnancy	• Naltrexone

Medication-assisted therapy

The preferred treatment options for OUD in pregnancy include 2 forms of medication-assisted treatment (MAT): methadone or buprenorphine.[12,23,24] The rationale for treatment with MAT includes the prevention of opioid withdrawal, the prevention of complications owing to nonmedical opioid use and relapse to use, improved compliance with prenatal care and comprehensive addiction treatment, and a reduced risk of obstetric complications.[8]

It is recommended that all obstetric providers be familiar with the federal guideline on emergency narcotic addiction treatment, 21 CFR 1306.07(b).[25] This exception, known as the "3-day rule" allows a practitioner who is not separately registered as a narcotic treatment provider to administer (but not prescribe) narcotic drugs to relieve acute withdrawal while arranging for a patient's referral for treatment. Treatment can be provided for no more than 72 hours, and should be performed in consultation or collaboration with a specialist comfortable with initiating treatment for OUD. This provision may be useful when a pregnant patient presents in withdrawal at a time of day when access to immediate OUD treatment is not available, such as evenings and weekends.

Methadone Methadone is a pure opioid receptor agonist that binds to and activates μ-opioid receptors. It is provided through federally regulated opiate treatment programs that dispense daily medication doses as a component of comprehensive addiction care. The dose is increased slowly over several weeks to reach a therapeutic level while minimizing the increased risk of overdose during treatment initiation. Methadone has long been used as a treatment for OUD in pregnancy, with clear evidence of improvement in obstetric outcomes.[26] Because treatment with methadone can only be continued through a federally regulated opiate treatment program, open communication between the opioid treatment program and the obstetric team is necessary for optimal care. However, this communication must be done while following special guidelines for disclosure of information regarding addiction and substance use treatment.[27]

Although long considered the standard of care for OUD in pregnancy, methadone treatment is not without its adverse effects. These effects include respiratory depression and risk of overdose, QTc interval prolongation, as well as interaction with other drugs, including antiretroviral agents.[23] In addition, as with all currently used MAT options for OUD in pregnancy, it is also associated with the risk of NAS.

Buprenorphine Buprenorphine is a partial μ-receptor agonist that binds with a high affinity to the μ-opioid receptor, but does not activate the receptor completely when bound. The partial agonistic activity makes overdose less likely when use is compared with other opioids.[28] However, owing to its high affinity for the opioid receptor, patients must demonstrate withdrawal symptoms before initiating treatment, to avoid precipitated withdrawal, which can be very difficult to treat.[23]

Buprenorphine is accessible through office-based maintenance therapy, which can be undertaken by a licensed provider who has obtained a DATA-2000 waiver from the US Drug Enforcement Agency. This process requires additional provider training, which can be obtained by several routes, the simplest of which is a full-day training program available on-line or in person. Buprenorphine has many advantages that allow for patient discretion and accessibility outside of areas where daily methadone treatment is an option. Buprenorphine treatment can be incorporated into a comprehensive obstetric treatment program if a waivered physician is available.

Most buprenorphine treatment programs outside of pregnancy use primarily a buprenorphine/naloxone combination medication.[23] Naloxone is added to help deter alternative administration of buprenorphine in an abuse/diversion setting. Although naloxone does not seem to have systemic absorption when taken correctly in a combination sublingual treatment, buprenorphine monotherapy is currently recommended in pregnancy.[8,12,15] However, recent data suggest that buprenorphine/naloxone combination therapy may be an additional option during pregnancy. At this time, no maternal, fetal, or neonatal adverse effects have been identified with the combination product.[29–31] It is expected that the use of this treatment in pregnancy will increase as more data become available.

If a patient maintained on combination therapy becomes pregnant, and she is unwilling or unable to change to monotherapy, informed consent on limited outcomes is recommended before continuing treatment.

A recently available buprenorphine implant is being used in addiction treatment,[32,33] as opposed to conventional sublingual therapy. However, there are currently no data on the use of this treatment in a pregnant population.

Methadone versus buprenorphine: initiating therapy in pregnancy Both methadone and buprenorphine are appropriate choices for initiating treatment in pregnancy. A personalized approach to treatment is required, because there are benefits and downfalls to both therapies (**Table 3**).[8,12,15] Data do indicate less severe manifestations of NAS with maternal treatment using buprenorphine,[19] and a recent systematic review and metaanalysis suggested that buprenorphine treatment was associated with a lower risk of preterm birth, greater birth weight, and larger neonatal head circumference, with no increase in adverse events.[34] However, methadone has been associated with a higher treatment retention rate[35] and individual patient characteristics must be considered when choosing the best treatment to minimize relapse risk.

It is important to note that, owing to physiologic and metabolic changes of pregnancy, dosages of methadone and buprenorphine often require multiple dose changes during pregnancy.[36–38] Patients can be reassured by their obstetricians that such changes are common in pregnancy and should be considered when patients report a return of or an increase in withdrawal symptoms. The decision for a dosage increase is determined by the opioid- agonist therapy provider, based on the presence of withdrawal symptoms or patient reported urges for illicit use, often in collaboration with the obstetric providers. Changes may include increasing the overall dose and/or increasing the frequency of dosing to control withdrawal symptoms.[39,40] It is of note that methadone and buprenorphine doses do not seem to have a consistent effect on the incidence and severity of NAS[41,42]; therefore, maternal treatment goals must be to manage withdrawal symptoms and prevent relapse and illicit use, rather than to minimize daily treatment dosages.

Patient often express concern about the long-term implications of prenatal exposure to MAT. Studies are complicated by substantial difficulties in isolating the effects of opioid treatment from other confounders often seen in women experiencing OUD.[43] However, limited data suggest the possibility of potential vision, motor, behavioral, and cognitive problems, as well as an increased rate of otitis media.[44,45] It is important that these families be identified early and be provided with additional support to optimize long-term outcomes.

Alternative treatment options Although methadone and buprenorphine are both recommended as first-line therapy for treatment of OUD in pregnancy, they may not be acceptable treatments for some patients for a variety of reasons, including financial, geographic, or stigma. Therefore, it is important that obstetric providers be familiar with alternative treatments that may be provided to their patients.[12,15]

Table 3
Medication specific issues: medication-assisted therapy in pregnancy

Treatment	Pros	Cons
Methadone	• Demonstrated safety and efficacy in pregnancy • Decreased medication diversion • More structured program • More effective for polysubstance abuse • Effective if failed buprenorphine treatment • Safe for breastfeeding	• Daily clinic treatment required • Higher risk of overdose • Interactions with other medication • Prolongation of QT interval • Neonatal abstinence syndrome
Buprenorphine	• Does not require proximity for daily clinic visits • Decreased overdose risk • Decreased interactions with other medications • Less severe, shorter neonatal abstinence • More discreet • Safe for breastfeeding	• Risk of precipitated withdrawal during initiation • Lack of long-term data on child outcomes • Increased diversion risk • Lower retention in treatment • Less effective if buprenorphine drug of abuse • Requires mild withdrawal to start treatment
Buprenorphine + naloxone	• Decreased diversion risk • Similar outcomes to buprenorphine alone • Limited breastfeeding data	• Severe withdrawal if used incorrectly (ie, injected) • Lack of long-term data on child outcomes
Naltrexone	• Requires completed opioid withdrawal to initiate • Limits overdose risk • No maternal withdrawal if treatment stopped • Minimal breastfeeding data	• Limited effectiveness of opioid treatment if required (eg, after a cesarean section) • Lack of long-term data on infant and child outcomes • Minimal data on pregnancy and breastfeeding • Minimal data on long-term maternal outcomes

Medically assisted withdrawal Although opioid withdrawal has historically been associated with a higher risk of miscarriage and fetal demise,[46] available recent data do not support a significantly increased risk of fetal complications with medically assisted withdrawal during pregnancy.[47,48] MAT is currently considered as the first-line treatment of OUD in pregnancy, but medically supervised withdrawal may be considered in situations in which a woman will not accept MAT, or MAT is not available.[8,12] Although recent studies have described successful outcomes after medically supervised withdrawal in pregnancy,[48,49] there remains a high risk of maternal relapse as well as NAS, likely related to relapse.[50] Significant ancillary services are often required, such as intensive outpatient therapy, for the successful maintenance of abstinence. In addition, there are no studies addressing the long-term outcomes for patients treated with medically supervised withdrawal during pregnancy.[51]

Owing to concerns and guilt related to the risk of NAS, women may request self-wean from MAT and abstinence from all treatment. It is important to educate patients that success is low with self-wean, and most patients end up maintaining or increasing their current dose.[52] In addition, with a clinical focus based on treatment of a chronic maternal disease, goals must be directed toward long-term success in recovery for the patient. Owing to the high relapse rate associated with maternal withdrawal and abstinence (90%), medically assisted withdrawal cannot currently be considered a recommended form of treatment.

Naltrexone Naltrexone therapy, in oral, injectable, and implant forms, has been gaining more attention as an alternative to opioid-based treatments.[53] Naltrexone is a pure opioid antagonist, similar to naloxone, and it seems to block most opioid receptors. Naltrexone has been shown to reduce the risk of relapse in nonpregnant populations.[23,54] Management of acute pain while using this medication has been found to be challenging, which would certainly complicate analgesia surrounding childbirth.[55] In addition, currently available data on use in pregnancy are limited, although no significant adverse outcomes have been noted when compared with other MAT.[56] Initiating naltrexone requires complete withdrawal from opioids, making the initiation of therapy difficult even outside of pregnancy. Data are currently limited on both the safety and effectiveness of naltrexone in pregnancy. If a pregnancy is identified in a woman currently undergoing naltrexone treatment, a significant discussion of possible benefits and unknown risks will need to be undertaken.[53]

COMPREHENSIVE OBSTETRIC CARE AND OPIOID USE DISORDERS

To best provide obstetric care for women experiencing OUD, a "whole-women" approach must be taken.[15] This means comprehensive management of the other medical and social issues often associated with OUD in pregnancy. A modified care schedule may include flexible appointments, grouping prenatal visits with ultrasound and social services, and offering convenient consultations with lactation specialists and pediatrics.[11,12] Even in women who are not engaged in treatment of substance use disorders, participation in prenatal care has been associated with significant reductions in prematurity and low birth weight infants.[57]

Antepartum Care

Communication
A vital component of obstetric care is adequate collaboration among all care providers. It is important for providers to obtain written permission from the patient to coordinate care and follow up with her substance use disorder and psychiatric providers, as well as with social services, as is required by federal law for patients undergoing addiction treatment.[27] Pregnant women with ongoing active substance use must be encouraged to continue to engage in prenatal care and legal action to address perinatal OUDs is strongly discouraged.[58] Supportive obstetric care without criminal ramifications for the mother with substance use will allow for the best outcomes for both mother and infant.

Owing to the ongoing risk of maternal relapse to illicit use, which carries an increased risk of overdose and death, prescription of naloxone, the opioid antagonist administered to rapidly reverse the effects of an opioid overdose, for emergency administration should be considered. A patient's family and caregivers should be instructed on use, with the fetal risks of acute maternal withdrawal clearly outweighed by the risk of maternal death from overdose.

Psychiatric disorders
Just fewer than one-half of individuals suffering from OUD have coexisting mental health concerns,[59] many of which are underdiagnosed and undertreated, and may be associated with increased psychological, social, and medical impairments.[60,61] The most common codiagnoses include depression and anxiety. It is important to take a thorough mental health history and to refer patients for additional services as indicated. This step also includes an assessment for the impact of victimization and trauma in the patient's life to best guide health care delivery, a principle termed trauma-informed care.[62] Patients should be scheduled for a follow-up phone call or visit before the routine postpartum visit, to assess for the risk of postpartum depression and psychosis.

Tobacco use disorders
Tobacco use in pregnancy has been associated with an increased risk of adverse pregnancy outcomes including poor fetal growth, placental abruption, preterm birth, and stillbirth.[63] Tobacco use disorders are much more prevalent in pregnant women experiencing OUD (95%) than in pregnant women without substance use concerns (15%).[64,65] This population also has much more limited success in quitting smoking during pregnancy. Recent studies suggest some success with incentive-based treatment programs.[66] Even a decrease in the amount of daily tobacco use, if cessation is unachievable, is associated with improved neonatal outcomes.[67] Tobacco use has also been shown to increase the duration and medication required for infants suffering from NAS.[68,69]

Infectious complications
Infectious disease is more common in women suffering from OUD.[70] In particular, 1 study suggested a rate of hepatitis C exposure of 53% and chronic infection of 37%.[71] Thus, women with identified OUD should be screened for hepatitis C at prenatal intake. In addition, testing for infections such as sexually transmitted infections, hepatitis B, and tuberculosis should be considered, and repeated in later pregnancy for women considered to be at ongoing risk of new exposure. Women not previously immunized should also be offered hepatitis A and B vaccination.[8,23]

Constipation
Patients using opioids including MAT for OUD are at significant risk of opioid-induced constipation and bowel dysfunction. Constipation-related issues should be addressed with patients at each visit. Medications including bisacodyl, Senna, and polyethylene glycol have been shown to be effective for opioid-induced constipation in nonpregnant patients,[72] although no data are currently available regarding the treatment of opioid-induced constipation in pregnancy.

Fetal surveillance
Although opioids are consistently associated with the risk of NAS, studies have demonstrated uncertainty regarding the association of opioid exposure and an increased risk of fetal anomalies.[73] A targeted anatomic survey should be considered to evaluate for possible fetal anomalies, which can be present in up to 2% to 3% of normal pregnancies. Given the increased risk of fetal growth abnormalities with OUDs,[74,75] fetal growth assessments may be considered, either through close clinical examination or via fetal ultrasound examination. For women who are stable in treatment, consideration should be given to sonographic evaluation of fetal growth in the

third trimester. In the absence of fetal growth restriction or any additional maternal complications, there are no current recommendations for additional fetal surveillance during the pregnancy. For women with ongoing illicit substance use, more frequent evaluation, including antepartum surveillance, may be considered. No late preterm or early term delivery is currently recommended for maternal OUD, and delivery should be facilitated as obstetrically indicated.[8,12]

It is important to note that antepartum surveillance, if indicated, may demonstrate such abnormalities as decreased fetal heart rate baseline, decreased variability, and fewer accelerations, likely owing to suppressed motor activity in the fetus.[76,77] Surveillance performed immediately before or immediately after medication is administered, thus avoiding peak effects, is recommended when possible.

Patient expectations

It is important to establish clear expectations for the patient to best optimize the patient–provider relationship. This process includes guidelines for best partnership for prenatal care, what to expect during labor and delivery, and how to best partner to prevent an increased risk of relapse after delivery. Prenatal consultations are suggested with anesthesia, pediatrics/neonatology, and lactation support, and delivery unit tours should be considered. In addition, it is recommended to discuss with the patient how her pain will be managed during labor as well as upon discharge.

Patients with OUD may experience substantial barriers to routine prenatal care, including an inability to attend consistent prenatal appointments owing to transportation or childcare issues. There remains an ongoing need for focused programming that allows for opportunities to overcome these issues.[78]

Peripartum Care

Intrapartum

Patients should be continued on MAT throughout labor and delivery to avoid withdrawal symptoms.[8,12] Although theoretic concerns about precipitated withdrawal have been raised with using buprenorphine in conjunction with pure opioid antagonists (which may be used for labor analgesia), buprenorphine can be safely continued without interruption through labor and delivery, as well as through the postpartum period.[79] Because patients may have hyperalgesia as a result of treatment, it is important to consider early epidural and to remember that MAT will not cover the pain associated with the childbirth process. Alternative pain management protocols such as transverse abdominus plane blocks or nitrous oxide may also be beneficial.[80] Finally, it is very important to avoid treatment with partial opioid antagonists such as nalbuphine and butorphanol during labor and delivery, because these agents can precipitate withdrawal symptoms.

Birthing center staff should be counseled on intrapartum fetal heart rate tracings for patients on methadone, including the potential for reduced variability and accelerations, and a lower baseline.[81] No data are currently available on the potential changes in intrapartum fetal monitoring with buprenorphine therapy.

Postpartum

Limited studies indicate that women with OUD on MAT who undergo cesarean section may require up to 70% more opioid analgesia than women without OUD to adequately treat their pain.[82,83] After delivery, women should continue with a pregnancy-level dosing of MAT, because most studies suggest that medication does not need to be reduced to prepregnancy levels for several weeks.[84] Patients may require a short course of narcotics at discharge after cesarean delivery, and this has not been shown to be a risk factor for relapse for postsurgical patients on methadone or buprenorphine therapy.[85] Higher nonopioid medication use may also be required.[86]

The importance of parental participation in reducing the sequelae of NAS for the infant and for the mother cannot be underestimated.[87] It is important to encourage women who are stable in treatment to consider breastfeeding, which has been shown to improve maternal bonding and potentially decrease the severity of NAS.[88] Contra-indications to breastfeeding include active relapse to illicit drug use and infectious complications such as with human immunodeficiency virus.[89] In addition, rooming-in, skin-to-skin care, and parenting education and support may further improve outcomes for the family unit. The addition of parenting support groups exclusively for women in MAT has also been found to be beneficial.[90]

It is important to address contraception during prenatal care and again at the time of discharge, because the majority of pregnancies are unplanned and women in MAT have lower use of contraception. In addition, they often lack information about effective long-acting reversible contraception.[91,92]

RESPONSIBLE OPIOID PRESCRIBING

Health care providers play an important role in reducing opioid overprescribing, which is an important contributor to the opioid epidemic.[2,3] This role includes limited prescriptions for opioids during pregnancy and at hospital discharge,[93,94] as well as adequate patient education at the time of postdelivery discharge.[95] When prescribing opioids outside of pregnancy to women of childbearing age, discussion of plans for pregnancy, use of reliable contraception, and risks of ongoing opiate use must be considered as primary prevention of both OUD and NAS.[96] Regular use of state-established prescription drug monitoring programs will also help to avoid duplicate prescriptions and doctor shopping, and may also facilitate the identification of women experiencing OUD. Outside of pregnancy, guidelines and best practice statements now exist to help limit the overuse of opioids for chronic pain disorders.[97,98]

Although women with chronic pain may experience physical opioid dependence, they often represent a subset of patients at risk of NAS, but without the other clinical issues associated with OUD. There are few data available on the effects of medically indicated chronic opioid use on pregnancy outcomes, other than the risk of NAS. Although new data and guidelines do not support the use of long-term opioids for chronic pain, many women have already been placed on long-term therapy before achieving pregnancy. There are currently limited data on this population and specific obstetric risks, including the incidence of NAS, that might be encountered. Best practice should include a discussion of limiting opioid use to the minimum required, supporting the use of alternative and complementary pain treatment, and consultations with anesthesia and pediatrics before delivery.[99,100]

SUMMARY

OUDs have significant implications in pregnancy, and outcomes are improved when patients are cared for in an environment that addresses both the treatment of OUD and focused obstetric care tailored to the unique issues that may arise. A personalized approach will identify the best treatment for each patient, with current recommendations focusing on MAT using methadone or buprenorphine. Focused obstetric care allows for appropriate and supportive pregnancy care during the pregnancy and after delivery, with special attention paid to contraception and postpartum depression. Providers must also take steps to minimize ongoing opioid prescribing, using currently accepted guidelines to limit excessive prescriptions.

REFERENCES

1. Rudd RA, Aleshire N, Zibbell JE, et al. Increases in drug and opioid overdose deaths – United States, 2000-2014. MMWR Morb Mortal Wkly Rep 2016; 64(50–51):1378–82.
2. Kozhimannil KB, Graves AJ, Jarlenski M, et al. Non-medical opioid use and sources of opioids among pregnant and non-pregnant reproductive-aged women. Drug Alcohol Depend 2017;174:201–8.
3. Kozhimannil KB, Graves AJ, Levy R, et al. Nonmedical use of prescription opioids among pregnant U.S. women. Womens Health Issues 2017;27(3):308–15.
4. Patrick SW, Davis MM, Lehman CU, et al. Increasing incidence and geographic distribution of neonatal abstinence syndrome: United States 2009 to 2012. J Perinatol 2015;35(8):650–5.
5. Corr TE, Hollenbeak CS. The economic burden of neonatal abstinence syndrome in the United States. Addiction 2017;112(9):1590–9.
6. American Psychiatric Association (APA). Diagnostic and statistical manual of mental disorders. 5th edition. Arlington (VA): APA; 2013.
7. Schauberger CW, Newbury EJ, Coburn JM, et al. Prevalence of illicit drug use in pregnant women in a Wisconsin private practice setting. Am J Obstet Gynecol 2014;211(3):255.e1-4.
8. American College of Obstetrics and Gynecology (ACOG) Committee on Obstetric Practice. ACOG practice bulletin no. 711. Opioid use and opioid use disorder in pregnancy. Obstet Gynecol 2017;130(2):e81–94.
9. American College of Obstetrics and Gynecology (ACOG) Committee on Ethics. ACOG committee opinion no. 633. Alcohol abuse and other substance use disorders: ethical issues in obstetric and gynecologic practice. Obstet Gynecol 2015;125(6):1529–37.
10. Chasnoff IJ, Wells AM, McGourty RF, et al. Validation of the 4Ps plus screen for substance use in pregnancy validation of the 4Ps plus. J Perinatol 2007;27(12): 744–8.
11. Jones HE, Deppen K, Hudak ML, et al. Clinical care for opioid-using pregnant and postpartum women: the role of obstetric providers. Am J Obstet Gynecol 2014;210(4):302–10.
12. Reddy UM, Davis JM, Ren X, et al. Opioid use in pregnancy, neonatal abstinence syndrome, and childhood outcomes: executive summary of a joint workshop by the Eunice Kennedy Shriver National Institute of Child Health and Human Development, American College of Obstetricians and Gynecologists, American Academy of Pediatrics, Society for Maternal-Fetal Medicine, Centers for Disease Control and Prevention, and the March of Dimes Foundation. Obstet Gynecol 2017;130(1):10–28.
13. Wright TE, Terplan M, Ondersma SJ, et al. The role of screening, brief intervention, and referral to treatment in the perinatal period. Am J Obstet Gynecol 2016; 215(5):539–47.
14. Mozurkewich EL, Rayburn WF. Buprenorphine and methadone for opioid addiction during pregnancy. Obstet Gynecol Clin North Am 2014;41(2):241–53.
15. Substance Abuse and Mental Health Services Administration (SAMHSA). A collaborative approach to the treatment of pregnant women with opioid use disorders. HHS Publication No. (SMA)16-4978. Rockville (MD): SAMHSA; 2016. Available at: https://ncsacw.samsha.gov/files/Collaborative_Approach_508.pdf. Accessed August 10, 2017.

16. Fullerton CA, Kim M, Thomas CP, et al. Medication-assisted treatment with methadone: assessing the evidence. Psychiatr Serv 2014;65(2):146–57.
17. Thomas CP, Fullerton CA, Kim M, et al. Medication-assisted treatment with buprenorphine: assessing the evidence. Psychiatr Serv 2014;65(2):158–70.
18. US Food and Drug Administration (FDA). What is the federal government doing to combat the opioid abuse epidemic? U.S. Food and Drug Administration; 2015. Available at: http://www.fda.gov/newsevents/testimony/ucm446076.htm. Accessed September 8, 2017.
19. Jones HE, Kaltenbach K, Heil SH, et al. Neonatal abstinence syndrome after methadone or buprenorphine exposure. N Engl J Med 2010;363(24): 2320–31.
20. Jones HE, Dengler E, Garrison A, et al. Neonatal outcomes and their relationship to maternal buprenorphine dose during pregnancy. Drug Alcohol Depend 2014; 334:414–7.
21. Bakstad B, Sarfi M, Welle-Strand GK, et al. Opioid maintenance treatment during pregnancy: occurrence and severity of neonatal abstinence syndrome. A national prospective study. Eur Addict Res 2009;15(3):128–34.
22. Huybrechts KF, Bateman BT, Desai RJ, et al. Risk of neonatal withdrawal after intrauterine co-exposure to opioids and psychotropic medications: cohort study. BMJ 2017;358:j3326.
23. Kampman K, Jarvis M. American Society of Addiction Medicine (ASAM) national practice guideline for the use of medications in the treatment of addiction involving opioid use. J Addict Med 2015;9(5):358–67.
24. World Health Organization (WHO). Guidelines for identification and management of substance use and substance use disorders in pregnancy. Geneva (Switzerland): World Health Organization; 2014.
25. Title 21 code of federal regulations. US Drug Enforcement Administration Web site. Available at: http://deadiversion.usdoj.gov/21cfr/cfr/1306/1306_07.htm. Accessed September 8, 2017.
26. Harper RG, Solish GI, Purow HM, et al. The effect of a methadone treatment program upon pregnant heroin addicts and their newborn infants. Pediatrics 1974; 54:300–5.
27. Substance abuse confidentiality regulations. Substance Abuse and Mental Health Services Administration Web. 2016. Available at: http://www.samhsa.gov/about-us/who-we-are/laws/confidentiality-regulations-faqs. Accessed August 10, 2017.
28. Bell JR, Butler B, Lawrance A, et al. Comparing overdose mortality associated with methadone and buprenorphine treatment. Drug Alcohol Depend 2009; 104(1–2):73–7.
29. Wiegand SL, Stringer EM, Stuebe AM, et al. Buprenorphine and naloxone compared with methadone treatment in pregnancy. Obstet Gynecol 2015; 125(2):363–8.
30. Lund IO, Fischer G, Welle-Strand GK, et al. A comparison of buprenorphine + naloxone to buprenorphine and methadone in the treatment of opioid dependence during pregnancy: maternal and neonatal outcomes. Subst Abuse 2013;6:61–74.
31. Debelak K, Morrone WR, O'Grady KE, et al. Buprenorphine + naloxone compared with methadone treatment during pregnancy – initial patient care and outcome data. Am J Addict 2013;22(3):252–4.
32. Chavoustie S, Frost M, Snyder O, et al. Buprenorphine implants in medical treatment of opioid addiction. Expert Rev Clin Pharmacol 2017;10(8):799–807.

33. Rosenthal RN, Lofwall MR, Kim S, et al. Effect of buprenorphine implants on illicit opioid use among abstinent adults with opioid dependence treated with sublingual buprenorphine: a randomized clinical trial. JAMA 2016;316(3):282–90.

34. Zedler BK, Mann AL, Kim MM, et al. Buprenorphine compared with methadone to treat pregnant women with opioid use disorder: a systematic review and meta-analysis of safety in the mother, fetus and child. Addiction 2016;111(12):2115–28.

35. Minozzi S, Amato L, Bellisario C, et al. Maintenance agonist treatments for opiate-dependent pregnant women. Cochrane Database Syst Rev 2013;(12):CD0006318.

36. Albright B, de la Torre L, Skipper B, et al. Changes in methadone maintenance therapy during and after pregnancy. J Subst Abuse Treat 2011;41(4):347–53.

37. Wolff K, Boys A, Rostami-Hodjegan A, et al. Changes to methadone clearance during pregnancy. Eur J Clin Pharmacol 2005;61(10):763–8.

38. Bastian JR, Chen H, Zhang H, et al. Dose-adjusted plasma concentrations of sublingual buprenorphine are lower during than after pregnancy. Am J Obstet Gynecol 2017;216(1):64.e1-7.

39. Caritis SN, Bastian JR, Zhang H, et al. An evidence-based recommendation to increase the dosing frequency of buprenorphine during pregnancy. Am J Obstet Gynecol 2017. https://doi.org/10.1016/j.ajog.2017.06.029.

40. McCarthy JJ, Leamon MH, Willits HN, et al. The effect of methadone dose regimen on neonatal abstinence syndrome. J Addict Med 2015;9(2):105–10.

41. Cleary BJ, Donnelly J, Strawbridge J, et al. Methadone dose and neonatal abstinence syndrome – systematic review and meta-analysis. Addiction 2010;105(12):2071–84.

42. O'Connor AB, O'Brien L, Alto WA. Maternal buprenorphine dose at delivery and its relationship to neonatal outcomes. Eur Addict Res 2016;22(3):127–30.

43. Logan BA, Brown MS, Hayes MJ. Neonatal abstinence syndrome: treatment and pediatric outcomes. Clin Obstet Gynecol 2013;56(1):186–92.

44. Maguire DJ, Taylor S, Armstrong K, et al. Long-term outcomes of infants with neonatal abstinence syndrome. Neonatal Netw 2016;35(5):277–86.

45. Oei JL, Melhuish E, Uebel H, et al. Neonatal abstinence syndrome and high school performance. Pediatrics 2017;139(2). https://doi.org/10.1542/peds.2016-2651.

46. Rementeria JL, Nunag NN. Narcotic withdrawal in pregnancy: stillbirth incidence with a case report. Am J Obstet Gynecol 1973;116:1152–6.

47. Luty J, Nikolaou V, Bearn J. Is opiate detoxification unsafe in pregnancy? J Subst Abuse Treat 2003;24(4):363–7.

48. Bell J, Towers CV, Hennessy MD, et al. Detoxification from opiate drugs during pregnancy. Am J Obstet Gynecol 2016;215(3):374.e1-6.

49. Stewart RD, Nelson DB, Adjikari EH, et al. The obstetrical and neonatal impact of maternal opioid detoxification in pregnancy. Am J Obstet Gynecol 2013;209(3):267.e1-5.

50. Jones HE, O'Grady KE, Malfi D, et al. Methadone maintenance vs. methadone taper during pregnancy: maternal and neonatal outcomes. Am J Addict 2008;17(5):372–86.

51. Jones HE, Terplan M, Meyer M. Medically assisted withdrawal (detoxification): considering the mother-infant dyad. J Addict Med 2017;11(2):90–2.

52. Welle-Strand GK, Skurtveit S, Tanum L, et al. Tapering from methadone or buprenorphine during pregnancy: maternal and neonatal outcomes in Norway 1996-2009. Eur Addict Res 2015;21(5):253–61.

53. Jones HE, Chisolm MS, Jansson LM, et al. Naltrexone in the treatment of opioid-dependent pregnant women: the case for a considered and measured approach to research. Addiction 2013;108(2):233–47.

54. Rea F, Bell JR, Young MR, et al. A randomised, controlled trial of low dose naltrexone for the treatment of opioid dependence. Drug Alcohol Depend 2004;75(1):79–88.

55. Vickers BP, Jolly A. Naltrexone and problems in pain management. BMJ 2006; 332(7534):132–3.

56. Kelty E, Hulse G. A retrospective cohort study of obstetric outcomes in opioid-dependent women treated with implant naltrexone, oral methadone or sublingual buprenorphine, and non-dependent controls. Drugs 2017;77(11): 1199–210.

57. El-Mohandes A, Herman AA, Nabil El-Khorazaty M, et al. Prenatal care reduces the impact of illicit drug use on perinatal outcomes. J Perinatol 2003;23(5): 354–60.

58. ACOG Committee on Health Care for Underserved Women. ACOG committee opinion no. 473. Substance abuse reporting and pregnancy: the role of the obstetrician-gynecologist. Obstet Gynecol 2011;117(1):200–1.

59. Zhang C, Brook JS, Leukefeld CG, et al. Associations between compulsive buying and substance dependence/abuse, major depressive episodes, and generalized anxiety disorder among men and women. J Addict Dis 2016; 35(4):298–304.

60. Benningfield MM, Arria AM, Kaltenbach K, et al. Co-occurring psychiatric symptoms are associated with increased psychological, social, and medical impairment in opioid dependent pregnant women. Am J Addict 2010;19(5):416–21.

61. Holbrook A, Kaltenbach K. Co-occurring psychiatric symptoms in opioid-dependent women: the prevalence of antenatal and postnatal depression. Am J Drug Alcohol Abuse 2012;38(6):575–9.

62. Torchalla I, Linden IA, Strehlau V, et al. "Like a lots happened in my whole childhood": violence, trauma and addiction in pregnant and postpartum women from Vancouver's Downtown Eastside. Harm Reduct J 2015;12:1.

63. Salihu HM, Wilson RE. Epidemiology of prenatal smoking and perinatal outcomes. Early Hum Dev 2007;83(11):713–20.

64. Chisolm MS, Fitzsimons H, Leoutsakos JM, et al. A comparison of cigarette smoking profiles in opioid-dependent pregnant patients receiving methadone or buprenorphine. Nicotine Tob Res 2013;15(7):1297–304.

65. Substance Abuse and Mental Health Services Administration (SAMHSA). Results from the 2012 National survey on drug use and health. Summary of national findings. NSDUH series H-46, HHS. Publication No. (SMA) 13-4795. Rockville (MD): SAMHSA; 2013.

66. Akerman SC, Brunette MF, Green AI, et al. Treating tobacco use disorder in pregnant women in medication-assisted treatment for an opioid use disorder: a systematic review. J Subst Abuse Treat 2015;52:40–7.

67. Winklbaur B, Baewert A, Jagsch R, et al. Association between prenatal tobacco exposure and outcomes of neonates born to opioid-maintained mothers. Implications for treatment. Eur Addict Res 2009;15(3):150–6.

68. Choo RE, Huestis MA, Schroeder JR, et al. Neonatal abstinence syndrome in methadone-exposed infants is altered by level of prenatal tobacco exposure. Drug Alcohol Depend 2004;75(3):253–60.

69. Jones HE, Heil SH, Tuten M, et al. Cigarette smoking in opioid-dependent pregnant women: neonatal and maternal outcomes. Drug Alcohol Depend 2013; 131(3):271–7.
70. Holbrook AM, Baxter JK, Jones HE, et al. Infections and obstetric outcomes in opioid-dependent pregnant women maintained on methadone or buprenorphine. Addiction 2012;107(S1):83–90.
71. Page K, Leeman L, Bishop S, et al. Hepatitis C cascade of care among pregnant women on opioid agonist pharmacotherapy attending a comprehensive prenatal program. Matern Child Health J 2017. https://doi.org/10.1007/s10995-017-2316-x.
72. Muller-Lissner S, Bassotti G, Coffin B, et al. Opioid-induced constipation and bowel dysfunction: a clinical guideline. Pain Med 2016. https://doi.org/10.1093/pm/pnw255.
73. Lind JN, Interrante JD, Ailes EC, et al. Maternal use of opioids during pregnancy and congenital malformations: a systematic review. Pediatrics 2017;139(6). https://doi.org/10.1542/peds.2016-4131.
74. Mactier H, Shipton D, Dryden C, et al. Reduced fetal growth in methadone-maintained pregnancies is not fully explained by smoking or socio-economic depravation. Addiction 2014;109(3):482–8.
75. Liu AJ, Sithamparanathan S, Jones MP, et al. Growth restriction in pregnancies of opioid-dependent mothers. Arch Dis Child Fetal Neonatal Ed 2010;95(4):F258–62.
76. Jansson LM, Velez M, McConnell K, et al. Maternal buprenorphine treatment and fetal neurobehavioral development. Am J Obstet Gynecol 2017;216(5):529.e1-8.
77. Jansson LM, Dipietro J, Elko A. Fetal response to maternal methadone administration. Am J Obstet Gynecol 2005;193(3 Pt 1):611–7.
78. Terplan M, Longinaker N, Appel L. Women-centered drug treatment services and need in the United States, 2002-2009. Am J Public Health 2015;105(11):e50–4.
79. Jones HE, Johnson RE, Milio L. Post-cesarean pain management of patients maintained on methadone or buprenorphine. Am J Addict 2006;15(3):528–9.
80. Pan A, Zakowski M. Peripartum anesthetic management of the opioid-tolerant of buprenorphine/suboxone-dependent patient. Clin Obstet Gynecol 2017;60(2):447–58.
81. Ramirez-Cacho WA, Flores S, Schrader RM, et al. Effect of chronic methadone therapy on intrapartum fetal heart rate patterns. J Soc Gynecol Investig 2006;13(2):108–11.
82. Meyer M, Wagner K, Benvenuto A, et al. Intrapartum and postpartum analgesia for women maintained on buprenorphine during pregnancy. Obstet Gynecol 2007;110(2Pt1):261–6.
83. Meyer M, Paranya G, Keefer Norris A, et al. Intrapartum and postpartum analgesia for women maintained on buprenorphine during pregnancy. Eur J Pain 2010;14(9):939–43.
84. Jones HE, Johnson RE, O'Grady KE, et al. Dosing adjustments in postpartum patients maintained on buprenorphine or methadone. J Addict Med 2008;2(2):103–7.
85. Alford DP, Compton P, Samet JH. Acute pain management for patients receiving maintenance methadone or buprenorphine therapy. Ann Intern Med 2006;144(2):127–34.

86. Jones HE, O'Grady K, Dahne J, et al. Management of acute postpartum pain in patients maintained on methadone or buprenorphine during pregnancy. Am J Drug Alcohol Abuse 2009;35(3):151–6.
87. Bagley SM, Wachman EM, Holland E, et al. Review of the assessment and management of neonatal abstinence syndrome. Addict Sci Clin Pract 2014;9(1):19.
88. O'Conner AB, Collett A, Alto WA, et al. Breastfeeding rates and the relationship between breastfeeding and neonatal abstinence syndrome in women being maintained on buprenorphine during pregnancy. J Midwifery Womens Health 2013;58(4):383–8.
89. American Academy of Pediatrics (AAP) Committee on Drugs. Transfer of drugs and other chemicals into human milk. Pediatrics 2001;108(3):776–89.
90. Kahn LS, Mendel WE, Fallin KL, et al. A parenting education program for women in treatment for opioid-use disorder at an outpatient medical practice. Soc Work Health Care 2017;56(7):649–65.
91. Terplan M, Hand DJ, Hutchinson M, et al. Contraceptive use and method choice among women with opioid and other substance use disorders: a systematic review. Prev Med 2015;80:23–31.
92. Matusiewicz AK, Melbostad HS, Heil SH. Knowledge of and concerns about long-acting reversible contraception among women in medication–assisted treatment for opioid use disorder. Contraception 2017. https://doi.org/10.1016/j.contraception.2017.07.167.
93. Bateman BT, Cole NM, Maeda A, et al. Patterns of opioid prescription and use after cesarean delivery. Obstet Gynecol 2017;130(1):29–35.
94. Osmundson SS, Schornack LA, Grasch JL, et al. Postdischarge opioid use after cesarean delivery. Obstet Gynecol 2017;130(1):36–41.
95. Prabhu M, McQuaid-Hanson E, Hopp S, et al. A shared decision-making intervention to guide opioid prescribing after cesarean delivery. Obstet Gynecol 2017;130(1):42–6.
96. Ko JY, Wolicki S, Barfield WD, et al. CDC grand rounds: public health strategies to prevent neonatal abstinence syndrome. MMWR Morb Mortal Wkly Rep 2017;66(9):242–5.
97. Wisconsin Medical Examining Board Opioid Prescribing Guideline – November 16, 2016. 2016. State of Wisconsin Department of Safety and Professional Services. Available at: www.dsps.wi.gov/Documents/Board%20Services/Other%20Resources/MEB/20161116_MEB_Guidelines_v4.pdf. Accessed August 11, 2017.
98. Centers for Disease Control and Prevention (CDC). CDC guidelines for prescribing opioids for chronic pain – United States, 2016. Centers for Disease Control and Prevention. 2016. Available at: www.cdc.gov/mmwr/volumes/65/rr/rr6501e1.htm. Accessed September 8, 2017.
99. Kallen B, Reis M. Ongoing pharmacological management of chronic pain in pregnancy. Drugs 2016;76(9):915–24.
100. Pritham UA, McKay L. Safe management of chronic pain in the pregnancy in an era of opioid misuse and abuse. J Obstet Gynecol Neonatal Nurs 2014;43(5):554–67.

Preventing Opioid Overdose in the Clinic and Hospital

Analgesia and Opioid Antagonists

Stephanie Lee Peglow, DO, MPH[a],*,
Ingrid A. Binswanger, MD, MPH, MS[b,c]

KEYWORDS

- Opioid overdose • Naloxone • Overdose education • Harm reduction
- Opioid prescribing • Prevention of overdose

KEY POINTS

- Tailor opioid overdose preventive efforts to patients' individual stage of opioid therapy or involvement; not all interventions are universally appropriate.
- Consider risk stratification when treating pain with opioids.
- Apply appropriate harm-reduction strategies, such as prescribing naloxone, to patients as risk for overdose.
- Consider treatment of opioid use disorders with pharmacotherapy in your own practice.

INTRODUCTION

North America has experienced an overdose epidemic linked across countries related to increased opioid pharmaceutical marketing, opioid prescribing, prescribed and illicit opioid use, and opioid trafficking.[1] As a result, greater than 2 million United States inhabitants met criteria for opioid use disorder (OUD) and nearly 5% of US adults reported nonmedical use of opioids in 2013.[2] US opioid advertising campaigns and

This article originally appeared in *Medical Clinics*, Volume 102, Issue 4, July 2018.
Disclosure Statement: Dr S.L. Peglow was supported by the Veterans Administration Mental Illness, Research, Education and Clinical Center and by Research in Addiction Medicine Scholars Program-R25DA033211. Dr I.A. Binswanger is supported by the National Institute On Drug Abuse of the National Institutes of Health under Award Number R01DA042059. The content is solely the responsibilities of the authors and does not necessarily represent the official views of the National Institutes of Health. Dr I.A. Binswanger is currently employed by the Colorado Permanente Medical Group.
^a Department of Psychiatry and Behavioral Sciences, Eastern Virginia Medical School, 825 Fairfax Avenue Suite 710, Norfolk, VA 23507, USA; ^b Institute for Health Research, Kaiser Permanente Colorado, 2550 South Parker Road, Suite 200, Aurora, CO 80014, USA; ^c Division of General Internal Medicine, Department of Medicine, University of Colorado, 12631 East 17th Avenue, Academic Office One, Campus Box B180, Aurora, CO 80045, USA
* Corresponding author.
E-mail address: Peglowsl@evms.edu

prescribing patterns have spread to Canada.[3] In 2012 it was estimated 75,000 to 125,000 Canadians injected drugs, and another 200,000 had OUDs because of pharmaceutical opioids.[4] In Mexico, estimates suggest that 100,000 people use illicit opioids and an increasing number of those use heroin.[1]

In the United States, a large proportion of individuals who use illicit pharmaceutical opioids (68%) report they received the prescription drug from a friend or family member who was prescribed it by their doctor.[5] Those that reported heavy, nonmedical opioid use reported that their primary source was direct physician prescribing.[6] Thus, physicians have the responsibility to prevent the potential harms of opioids by using sound preventive strategies.

This article describes opioid overdose preventive strategies for medical providers (**Fig. 1**), with a particular focus on special populations, such as youth and pregnant women. Opioid overdose can occur in any point along the continuum of use, from opioid naivety to long-term opioid use for pain to OUD (**Box 1**). Furthermore, overdose is caused by a range of factors, including drug interactions, use via injection route, and intentional overdose. We summarize current preventive strategies medical providers in primary care may use to reduce risk throughout the continuum of opioid use and across a range of contributing factors.

We highlight opioid prescribing guidelines from the Veterans Affairs/Department of Defense, Centers for Disease Control and Prevention (CDC), and Canadian Guidelines, last updated February 2017, March 2016, and 2017, respectively.[7–9] The recommendations within these guidelines are largely based on observational data; hence the quality of the evidence supporting many recommendations is still moderately weak.[10] In addition, overdose prevention research is evolving and recommendations may change based on results from ongoing and new studies. Importantly, existing guidelines focus heavily on limiting prescribing, but a one-size-fits-all approach may not be appropriate or feasible, nor address other facets of the opioid epidemic, such as increasing heroin and nonprescribed fentanyl use. Furthermore, we acknowledge that counseling patients about overdose risk and meeting all opioid prescribing

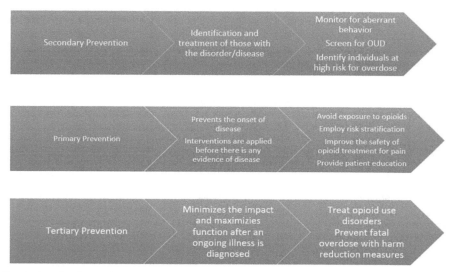

Fig. 1. Levels of overdose prevention.

Box 1
Definitions

Chronic opioid use: "Daily or near-daily use of opioids for at least 90 days, often indefinitely."[12] Chronic opioid use should be distinguished from an OUD; although it may be associated with tolerance and/or physiologic withdrawal, it does not necessarily involve the other social, behavioral, and compulsive characteristics of an OUD.

Nonmedical use of opioids (or misuse): "Use of a medication (for a medical purpose) other than as directed or as indicated, whether willful or unintentional, and whether harm results or not."[12] Nonmedical use may occur in individuals with or without an OUD.

Aberrant use: "A behavior outside the boundaries of the agreed on treatment plan which is established as early as possible in the doctor-patient relationship."[12] Aberrant use by someone prescribed opioids does not necessarily define an OUD but may raise a provider's concerns that that individual is developing an OUD.

Diversion: "The intentional transfer of a controlled substance from legitimate distribution and dispensing channels."[12] Individuals with and without OUDs may engage in diversion.

---

guidelines may be difficult in busy primary care practices, particularly in the face of other competing demands.[11]

PRIMARY PREVENTION MEASURES
Minimizing Exposure to Opioids Among People Who Are Opioid Naive or Do Not Have an Opioid Use Disorder

Prescribed opioids are associated with an overall 5.5% risk of addiction[8] and a 0.2% risk of fatal overdose at a mean of 2.6 years after initial opioid prescription.[13] Even opioids prescribed at hospital discharge are associated with an increased risk of chronic opioid use 1 year later.[14] Avoiding exposure to opioids may reduce incidence of addiction and death from overdose, hence the first strong recommendation in all three guidelines is nonpharmacologic therapy for pain, such as physical therapy, and, when medications are needed, nonopioid pharmacotherapy, such as acetaminophen or nonsteroidal anti-inflammatory drugs.[7–9,15]

History Taking and Risk Evaluation and Mitigation

If opioids are needed for pain, then providers should conduct a thorough history and evaluate the risk of aberrant behavior and overdose (**Box 2**). The Substance Abuse and Mental Health Services Administration[5] toolkit for providers suggests including specific questions about alcohol and over-the-counter medications.[5] To help evaluate the risk of aberrant behavior, commonly used tools are the Screener and Opioid Assessment for Patients with Pain[16] and the Opioid Risk Tool.[9] Prescription opioids taken in combination with benzodiazepines were found in 30% of opioid overdoses,[6] and coprescribing increases the risk of fatal and nonfatal overdose.[17] Thus, to mitigate risk, providers should consider alternatives to either benzodiazepines or opioids when coprescribing both medications.[8,15]

Patient Education and Informed Consent

If opioids are used, it is helpful to establish treatment goals, discuss risks and realistic benefits, and consider how opioids will be discontinued if benefits do not outweigh risks.[8,9] This discussion should include the responsibilities of the patient and the doctor; potential side effects including sedation, addiction, motor vehicle accidents, and

---

Box 2
Risk groups for overdose

- Chronic medical illness (pulmonary, renal, or hepatic)[18]
- History of substance use disorder[19]
- History of psychiatric disorder[20]
- Controlled substance prescriptions from multiple providers[21]
- Prescribed a combination of opioids and benzodiazepines[21]
- High daily dosages of opioids[21]
- Long-acting and extended-released opioid formulations[22]
- Illicit drug use[23]
- Recent history of incarceration[24]
- History of prior overdose[23]

---

death; limited evidence showing long-term benefits for chronic pain; and the risk of respiratory depression when combined with sedatives.[8,9]

Considerations on Prescribing Practices to Reduce Overdose Risk

Both dose and duration have a dose-dependent effect on development of overdose, but duration seems to be a stronger predictor of OUD.[8,25] Partially because of this, Canadian, Veterans Affairs/Department of Defense, and CDC recommend an upper limit to opioid prescribing (90-mg morphine equivalent dosing). Although research consensus is lacking, there is some evidence that extended-release or long-acting formulations may increase risk of unintentional overdose[22]; thus the Veterans Affairs and CDC guidelines advise against using longer acting formulations.[9] A recent intervention that combined nursing care management, an electronic registry, academic detailing, and electronic decision support tools demonstrated increased adherence to opioid guidelines compared with the group receiving electronic decision support only.[26]

Safe Storage Practices and Reducing Household Exposure

Parents are an important source of pharmaceutical opioids to children. Exposure may occur through two routes: intentional sharing of opioids for a treatment of a child's minor aches and pains, or by diversion of pills by an adolescent from their parent's prescription.[27] Counseling on safe storage and disposal practices when providing opioids to an adult with children in the home is also important to protect household members from risky, inadvertent, or recreational exposure.[27]

Educational Strategies to Prevent Risky Use in Adolescents

Brief universal preventive interventions administered during middle school have been shown to reduce prescription drug misuse among adolescents and young adults.[28] The American Academy of Pediatrics suggests providers echo these clear and consistent nonuse messages and provide Screening, Brief Intervention, and Referral to Treatment to their adolescent patients.[29] CRAFFT, an age-appropriate Screening, Brief Intervention, and Referral to Treatment intervention, can be used as a screener.[30] In those found to be of low risk, brief negotiated interviews may be helpful to reduce risky use of opioids; those of higher risk should be referred to treatment.[29]

SECONDARY PREVENTION MEASURES
Urine Drug Test

Substance misuse has been shown to be 30% or greater in patients prescribed long-term opiates.[31] Although urine drug testing has not been robustly shown to reduce opioid misuse as a stand-alone intervention,[31] urine toxicology at initiation of opioids and periodically throughout treatment with appropriate confirmatory testing can help identify patients who warrant further education about opioid safety, evaluation for a substance use disorder (SUD), and referral for treatment.[32] Barriers to use of urine toxicology include provider discomfort discussing results, lack of access to testing, inadequate knowledge on how to interpret results, and belief that one's patients are not at risk of misuse or illicit use.[31] In addition, misinterpretation of results or lack of confirmatory testing may lead to falsely accusing patients of diversion or illicit use, hence restricting care to patients and breaking down the therapeutic alliance.[31]

Prescription Monitoring Programs

Evidence on state-wide prescription monitoring programs (PMP) suggests that they have potential to change prescribing behaviors and identify patients at risk for overdose.[15] Although it is still not known if implementation or use decreases overdose deaths, research has suggested some positive effects in isolated states.[33–35] Thus, the CDC guidelines suggest checking PMP at the initiation of opioid therapy and at intervals of no greater than 3 months while on treatment.[9] The utility of PMPs can be limited. Providers may be unaware of their existence and have difficulty accessing data from other states. In addition, reporting to these systems can be limited.[36] These systems also have the potential to lead to inadequate pain care. For example, providers may inappropriately label patients as "doctor shoppers" or become uncomfortable prescribing opioids because they are required to access the system and face risks of criminal sanctions for overprescribing.[36]

Identifying Nonmedical Opioid Use and Opioid Use Disorders

Aberrant behavior has an estimated prevalence of 11.5% among patients prescribed chronic opioid therapy,[37] but patients on chronic opioid therapy may be reluctant to disclose risk behavior to their prescribing providers.[38] Integrating loved ones into follow-up can bring the provider's attention to worrisome behaviors and medication use practices. Two screeners have been shown to help identify potential nonmedical use, the Pain Assessment and Documentation Tool and the Current Opioid Misuse Measure.[39,40] Providers should evaluate those patients identified with nonmedical or aberrant use for OUD and refer those with OUD to treatment, or initiate OUD treatment in their practices.

Continued Evaluation of Opioid Risk/Benefit Profile and Considering Tapering

The CDC suggests that the marker of clinical improvement is a 30% improvement in both pain and function.[9] If these milestones are not achieved with opioid treatment optimization, the physician may consider opioid discontinuation.[9] These functional outcomes can be measured with the Pain Average, Interference with Enjoyment of Life[41] and Interference with General Activity Assessment Scale.[42]

When the risks of long-term opioid therapy outweigh benefits, opioid tapering may be considered. Although there are concerns about patients transitioning to heroin after being discontinued or rapidly tapered from opioids,[43] several strategies are successful in tapering opioids, such as weekly dose reductions of 10% to 50% of total daily dose.[9] To address patients' concerns of increased pain and withdrawal, support from a trusted health care provider and social support can facilitate a successful opioid taper.[44] One review suggested improvement in pain severity, function, and quality of life after dose tapering.[45]

TERTIARY PREVENTION
Naloxone

Naloxone is an effective, short-acting opioid antagonist that is used for overdose reversal. Based on the successful experience of community-based overdose education and naloxone distribution programs,[18,46] which have traditionally targeted people using heroin and other illicit opioids, naloxone is increasingly being prescribed to patients at risk in medical settings. There is evidence to support community-based overdose education and naloxone distribution programs.[18] For example, in Massachusetts, communities with high concentrations of naloxone distribution to lay bystanders seemed to have reduced overdose rates.[47] Studies have shown that educating lay bystanders about naloxone increases knowledge about how to identify and treat an opioid overdose, with scores that were similar to those of medical experts.[48,49] Trained individuals have been able to successfully diffuse this information within their communities.[50] Outside of community settings, naloxone has been feasibly implemented in community emergency department settings[51] and primary care.[41,52]

Although the optimal patient groups for naloxone prescription have not yet been determined, naloxone may be considered for patients started on chronic opioid therapy and those who are in the process of tapering or have recently discontinued opioid therapy. Providers may opt to prescribe naloxone to individuals with risk factors for opioid overdose (see **Box 2**). **Table 1** shows groups suggested for naloxone by recent guidelines. In US states where laws allow for it, physicians may prescribe naloxone to family members and lay persons (**Fig. 2**). For medical providers, the liability risks of prescribing naloxone seem limited.[53] Furthermore, some states have implemented standing orders, under which individuals can obtain naloxone from a pharmacy without getting an individual prescription from their provider.

Providers may be concerned about increasing risk behavior as a result of naloxone prescribing,[11] whereas patients may be concerned about the stigma associated with receiving naloxone.[38] In one study, coprescribing naloxone with chronic opioid therapy for noncancer pain was associated with reduced opioid-related emergency department visits.[52] Although the reasons for this reduction are unknown, it may be partially caused by the education provided with naloxone, because overdose education combined with motivational interviewing has been shown to reduce self-reported opioid overdose risk behaviors and nonmedical use of prescription opioids.[54]

Naloxone is available in different formulations. Although the auto-injector and nasal spray are easy to use and avoid the risk of needle stick injuries, the auto-injector is costly and both have variable insurance coverage.[55] Substance Abuse and Mental Health Services Administration has issued an Opioid Overdose Prevention Toolkit[56] and Prescribe to Prevent (prescribetoprevent.org) provides Continuing Medical Education for medical providers.

Treatment of Opioid Use Disorders

Opioid agonist treatment (including methadone and buprenorphine) effectively decreases opioid use and reduces the risk of overdose and death in those with OUDs.[57] However, these modalities are vastly underused.[58] For buprenorphine, management may occur in primary care settings. In the United States, a buprenorphine

Table 1
Patient groups to consider for naloxone prescribing, by guidelines

CDC[9]	Veterans Affairs/ Department of Defense[7]	Canadian[8]
• Prescribed doses of greater or equal to 50-mg morphine equivalents • Personal history of previous overdose • History of substance use disorder or concurrent use of benzodiazepines • Relatives of family members with OUD in states where third party prescribing is allowed	• Starting chronic opioid therapy • Tapering or have recently discontinued opioid therapy	• High-dose opioid therapy • Comorbidities • During opioid rotation • OUD • Recreational opioid use • Intravenous drug use

Drug Enforcement Administration[28] waiver is required for health care practitioners. In Canada, specialized training is suggested but not required.[59] Buprenorphine provided in primary care has been shown to be safe and effective.[60] In the United States, providers have to refer to specialized methadone treatment centers for their patients to access methadone for addiction.[61] Primary care providers can prescribe the opioid antagonist naltrexone in daily oral or monthly injectable form without special licenses, although evidence for reduced overdose rates with naltrexone is currently lacking.

Reducing Risk After Nonfatal Overdose

Those with a previous overdose are commonly considered a high-risk group for repeat overdose; of those prescribed opioids, most continue to be prescribed opioids after overdose.[62] The CDC recommends clinicians work with these patients to reduce

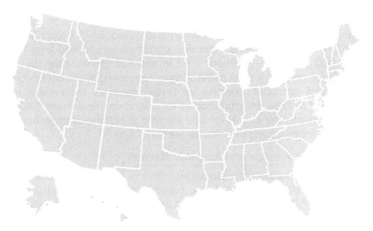

Fig. 2. States that give immunity to prescribers for prescribing naloxone to lay persons (in *green*) as of July 1, 2017. This figure was created under a Creative Commons Attribution-4.0 International License. (*Adapted from* Prescription drug abuse policy system (PDAPS). Legal Science, LLC. Naloxone overdose prevention laws. Available at: http://j.mp/2hDyf2N. Accessed September 30, 2017; with permission.)

opioid dosage and prescribe naloxone.[9] If opioids are continued, providers should consider incorporating risk mitigation strategies and carefully considering the risks versus benefits of ongoing opioid therapy.[9]

SPECIAL POPULATIONS
Patients with Psychiatric Disorders

Patients with comorbid psychiatric disorders are more likely to receive an opioid for pain than those without mental health diagnoses,[63] and are more likely to receive higher dose opioids, multiple opioids, and benzodiazepines with opioids.[64,65] Patients with psychiatric disorders are also less likely to benefit from opioids,[66] are more likely to misuse opioids and develop an OUD,[67] and are more likely to attempt suicide.[68] Guidelines suggest caution in prescribing opioids to those with active, uncontrolled psychiatric illness.[7–9] Alternative therapies are preferred, such as tricyclic or serotonin and norepinephrine reuptake inhibitor antidepressants for patient with chronic pain and depression/anxiety. Opioid therapy in this population necessitates more frequent follow-up, monitoring, and observation.[8,9] When available, consider referring patients with psychiatric conditions to addiction medicine/psychiatry or other behavioral health specialists.[7] Complimentary treatment of chronic pain with movement, exercise, and cognitive-behavioral therapy for pain may help pain and mood outcomes and reduce suicide risk.[69]

Adolescents and Young Adults

Opioid use is common among adolescents.[61,70] Adolescents prescribed opioids had a 33% increase in misuse of opiates after high school[71]; the earlier the exposure to opioids the higher the risk of developing misuse and dependence.[7,25,72] All guidelines suggest avoiding opioids in adolescents when possible, and when it is not possible, frequent monitoring and dispensing, close monitoring for aberrancies, and tapering as early as clinically appropriate.[7–9]

Elderly Patients

Pain management is difficult in the elderly because of increased risks of opioid and nonopioid therapies.[73] Because of physiologic changes, opioids may accumulate and increase risk of respiratory depression and overdose.[74] Polypharmacy may increase risk of medication interactions and cognitive errors may lead to medication dosages beyond what is prescribed.[9,59,75] In patients greater than 65 years of age, additional caution and increased monitoring is suggested when prescribing opioids.[9] Prescribers might consider exercise or bowel regimes to prevent constipation, assessing for risk of falls, and monitoring for cognitive impairment.[9] Suggestions to improve safety among the elderly include starting at half the starting dose of younger populations, and considering codeine or tramadol first.[7,8]

Women of Reproductive Age and Pregnant Women

Opioids used in pregnancy are associated with low birth weight, stillbirth, poor fetal growth, preterm delivery, birth defects, cardiac abnormalities, and neonatal abstinence syndrome.[76] Severe withdrawal from opioids has been associated with premature labor and spontaneous abortion.[8] If a woman is planning to become pregnant, providers may consider opioid tapering and discontinuation before pregnancy.[8] For women already taking opioids and pregnant, providers may consider referral or specialized consultation before considering tapering/discontinuing opioids because of potential fetal risks. If a pregnant woman is determined to have an OUD, urgent referral to buprenorphine or methadone management is especially important because these therapies have been associated with improved outcomes.[77] However, naltrexone is not recommended.[9,78] Codeine is be avoided in breastfeeding mothers, because of possibility of neonatal toxicity and death,[8] but breastfeeding is encouraged in mothers prescribed buprenorphine or methadone.[79]

Patients with Active Substance Use Disorders

Patients with untreated SUDs have significant risk of developing an OUD or experiencing and overdose, suicide, and other cause of mortality.[8,19,63,80] Patients with past SUD history, especially if recent, prolonged, or severe, also have elevated risk.[8,80,81] Screening for recent SUDs is as simple as a single question "How many times in the past year have you used an illegal drug or used a prescription medication for nonmedical reasons?"[82] Other options for screening include the Drug Abuse Screening Test or the Alcohol Use Disorders Identification Test.[9,59,83,84] Guidelines strongly suggest against opioids for chronic noncancer pain in people with an active SUD[7,8] because of the risk of addiction to opioids. After nonpharmacologic or nonopioid options, codeine and tramadol are first line for patients with SUD. If higher potency is required, morphine is preferred to oxycodone or hydromorphone.[8,59] Referrals are encouraged for patients with continued pain despite buprenorphine and minimal counseling in the primary care setting and for those with comorbid active SUDs when available.[7] Unfortunately, successful referral is difficult in clinical practice because access to these services is limited.[85]

SUMMARY

Prescribers have an important role in prevention of OUDs and opioid overdose. These strategies include minimizing opioid exposure for opioid-naive patients, using risk-mitigation and harm-reduction strategies, and treating OUD. Given that not all interventions are universally appropriate, it is important to consider tailoring preventive efforts to match the individual's stage of opioid involvement.

ACKNOWLEDGMENT

The editors thank Antonio Quidgley-Nevares, Eastern Virginia Medical School, for providing a critical review of this article.

REFERENCES

1. Vashishtha D, Mittal ML, Werb D. The North American opioid epidemic: current challenges and a call for treatment as prevention. Harm Reduct J 2017;14(1):7.
2. Han B, Compton WM, Jones CM, et al. Nonmedical prescription opioid use and use disorders among adults aged 18 through 64 years in the United States, 2003-2013. JAMA 2015;314(14):1468–78.
3. Van Zee A. The promotion and marketing of oxycontin: commercial triumph, public health tragedy. Am J Public Health 2009;99(2):221–7.
4. Nosyk B, Anglin MD, Brissette S, et al. A call for evidence-based medical treatment of opioid dependence in the United States and Canada. Health Aff (Millwood) 2013;32(8):1462–9.
5. Administration SAaMHS. SAMSHA opioid overdose prevention toolkit: opioid overdose prevention TOOLKIT: information for prescribers. 2013. Available at: https://store.samhsa.gov/product/SAMHSA-Opioid-Overdose-Prevention-Toolkit/ SMA16-4742. Accessed August 1, 2017.

6. Jones CM, Mack KA, Paulozzi LJ. Pharmaceutical overdose deaths, United States, 2010. JAMA 2013;309(7):657–9.
7. The Opioid Therapy for Chronic Pain Work Group. VA/DoD Clinical Practice Guidelines for Opioid Therapy for Chronic Pain. Version 3.0- February 2017. Available at: https://www.healthquality.va.gov/guidelines/Pain/cot/VADoDOTCPG022717.pdf. Accessed August 1, 2017.
8. Busse JW, Craigie S, Juurlink DN, et al. Guideline for opioid therapy and chronic noncancer pain. CMAJ 2017;189(18):E659–66.
9. Dowell D, Haegerich TM, Chou R. CDC guideline for prescribing opioids for chronic pain: United States, 2016. JAMA 2016;315(15):1624–45.
10. Chou R, Turner JA, Devine EB, et al. The effectiveness and risks of long-term opioid therapy for chronic pain: a systematic review for a National Institutes of Health Pathways to Prevention Workshop. Ann Intern Med 2015;162(4):276–86.
11. Binswanger IA, Koester S, Mueller SR, et al. Overdose education and naloxone for patients prescribed opioids in primary care: a qualitative study of primary care staff. J Gen Intern Med 2015;30(12):1837–44.
12. Chou R, Fanciullo GJ, Fine PG, et al. Clinical guidelines for the use of chronic opioid therapy in chronic noncancer pain. J Pain 2009;10(2):113–30.
13. Kaplovitch E, Gomes T, Camacho X, et al. Sex differences in dose escalation and overdose death during chronic opioid therapy: a population-based cohort study. PLoS One 2015;10(8):e0134550.
14. Calcaterra SL, Yamashita TE, Min SJ, et al. Opioid prescribing at hospital discharge contributes to chronic opioid use. J Gen Intern Med 2016;31(5):478–85.
15. Office of he Assistant Secretary for Planning and Evaluation; US Department of Health & Human Services. Opioid abuse in the US and HHS actions to address opioid-drug related overdoses and death 2015. Available at: https://aspe.hhs.gov/basic-report/opioid-abuse-us-and-hhs-actions-address-opioid-drug-related-overdoses-and-deaths. Accessed August 1, 2017.
16. Butler SF, Budman SH, Fernandez K, et al. Validation of a screener and opioid assessment measure for patients with chronic pain. Pain 2004;112(1–2):65–75.
17. Turner BJ, Liang Y. Drug overdose in a retrospective cohort with non-cancer pain treated with opioids, antidepressants, and/or sedative-hypnotics: interactions with mental health disorders. J Gen Intern Med 2015;30(8):1081–96.
18. Mueller SR, Walley AY, Calcaterra SL, et al. A review of opioid overdose prevention and naloxone prescribing: implications for translating community programming into clinical practice. Subst Abus 2015;36(2):240–53.
19. Bohnert AS, Valenstein M, Bair MJ, et al. Association between opioid prescribing patterns and opioid overdose-related deaths. JAMA 2011;305(13):1315–21.
20. Toblin RL, Paulozzi LJ, Logan JE, et al. Mental illness and psychotropic drug use among prescription drug overdose deaths: a medical examiner chart review. J Clin Psychiatry 2010;71(4):491–6.
21. U S Department of Health And Human Services. Opioid abuse in the United States and Department of Health and Human Services actions to address opioid-drug-related overdoses and deaths. J Pain Palliat Care Pharmacother 2015;29(2):133–9.
22. Miller M, Barber CW, Leatherman S, et al. Prescription opioid duration of action and the risk of unintentional overdose among patients receiving opioid therapy. JAMA Intern Med 2015;175(4):608–15.
23. Coffin PO, Tracy M, Bucciarelli A, et al. Identifying injection drug users at risk of nonfatal overdose. Acad Emerg Med 2007;14(7):616–23.

24. Binswanger IA, Stern MF, Deyo RA, et al. Release from prison: a high risk of death for former inmates. N Engl J Med 2007;356(2):157–65.
25. Edlund MJ, Martin BC, Russo JE, et al. The role of opioid prescription in incident opioid abuse and dependence among individuals with chronic noncancer pain: the role of opioid prescription. Clin J Pain 2014;30(7):557–64.
26. Liebschutz JM, Xuan Z, Shanahan CW, et al. Improving adherence to long-term opioid therapy guidelines to reduce opioid misuse in primary care: a cluster-randomized clinical trial. JAMA Intern Med 2017;177(9):1265–72.
27. Binswanger IA, Glanz JM. Pharmaceutical opioids in the home and youth: implications for adult medical practice. Subst Abus 2015;36(2):141–3.
28. Spoth R, Trudeau L, Shin C, et al. Longitudinal effects of universal preventive intervention on prescription drug misuse: three randomized controlled trials with late adolescents and young adults. Am J Public Health 2013;103(4):665–72.
29. Levy SJ, Kokotailo PK. Substance use screening, brief intervention, and referral to treatment for pediatricians. Pediatrics 2011;128(5):e1330–40.
30. Knight JR, Sherritt L, Shrier LA, et al. Validity of the CRAFFT substance abuse screening test among adolescent clinic patients. Arch Pediatr Adolesc Med 2002;156(6):607–14.
31. Starrels JL, Becker WC, Alford DP, et al. Systematic review: treatment agreements and urine drug testing to reduce opioid misuse in patients with chronic pain. Ann Intern Med 2010;152(11):712–20.
32. Jarvis M, Williams J, Hurford M, Lindsay D, Lincoln P, Giles L, Luongo P, Safarian T. Appropriate use of drug testing in clinical addiction medicine. J addict med. 2017;11(3):163–73.
33. Brown R, Riley MR, Ulrich L, et al. Impact of New York prescription drug monitoring program, I-STOP, on statewide overdose morbidity. Drug Alcohol Depend 2017;178:348–54.
34. Haegerich TM, Paulozzi LJ, Manns BJ, et al. What we know, and don't know, about the impact of state policy and systems-level interventions on prescription drug overdose. Drug Alcohol Depend 2014;145:34–47.
35. Paulozzi LJ, Kilbourne EM, Desai HA. Prescription drug monitoring programs and death rates from drug overdose. Pain Med 2011;12(5):747–54.
36. Deyo RA, Irvine JM, Millet LM, et al. Measures such as interstate cooperation would improve the efficacy of programs to track controlled drug prescriptions. Health Aff (Millwood) 2013;32(3):603–13.
37. Fishbain DA, Cole B, Lewis J, et al. What percentage of chronic nonmalignant pain patients exposed to chronic opioid analgesic therapy develop abuse/addiction and/or aberrant drug-related behaviors? A structured evidence-based review. Pain Med 2008;9(4):444–59.
38. Mueller SR, Koester S, Glanz JM, et al. Attitudes toward naloxone prescribing in clinical settings: a qualitative study of patients prescribed high dose opioids for chronic non-cancer pain. J Gen Intern Med 2017;32(3):277–83.
39. Meltzer EC, Rybin D, Saitz R, et al. Identifying prescription opioid use disorder in primary care: diagnostic characteristics of the current opioid misuse measure (COMM). Pain 2011;152(2):397–402.
40. Passik SD, Kirsh KL, Whitcomb L, et al. Monitoring outcomes during long-term opioid therapy for noncancer pain: results with the pain assessment and documentation tool. J Opioid Manag 2005;1(5):257–66.
41. Spelman JF, Peglow S, Schwartz AR, et al. Group visits for overdose education and naloxone distribution in primary care: a pilot quality improvement initiative. Pain Med 2017;18(12):2325–30.

42. Krebs EE, Lorenz KA, Bair MJ, et al. Development and initial validation of the PEG, a three-item scale assessing pain intensity and interference. J Gen Intern Med 2009;24(6):733–8.
43. Compton WM, Jones CM, Baldwin GT. Relationship between nonmedical prescription-opioid use and heroin use. N Engl J Med 2016;374(2):154–63.
44. Frank JW, Levy C, Matlock DD, et al. Patients' perspectives on tapering of chronic opioid therapy: a qualitative study. Pain Med 2016;17(10):1838–47.
45. Frank JW, Lovejoy TI, Becker WC, et al. Patient outcomes in dose reduction or discontinuation of long-term opioid therapy: a systematic review. Ann Intern Med 2017;167(3):181–91.
46. Wheeler E, Jones TS, Gilbert MK, et al. Opioid overdose prevention programs providing naloxone to laypersons—United States, 2014. MMWR Morb Mortal Wkly Rep 2015;64(23):631–5.
47. Walley AY, Xuan Z, Hackman HH, et al. Opioid overdose rates and implementation of overdose education and nasal naloxone distribution in Massachusetts: interrupted time series analysis. BMJ 2013;346:f174.
48. Strang J, Manning V, Mayet S, et al. Overdose training and take-home naloxone for opiate users: prospective cohort study of impact on knowledge and attitudes and subsequent management of overdoses. Addiction 2008;103(10):1648–57.
49. Green TC, Heimer R, Grau LE. Distinguishing signs of opioid overdose and indication for naloxone: an evaluation of six overdose training and naloxone distribution programs in the United States. Addiction 2008;103(6):979–89.
50. Sherman SG, Gann DS, Tobin KE, et al. "The life they save may be mine": diffusion of overdose prevention information from a city sponsored programme. Int J Drug Policy 2009;20(2):137–42.
51. Dwyer K, Walley AY, Langlois BK, et al. Opioid education and nasal naloxone rescue kits in the emergency department. West J Emerg Med 2015;16(3):381–4.
52. Coffin PO, Behar E, Rowe C, et al. Nonrandomized intervention study of naloxone coprescription for primary care patients receiving long-term opioid therapy for pain. Ann Intern Med 2016;165(4):245–52.
53. Davis CS, Burris S, Beletsky L, et al. Co-prescribing naloxone does not increase liability risk. Subst Abus 2016;37(4):498–500.
54. Bohnert AS, Bonar EE, Cunningham R, et al. A pilot randomized clinical trial of an intervention to reduce overdose risk behaviors among emergency department patients at risk for prescription opioid overdose. Drug Alcohol Depend 2016; 163:40–7.
55. Kerensky T, Walley AY. Opioid overdose prevention and naloxone rescue kits: what we know and what we don't know. Addict Sci Clin Pract 2017;12(4):1–7.
56. Substance Abuse and Mental Health Services Administration. SAMHSA opioid overdose prevention toolkit. Rockville (MD): US Department of Health and Human Services; 2013. HHS Publication No. (SMA) 13-4742.
57. Potter JS, Marino EN, Hillhouse MP, et al. Buprenorphine/naloxone and methadone maintenance treatment outcomes for opioid analgesic, heroin, and combined users: findings from Starting Treatment With Agonist Replacement Therapies (START). J Stud Alcohol Drugs 2013;74(4):605–13.
58. Volkow ND, Frieden TR, Hyde PS, et al. Medication-assisted therapies: tackling the opioid-overdose epidemic. N Engl J Med 2014;370(22):2063–6.
59. Kahan M, Wilson L, Mailis-Gagnon A, et al, National Opioid Use Guideline Group. Canadian guideline for safe and effective use of opioids for chronic noncancer pain: clinical summary for family physicians. Part 2: special populations. Can Fam Physician 2011;57(11):1269–76, e1419–28.

60. Fiellin DA, Pantalon MV, Pakes JP, et al. Treatment of heroin dependence with buprenorphine in primary care. Am J Drug Alcohol Abuse 2002;28(2):231–41.
61. McCabe SE, West BT, Boyd CJ. Leftover prescription opioids and nonmedical use among high school seniors: a multi-cohort national study. J Adolesc Health 2013;52(4):480–5.
62. Larochelle MR, Liebschutz JM, Zhang F, et al. Opioid prescribing after nonfatal overdose and association with repeated overdose. Ann Intern Med 2016;165(5):376–7.
63. Edlund MJ, Martin BC, Devries A, et al. Trends in use of opioids for chronic non-cancer pain among individuals with mental health and substance use disorders: the TROUP study. Clin J Pain 2010;26(1):1–8.
64. Nielsen S, Lintzeris N, Bruno R, et al. Benzodiazepine use among chronic pain patients prescribed opioids: associations with pain, physical and mental health, and health service utilization. Pain Med 2015;16(2):356–66.
65. Seal KH, Shi Y, Cohen G, et al. Association of mental health disorders with prescription opioids and high-risk opioid use in US veterans of Iraq and Afghanistan. JAMA 2012;307(9):940–7.
66. Wasan AD, Davar G, Jamison R. The association between negative affect and opioid analgesia in patients with discogenic low back pain. Pain 2005;117(3):450–61.
67. Edlund MJ, Steffick D, Hudson T, et al. Risk factors for clinically recognized opioid abuse and dependence among veterans using opioids for chronic non-cancer pain. Pain 2007;129(3):355–62.
68. Im JJ, Shachter RD, Oliva EM, et al. Association of care practices with suicide attempts in US veterans prescribed opioid medications for chronic pain management. J Gen Intern Med 2015;30(7):979–91.
69. Davidson CL, Babson KA, Bonn-Miller MO, et al. The impact of exercise on suicide risk: examining pathways through depression, PTSD, and sleep in an inpatient sample of veterans. Suicide Life Threat Behav 2013;43(3):279–89.
70. Mazer-Amirshahi M, Mullins PM, Rasooly IR, et al. Trends in prescription opioid use in pediatric emergency department patients. Pediatr Emerg Care 2014;30(4):230–5.
71. Miech R, Johnston L, O'Malley PM, et al. Prescription opioids in adolescence and future opioid misuse. Pediatrics 2015;136(5):e1169–77.
72. McCabe SE, West BT, Morales M, et al. Does early onset of non-medical use of prescription drugs predict subsequent prescription drug abuse and dependence? Results from a national study. Addiction 2007;102(12):1920–30.
73. Bernabei R, Gambassi G, Lapane K, et al. Management of pain in elderly patients with cancer. SAGE Study Group. Systematic Assessment of Geriatric Drug Use via Epidemiology. JAMA 1998;279(23):1877–82.
74. Wilder-Smith OH. Opioid use in the elderly. Eur J Pain 2005;9(2):137–40.
75. Le Roux C, Tang Y, Drexler K. Alcohol and opioid use disorder in older adults: neglected and treatable illnesses. Curr Psychiatry Rep 2016;18(9):87.
76. Broussard CS, Rasmussen SA, Reefhuis J, et al. Maternal treatment with opioid analgesics and risk for birth defects. Am J Obstet Gynecol 2011;204(4):314.e1-11.
77. ACOG Committee on Health Care for Underserved Women, American Society of Addiction Medicine. ACOG committee opinion no. 524: opioid abuse, dependence, and addiction in pregnancy. Obstet Gynecol 2012;119(5):1070–6.
78. Administration SAaMHS. Clinical use of extended-release injectable naltrexone in the treatment of opioid use disorder: a brief guide. Rockville (MD): US

Department of Health and Human Services; 2015. HHS Publication No. (SMA) 14-4892R.

79. American College of Obstetricians and Gynecologists. Patient education Fact Sheet: Important information about opioid use disorder and pregnancy 2016. Available at: https://www.acog.org/Patients/FAQs/Important-Information-About-Opioid-Use-Disorder-and-Pregnancy. Accessed August 4, 2017.
80. Huffman KL, Shella ER, Sweis G, et al. Nonopioid substance use disorders and opioid dose predict therapeutic opioid addiction. J Pain 2015;16(2):126–34.
81. Hser YI, Evans E, Grella C, et al. Long-term course of opioid addiction. Harv Rev Psychiatry 2015;23(2):76–89.
82. Smith PC, Schmidt SM, Allensworth-Davies D, et al. A single-question screening test for drug use in primary care. Arch Intern Med 2010;170(13):1155–60.
83. Yudko E, Lozhkina O, Fouts A. A comprehensive review of the psychometric properties of the drug abuse screening test. J Subst Abuse Treat 2007;32(2):189–98.
84. Reinert DF, Allen JP. The alcohol use disorders identification test: an update of research findings. Alcohol Clin Exp Res 2007;31(2):185–99.
85. Jones CM, Campopiano M, Baldwin G, et al. National and state treatment need and capacity for opioid agonist medication-assisted treatment. Am J Public Health 2015;105(8):e55–63.

Safe Opioid Use

Management of Opioid-Related Adverse Effects and Aberrant Behaviors

Joseph Arthur, MD[a],*, David Hui, MD, MSc[a,b]

KEYWORDS

- Opioid • Cancer • Aberrant behavior • Adverse effects • Nausea • Constipation
- Tolerance • Sedation

KEY POINTS

- Successful opioid therapy requires the use of opioids in a safe and appropriate way to achieve optimal pain control while minimizing unintended adverse effects and opioid misuse, abuse, or diversion.
- A general approach to the management of opioid-related side effects involves opioid dose reduction, opioid rotation, a change in opioid route of administration, and symptomatic management of the side effects.
- A detailed patient history, risk assessment tools, prescription drug monitoring programs, and urine drug screens are important elements of a comprehensive strategy in the management of aberrant behavior.
- Measures taken to ensure safe opioid use include decreasing the time interval between follow-ups for refills, limiting the opioid quantity and doses at each visit, setting boundaries or limitations, or referring to specialist teams for comanagement.

INTRODUCTION

Opioid analgesics play a central role in the management of cancer pain and other symptoms such as dyspnea and cough; however, the benefits conferred by opioids must be carefully balanced against their potential adverse effects, which could

This article originally appeared in *Hematology/Oncology Clinics*, Volume 32, Issue 3, June 2018.
Financial and Competing Interest Disclosure: No relevant conflict of interest. D. Hui is supported in part by National Institutes of Health grants (1R01CA214960-01A1, R21NR016736), an American Cancer Society Mentored Research Scholar grant in Applied and Clinical Research (MRSG-14-1418-01-CCE), and the Andrew Sabin Family Fellowship Award.
[a] Department of Palliative Care, Rehabilitation and Integrative Medicine, The University of Texas MD Anderson Cancer Center, Unit 1414, 1515 Holcombe Boulevard, Houston, TX 77030, USA; [b] Department of General Oncology, The University of Texas MD Anderson Cancer Center, 1515 Holcombe Boulevard, Houston, TX 77030, USA
* Corresponding author.
E-mail address: jaarthur@mdanderson.org

Clinics Collections 9 (2020) 149–166
https://doi.org/10.1016/j.ccol.2020.07.031
2352-7986/20/

negatively affect symptom management, treatment adherence, psychological well-being, quality of life, and even survival. Many of the adverse effects can be anticipated and mitigated by clinicians with a good working knowledge of the opioid-related adverse effects, and by the provision of skilled patient education, proper monitoring, and timely management. This article provides an up-to-date synopsis on the management of various opioid-related adverse effects. It also discusses the strategies to minimize aberrant opioid use in patients with cancer, which is particularly important during this era of the opioid epidemic.

OPIOID-RELATED ADVERSE EFFECTS

The key determinants of opioid-related adverse effects include both patient-related (genetic variations,[1] age,[2,3] and renal[4,5] and liver dysfunction[6]) and medication-related factors. Medications that alter opioid absorption, metabolism, or clearance may increase their side effects.[7] Moreover, concurrent use of some medications may exacerbate side effects. For example, using opioids and benzodiazepines together could significantly worsen the patient's cognitive function and may precipitate respiratory depression.

Recommendations for management of opioid-related side effects in the literature are mainly based on consensus opinion and clinical experience.[8] There are 4 key strategies to address these adverse effects, including:

1. Opioid dose reduction
2. Opioid rotation
3. Changing the route of opioid administration
4. Symptomatic management of adverse effects.[9]

The prevalence, pathophysiology, and management strategies for several important opioid-related adverse effects, including nausea and vomiting, constipation, sedation, neurotoxicity, pruritus, and respiratory depression, are briefly reviewed (**Table 1**).

Opioid-Induced Nausea and Vomiting

Opioid-induced nausea and vomiting (OINV) occur in approximately 26% of patients treated with opioids.[10] Opioids cause nausea by stimulating receptors in the chemoreceptor trigger zone (CTZ), the gastrointestinal (GI) tract, or the vestibular apparatus to send impulses to the vomiting center located in the medulla oblongata, or by reducing GI motility, resulting in gastroparesis and constipation. Symptomatic management of OINV includes the use of antiemetics (**Table 2**) and treatment of any other coexisting conditions that may contribute to nausea (eg, constipation). See later discussion of the main classes of antiemetics used in the management of OINV.

Antipsychotics are dopamine-2 receptor antagonists that work centrally to block dopamine receptors in the CTZ and the vomiting center. They include butyrophenones (eg, droperidol, and haloperidol) and phenothiazines (eg, prochlorperazine, perphenazine, and promethazine), as well as atypical antipsychotics such as olanzapine, aripiprazole, and risperidone.[9,11] Common adverse effects include sedation, orthostatic hypotension, and extrapyramidal symptoms such as akathisia and dystonic reactions. Olanzapine has a higher affinity for the serotonin receptor than the dopamine receptor and hence has less propensity to cause extrapyramidal symptoms.

Metoclopramide is a unique medication because, apart from being a prokinetic agent by increasing gut motility via acetylcholine release, it can block dopamine receptors both centrally in the CTZ and peripherally in the GI tract. Thus, it is a drug of choice for the management of OINV. At high doses it is capable of blocking both

Table 1 Opioid-related adverse effects	
Type of Adverse Effect	**Example**
Gastrointestinal	Nausea
	Vomiting
	Constipation
	Gastroparesis
Central nervous system	Respiratory depression
	Drowsiness
	Cognitive impairment
	Hallucination
	Allodynia
	Hyperalgesia
	Myoclonus
	Seizure disorder
Cardiovascular	Hypotension
	Bradycardia
	QT prolongation or Torsade des pointes[a]
Autonomic nervous system	Urinary retention
	Xerostomia
Dermatologic	Pruritus
	Sweating
Hormonal or immunologic	Decreased libido
	Sexual dysfunction
	Decreased energy levels
	Osteoporosis
	Amenorrhea or oligomenorrhea
	Depression
	Immunosuppression

[a] In the case of methadone.

dopamine and serotonin receptors.[12] Known side effects include drowsiness, diarrhea, and rarely extrapyramidal symptoms.

Serotonin receptor antagonists act both centrally and peripherally by binding to 5-hydroxytryptamine-3 (5-HT3) receptors in the CTZ and the GI tract. Examples include dolasetron, granisetron, and ondansetron, which are first generation serotonin receptor antagonists; and palonosetron, a second-generation serotonin receptor antagonist. The major side effects of these agents are constipation and headache. Other classes of antiemetics that may be occasionally used include antihistamines, anticholinergics, and corticosteroids (see **Table 2**).

Opioid-Induced Constipation

Opioid-induced constipation (OIC) is the most common opioid-related side effect in cancer pain management, affecting 40% to 80% of patients on opioids. Opioids cause constipation by binding to peripheral receptors in the GI tract; decreasing gastric motility, intestinal water secretion, and blood flow; and increasing anal sphincter tone.[13] OIC is believed to be dose-dependent. Nonpharmacological approaches used in management include increasing hydration, soluble dietary fiber intake, and physical activity.

Due to the paucity of research, there is no established first-line therapy for OIC prevention or treatment. A stimulant is often recommended as part of the initial

Table 2
Common antiemetic medications used in the management of opioid-induced nausea and vomiting

Class	Medication	Common Doses	Comments
Prokinetic agents	Metoclopramide	5–10 mg orally or IV 4/d	Increases peristalsis via acetylcholine release; also blocks both dopamine and serotonin receptors at high doses
	Domperidone (not available in the United States)	10 mg orally every 6 h	Has fewer and less severe extrapyramidal side effects because it crosses the blood–brain barrier to a lesser extent
Antipsychotics	Haloperidol	0.5–2 mg orally 2 to 4/d	—
	Prochlorperazine	5–10 mg orally or IV every 6–8 h or 25 mg rectally every 12 h	Has both antidopaminergic and antihistaminic properties; less sedating than promethazine
	Promethazine	12.5–25 mg orally, IV, or rectally every 4–6 h	Has less dopamine-blocking properties than prochlorperazine; also has antihistaminic properties
	Olanzapine	2.5 to 5 mg orally 2/d	2nd generation antipsychotic; binds to a wide variety of receptors, including dopaminergic, serotonergic, histaminic, and muscarinic receptors
Serotonin antagonists	Ondansetron	4–8 mg orally or IV every 6–8 h	Class is relatively more expensive than other classes of antiemetics and hence considered as second-line agents
	Granisetron	1 mg orally or IV 2/d or 3.1 mg transdermal every 24 h	First-generation agent similar to ondansetron but longer acting
Anticholinergics	Scopolamine	0.3 mg orally every 8 h or 1.5 mg transdermal every 72 h	Can cross the blood–brain barrier and cause central nervous system side effects
Antihistamines	Diphenhydramine	25–50 mg orally or IV every 4–6 h	Very sedating
	Meclizine	12.5–25 mg orally every 6 to 8 h	More effective if nausea is related to motion
Corticosteroids	Dexamethasone	1–4 mg every 6 h	Usually used for short period of time due to the side effects with prolonged use
	Prednisone	5–15 mg every 6–8 h	Similar side effect profile to dexamethasone

Abbreviation: IV, intravenous.

prophylactic bowel regimen.[9] Patients are encouraged to take laxatives on a scheduled basis to ensure regular bowel movements at least every day or every other day.[14] Commonly used laxatives are shown in **Table 3**. Some experts have recommended the use of 2 or more laxatives with different mechanisms of action.[14] Docusate was found in a double-blind randomized control trial to provide limited additional benefit when combined with sennosides.[15] Although some studies have reported that transdermal fentanyl induces less OIC than other opioids, this remains to be confirmed.[16]

Because OIC is mediated predominantly by the peripheral mu-opioid receptors lining the GI tract, selective blockade of these receptors by peripherally acting mu-opioid receptor antagonist (PAMORA), medications such as methylnaltrexone, naloxegol, naldemedine, and alvimopan can relieve constipation without affecting the centrally mediated analgesic effects of opioids or precipitating withdrawal symptoms. A systematic review and meta-analysis on the efficacy of pharmacologic therapies for the treatment of OIC concluded that mu-opioid receptor antagonists are safe and effective for the treatment of OIC.[17]

Methylnaltrexone
In a double-blind, randomized, placebo-controlled trial involving 133 subjects with OIC refractory to other laxatives, 48% of subjects had a bowel movement within 4 hours after the first dose and 52% within 4 hours after 2 or more of the first 4 doses of methylnaltrexone, as compared with 15% and 8% in the placebo group, respectively ($P<.001$). The treatment did not seem to affect central analgesia or cause opioid withdrawal.[18] Methylnaltrexone has been commercially available in subcutaneous formulation at a dosage of 12 mg daily since 2008 and recently received US Food and Drug Administration (FDA) approval for the oral preparation at a dosage of 450 mg daily in 2016.[19] However, clinicians should avoid using this medication in patients with bowel obstruction and GI malignancies because they may develop bowel perforation.

Naloxegol
Naloxegol, a pegylated derivative of naloxone, is approved by the FDA at a dosage of 25 mg daily.[13]

Alvimopan
Alvimopan, the first PAMORA studied for OIC ,was found to potentially cause myocardial infarction with long-term use, resulting in the early termination of a phase III study. It is currently approved only for short-term use in the inpatient setting.[20]

Sedation
Sedation or decreased cognition occurs especially during the initial dosing or at higher doses.[21] The prevalence of opioid-induced cognitive dysfunction is 14% to 77%, depending on the population, opioid doses, and methods and duration of assessment.[22] The effect may be transient in some patients but persistent in others. The first step is to identify and minimize or discontinue any concomitant sedating medications such as antihistamines, anxiolytics, or antidepressants. Opioid dose reduction, opioid rotation, and the use of pharmacologic agents, such as methylphenidate, dextroamphetamine, donepezil, modafinil, and caffeine, have been suggested. Methylphenidate is the most widely studied psychostimulant in randomized clinical trials[23] and is considered the first-line therapy for opioid-induced sedation.[24]

Table 3
Laxatives used for the management of opioid-induced constipation

Class	Medication	Mechanism of Action	Comments
Surfactants	Docusate	Act as detergents to soften fat and increase water penetration to soften stool	Not effective as monotherapy; often used in combination with other laxatives
Emollients	Mineral oil	Act as lubricants to soften stool	May cause lipid pneumonitis if aspiration occurs
Bulk-forming agents	Psyllium Methylcellulose Wheat dextrin (Benefiber)	Absorb water into the intestine, increasing stool bulk, thereby promoting peristalsis	Psyllium and methylcellulose require at least 300–500 mL of water intake, otherwise impaction may occur; not recommended in very sick patients
Stimulants	Bisacodyl Senna	Stimulate peristalsis by irritating the smooth muscle and intramural plexus; increase secretion by inhibiting Na+ and K+ ATPase activity	Activation in colon by bacterial action; side effects include abdominal cramping
Hyperosmolar agents	Lactulose Polyethylene glycol Sorbitol	Increase intestinal fluid retention	Indigestible, unabsorbable compounds; side effects include abdominal bloating, colic, and flatulence; lactulose contraindicated in lactose-deficient patients
Saline laxatives	Magnesium hydroxide Magnesium citrate	Draw fluid into the intestine by osmosis	Avoid in renal or heart failure
Opioid antagonists	Methylnaltrexone Naloxegol	Peripherally acting mu-opioid receptor antagonist	Only works for OIC; contraindicated in bowel obstruction, bowel perforation, pelvic masses; side effects include abdominal pain, nausea, diarrhea
Rectal preparations	Mineral oil enema Sorbitol enema Lactulose enema Saline enema Sodium phosphate enema Glycerin suppository Bisacodyl suppository	In addition to their specific mechanisms of action, they stimulate the anocolonic reflex to induce defecation	Usually used in intractable constipation; contraindicated in thrombocytopenia and neutropenia; repeated saline enemas may cause electrolyte disturbances; glycerin can cause local irritation; sodium phosphate enema is considered the most potent

Investigational and new agents	Agent	Mechanism	Comments
	Naldemedine	Peripherally acting mu-opioid receptor antagonist	Currently investigational; side effects include diarrhea and abdominal pain
	Alvimopan	Peripherally acting mu-opioid receptor antagonist	Approved only for short-term use (<16 doses) in a hospital inpatient setting; a phase III trial was terminated early due to potential myocardial infarction with long-term use
	Lubiprostone	Secretagogue; activate chloride receptors on enterocytes to increase intestinal fluid secretion and gut motility	The only secretagogue approved for OIC; not recommended in patients on methadone because its activity is potentially inhibited by methadone; avoid in pregnancy; side effects include nausea, diarrhea, and abdominal pain
	Linaclotide Dolcanatide	Secretagogue; activate guanylate cyclase C receptors on enterocytes to increase intestinal secretion	Currently investigational; side effects include diarrhea

Opioid-Induced Neurotoxicity

Opioid-induced neurotoxicity (OIN) refers to the constellation of neurologic symptoms that may occur due to accumulation of toxic opioid metabolites. Symptoms include confusion, hallucinations, myoclonus, allodynia, or hyperalgesia.[25] Diagnosis of OIN is complicated by concomitant presence of other causes of delirium, such as infection, dehydration, metabolic abnormalities, or advanced cancer.[26] OIN is managed by treating the other precipitating causes of delirium, reducing the dose of opioids, or (most important) switching to a different opioid to prevent further accumulation of toxic metabolites. Some patients with severe or persistent symptoms may require further symptomatic treatment, such as antipsychotics for delirium or benzodiazepines for myoclonic jerks and seizures.[21]

Respiratory Depression

Respiratory depression is the most life-threatening opioid-related side effect. This is due to the effect of opioids on the respiratory centers in the brain stem leading to hypoventilation to the point of apnea. The effect is dose-dependent but tolerance may develop with prolonged opioid use. Hence, it is highly uncommon in patients on chronic opioid therapy with good adherence. Importantly, coadministration with benzodiazepines[27]; alcohol; or the presence of other comorbidities, such as pulmonary embolism, pneumonia, or cardiomyopathy, may precipitate respiratory depression. In addition to decreased respiratory rate (<8 times per minute), pupillary constriction and decreased level of consciousness are often observed. Naloxone, the preferred treatment, should be used only in unresponsive patients breathing less than 8 times per minute because it causes severe opioid withdrawal, even when titrated carefully.[21] It has a relatively short duration of action, so symptomatic patients who were receiving long-acting opioids require careful monitoring to determine the need for repeated naloxone boluses or a naloxone infusion.

Pruritus

Pruritus occurs in less than 10% of patients on oral opioids[9] but in 35% to 90% of those receiving epidural or intrathecal opioids.[28,29] The most compelling pathophysiologic evidence favors the centrally mediated mu-receptor pathway.[30] Others implicated include the histaminic, serotonergic, and the dopaminergic pathways.[31] Opioid-related pruritus is considered an adverse effect rather than an allergic reaction. It is self-limiting and not life-threatening. It is usually managed by reducing the opioid dose, switching to a different opioid, or treating with other medications. In a systematic review, nalbuphine, a mixed opioid agonist-antagonist, was found to be superior to placebo, diphenhydramine, naloxone, or propofol in treating pruritus from neuraxial opioids.[32] Other pharmacologic agents, such as serotonin 5-HT3 receptor antagonists, propofol, nonsteroidal antiinflammatory drugs, and dopamine D2 receptor antagonists, have also been found to be useful.[31]

Physical Dependence and Tolerance

Physical dependence is a physiologic state characterized by the onset of withdrawal symptoms after sudden opioid cessation, dose reduction, or administration of an opioid antagonist. Withdrawal symptoms (eg, piloerection, chills, insomnia, diarrhea, nausea, vomiting, and muscle aches) vary in severity and duration depending on the type, dose, and duration of opioid prescribed.[33] The symptoms are reduced by a gradual taper of opioids.

Tolerance is characterized by the need to use increasing opioid doses to maintain the same effects. It is a form of neuroadaptation to the effects of long-term adminis-tration of opioids. Neither physical dependence nor tolerance necessarily indicates addiction.[34] Discontinuing the opioid reverses tolerance and physical dependence within days to weeks, whereas the changes associated with addiction persist for months to years, even after the opioids are stopped. Addicted patients are, therefore, extremely vulnerable to overdosing after a period of abstinence because, although they may still have a persistent desire for opioids, they lose the opioid tolerance which previously protected them from overdosing.[33]

ABERRANT OPIOID-RELATED BEHAVIORS

Aberrant opioid use presents a significant challenge to helping patients with cancer manage their pain. Patients with cancer were previously thought to be less at risk for opioid abuse.[35,36] In 1 study, less than 5% of ambulatory patients with cancer met the criteria for a substance use disorder.[36] The most recent Centers for Disease Control and Prevention guideline for opioid prescriptions exempted patients with can-cer pain.[37] However, a more recent study found that chemical coping was diagnosed in 18% of outpatients with cancer.[38] Patients with cancer are also at a risk for aberrant use of prescription drugs if they have a preexisting issue with drug and substance abuse.[39] Clinicians are, therefore, faced with the challenge of helping patients who need to use opioids safely while minimizing opioid misuse and addiction.

Aberrant Behavior: A Spectrum of Conditions

There is a gradation of opioid-related aberrant behaviors from seemingly normal drug-taking behavior to a clear demonstration of addictive behavior (**Fig. 1**). Many patients exhibit different behaviors that fall in between these extremes (**Table 4**). Notably, not all patients who misuse or abuse drugs are addicts. Moreover, some behaviors, such as losing medications, may be relatively less serious than others, such as self-injecting or shooting oral formulations.

Risk Assessment and Monitoring of Aberrant Behaviors

Guidelines that provide specific recommendations for safe opioid prescribing in pa-tients with cancer are limited and, therefore, much of the information is based on the literature about patients who have noncancer pain. **Fig. 2** outlines a recommended

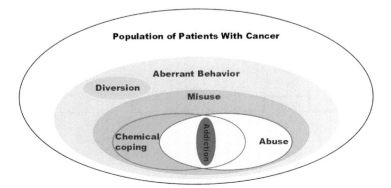

Fig. 1. Spectrum of aberrant opioid-related behavior.

Table 4 Definition of common terms to describe aberrant opioid use	
Misuse	The use of a medication for a medical purpose other than as directed or indicated, whether intentionally or unintentionally[63]
Abuse	The intentional self-administration of a medication for a nonmedical purpose, such as altering one's state of consciousness, or the use of any illegal drug[63]
Diversion	The intentional transfer of a controlled substance from legitimate distribution and dispensing channels[63]
Chemical coping	The inappropriate and/or excessive use of opioids to cope with the various stressful events associated with the diagnosis and management of cancer[66,67]
Addiction	A primary chronic neurobiological disease that occurs as result of genetic, psychosocial, and environmental factors It is characterized by 1 or more of the following: • Impaired control during use • Compulsive use • Continued use despite harm • Craving[68]
Pseudoaddiction	The apparent demonstration of a drug-seeking behavior in the setting of undertreated or poorly treated pain[69] It may be erroneously interpreted as addiction but the behavior resolves once adequate pain control is achieved

approach to patients with cancer on chronic opioid therapy. During the initial visit or before starting opioids, the clinician should carefully screen all patients using a comprehensive clinical history, including psychosocial, substance abuse, and family histories[40]; as well as risk assessment tools (see later discussion). Patients may then be stratified into low risk or high risk for opioid abuse. High-risk patients will

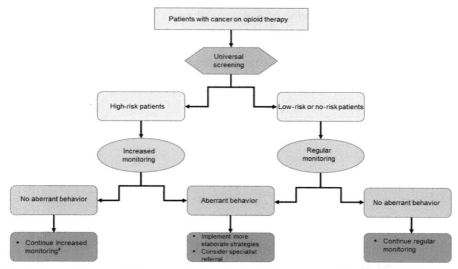

Fig. 2. General approach to managing patients with cancer on chronic opioid therapy. [a] Consider changing to regular monitoring if adherent pattern observed over a long time.

require increased monitoring during subsequent clinic visits. Studies have found that patients who are younger, male, have mental health or substance abuse disorders, or have alcohol or tobacco use are at a higher risk of aberrant opioid use.[41]

All patients should give informed consent, detailing the potential risks and benefits of opioid therapy; possible adverse effects; and education on safe opioid use, storage, and disposal strategies.[42] Clinicians should consider using a written opioid management plan, also known as opioid treatment agreement or contract. The plan helps define the goals and expectations of therapy and the responsibilities of both the clinician and patient about how opioids will be prescribed and taken, clinical follow-up, and monitoring.[43] Plans vary, but usually include obtaining opioids from 1 prescriber, filling prescriptions at 1 designated pharmacy, keeping one's scheduled appointments, random urine drug screens (UDS), and the actions that the clinician may take if the patient fails to adhere to the plan.

At every patient visit, monitor for evidence of maladaptive opioid-related behavior, otherwise known as red flags[44,45] (**Box 1**). Also, use prescription monitoring programs, pain medication diaries, pill counts, and periodic UDS. Routinely conducting and documenting this risk evaluation and monitoring process will allow the clinician to detect when a patient who initially seemed to demonstrate opioid-adherent behavior moves into a pattern of aberrant opioid use.

Risk assessment tools
Examples of validated risk assessment tools for patient screening include the Cut down, Annoyed, Guilty, and Eye-opener (CAGE) questionnaire; Screener and Opioid

---

Box 1
Behaviors suggestive of aberrant opioid use

Frequent unscheduled clinic appointments or telephone calls for early opioid refills

Self-escalation or request for excessive increase in the opioid dosage not consistent with patient's pain syndrome

Reports of lost or stolen opioid prescription or medication

Frequent emergency room visits for opioids

Seeking opioids from multiple providers (doctor shopping)

Requests for a specific opioid

Resistance to changes in the opioid regimen even when clinically indicated

Use of nonprescribed restricted medications or illicit drugs

Requesting opioids for its euphoric effect or for symptoms such as anxiety or insomnia

Reports of impaired functioning in daily activities due to opioid use

Family members expressing concern about patient's use of opioids

Reports of hoarding drugs

Reports of stealing or selling prescription drugs

Obtaining opioids from nonmedical sources

Reports of stealing, tampering, or forging opioid prescriptions

Discrepancy in pill counts without good explanation

Adapted from Arthur JA, Edwards T, Lu Z, et al. Frequency, predictors, and outcomes of urine drug testing among patients with advanced cancer on chronic opioid therapy at an outpatient supportive care clinic. Cancer 2016;122(23):3734; with permission.

Assessment for Patients with Pain (SOAPP) form; the Opioid Risk Tool (ORT); and the Diagnosis, Intractability, Risk, and Efficacy (DIRE) inventory.[46] Although risk assessment and monitoring tools may reveal the possibility of maladaptive behavior, they are based on patient self-reporting, which limits their usefulness.

The CAGE is a clinician-administered 4-item questionnaire that asks about a patient's perceived need to:

1. Cut down on alcohol use
2. Annoyance with questions about alcohol abuse
3. Guilt over drinking habits
4. Use of eye-opener drinks.[47]

Patients score 1 point for every "Yes" answer. A cut-off score of 2 or greater is considered positive and has a sensitivity of 0.93 and a specificity of 0.76 for identifying excessive alcohol use.[48] A positive CAGE may indicate an increased risk of maladaptive opioid use. The CAGE questionnaire was not specifically created for patients with pain; it is also commonly used in other settings. An updated version of the CAGE questionnaire, the CAGE-Adapted to Include Drugs (CAGE-AID) questionnaire, which substitutes "drink" with "drink or drugs," has also been evaluated for the detection of substance use disorder and found to have a sensitivity of 0.88 and a specificity of 0.55 for a score of 2 or greater.[49]

The SOAPP is a patient self-administered screening questionnaire used to help identify patients who may be at risk for aberrant drug-related behavior.[46,50] There are 3 different available versions. The SOAPP-Original, SOAPP-Revised, and SOAPP-Short Form are questionnaires with 14, 24, and 5 items, respectively, and with sensitivity, specificity scores of 0.86, 0.67; 0.81, 0.68; and 0.86, 0.67 for cut-off scores of greater than or equal to 7, greater than or equal to 18, and greater than or equal to 4, respectively.

ORT is a patient self-administered questionnaire that assesses 5 risk factor categories:

1. Family history of substance abuse
2. Personal history of substance abuse
3. Age 16 to 45 years
4. History of preadolescent sexual abuse
5. Psychological disease.[51]

It is a 10-item questionnaire with a possible score ranging from 0 to 26. A score of 0 to 3 is low risk, 4 to 7 is moderate risk, and greater than or equal to 8 is high risk.[52] The ORT has demonstrated excellent discrimination for both the male (c-statistic = 0.82) and the female (c-statistic = 0.85) prognostic models.

The DIRE is a clinician-administered questionnaire that predicts the possibility of patient compliance with long-term opioid therapy and the efficacy of analgesia. It consists of 4 categories of risk factors.[46] Total scores range from 7 to 21, with lower scores indicating greater risk. A cut-off score of 13 has a sensitivity of 0.94 and a specificity of 0.87.

Other tools that are used solely for continued monitoring of patients currently receiving opioid therapy include the Current Opioid Misuse Measure (COMM)[53] and the Addiction Behavior Checklist (ABC).[54]

Prescription drug monitoring programs

Prescription drug monitoring programs (PDMPs) collect data from pharmacies that dispense controlled substances and use it to create secure state-run electronic databases that are made available to authorized users. They provide key information about the patient's prescription history and document when and where patients received opioid prescriptions and who prescribed them.[55] PDMPs are particularly useful in providing objective data on patients who seek opioids from multiple prescribers (doctor shopping) and fill multiple prescriptions at different pharmacies (pharmacy shopping). As of August 24, 2017, every state in the United States had an extensive operational PDMP, except for Missouri, where the PDMP program is not state-wide.[56] PDMPs are effective in reducing aberrant opioid use by facilitating clinical decision-making and improving opioid prescribing practices.[57]

Urine drug screens

Two main types of UDS are used in clinical practice. The immunoassays use antibodies to detect the presence of a particular drug or its metabolite. They are more economical and have a quick turnaround time but are unable to distinguish between different drugs in the same class or detect synthetic opioids. The confirmatory or laboratory-based specific drug identification tests use gas or liquid chromatography or mass spectrometry. They can detect specific drugs but are more expensive and have a slower turnaround time.[58] The 3 types of abnormal UDS results are:

1. Absence of prescribed opioids (suggestive of diversion)
2. Presence of unprescribed opioids (suggestive of multiple prescriber involvement or obtaining opioids from unapproved sources)
3. Presence of illicit drugs.

Even these laboratory tests have pitfalls because of the complexity of opioid metabolic pathways. A normal UDS result does not necessarily rule out aberrant behavior. For example, patients who are using opioids for chemical coping may have a normal UDS but may still be using opioids in an excessive or maladaptive manner.

Best practice in the use of UDS in patients with cancer, who have unique symptom burdens and expectations, is not yet defined. UDS seems to be underutilized in patients with cancer as compared with noncancer patients with chronic pain. At the authors' facility, for example, UDS was conducted in only 6% of patients with cancer seen at the palliative care clinic and 54% of these were abnormal.[44]

Management of Detected Aberrant Behavior

When patients demonstrate aberrant behavior, the clinical team needs to have open and nonjudgmental discussions with them, communicating their concerns about patient safety. Measures that should be implemented to ensure that they adhere to safe opioid use include decreasing the time interval between follow-ups for refills, limiting the opioid quantity and dose of refills, setting boundaries or limitations, weaning off the opioids when possible, or referring to a pain or palliative medicine or drug addiction specialist for comanagement. Specific education regarding safe opioid use, storage, and disposal should be provided frequently to the patients and their caregivers.[59] In some patients, complete behavioral change is achievable but not in others. Goals for these patients can, therefore, focus on minimizing harm.

Use nonopioids and adjuvant analgesics

The World Health Organization ladder for management of cancer pain recommends starting pain management with nonopioid and adjuvant analgesics, especially in patients with mild pain. Clinicians should only consider opioids for patients with moderate to severe cancer pain or pain that is unresponsive to nonopioid therapies because these are the populations shown to benefit from opioids in randomized trials.[60]

Consider switching patients who demonstrate aberrant behaviors from opioids to non-opioid analgesics or use interventional techniques when possible.

Treat underlying comorbid psychiatric conditions

The prevalence of common psychiatric conditions, such as personality disorder, depression, and anxiety disorders, is extremely high in patients with a history of substance abuse.[61] During the initial, as well as subsequent, patient screenings, evaluate and treat any underlying comorbid psychiatric conditions. Psychological interventions, such as cognitive behavioral therapy, relaxation techniques, biofeedback, distraction techniques, problem-solving techniques, and other coping strategies, in appropriate patients are useful adjunctive therapies.[62] Treatment facilitates recovery from drug addiction and helps minimize the likelihood of relapse.

Adopt an interdisciplinary approach

Management of patients with aberrant opioid-related behavior requires a sound understanding of multiple domains, including biomedical, psychosocial, financial, and legal factors. An interprofessional team is better able to address these multi-dimensional care needs comprehensively while supporting each other to minimize burnout.[63]

The authors' supportive oncology team recently developed and implemented a specialized interdisciplinary team intervention to standardize care for patients with cancer with aberrant behavior. Using a quasi-experimental design, the intervention resulted in a significant reduction in the frequency of aberrant behaviors from a median of 3 per month before the intervention to 0.4 postintervention ($P<.0001$). There was also a significant reduction in opioid utilization from a median morphine equivalent dose of 165 mg daily at the first intervention visit to 112 mg daily at the last clinic follow-up ($P = .02$), despite that pain intensity did not change ($P = .98$).[64]

Consider prescribing intranasal naloxone

Coprescribing naloxone, a short-acting opioid antagonist, to patients on chronic opioids may help reduce opioid-related adverse effects without causing an increase in the dose of prescribed opioids.[65] Patients with a history of drug overdose, a history of a substance use disorder, requiring large opioid doses, or concurrently receiving benzodiazepines may particularly benefit from prescribed intranasal naloxone with instructions for administration by relatives and caregivers.[37]

SUMMARY

Successful opioid therapy requires that opioids be used in a safe and appropriate way to achieve optimal pain control while minimizing unintended adverse effects and aberrant use. A general approach to the management of opioid-related side effects involves opioid dose reduction, opioid rotation, a change in opioid route of administration, and symptomatic management of the side effects. Successful prevention of aberrant opioid use, early identification, and effective management are invaluable practices in managing patients with cancer pain, especially during this era of the opioid epidemic.

REFERENCES

1. Poulsen L, Brosen K, Arendt-Nielsen L, et al. Codeine and morphine in extensive and poor metabolizers of sparteine: pharmacokinetics, analgesic effect and side effects. Eur J Clin Pharmacol 1996;51:289–95.

2. Macintyre PE, Jarvis DA. Age is the best predictor of postoperative morphine requirements. Pain 1996;64:357–64.
3. Vigano A, Bruera E, Suarez-Almazor ME. Age, pain intensity, and opioid dose in patients with advanced cancer. Cancer 1998;83:1244–50.
4. Hagen NA, Foley KM, Cerbone DJ, et al. Chronic nausea and morphine-6-glucuronide. J Pain Symptom Manage 1991;6:125–8.
5. Osborne R, Joel S, Grebenik K, et al. The pharmacokinetics of morphine and morphine glucuronides in kidney failure. Clin Pharmacol Ther 1993;54:158–67.
6. Hasselstrom J, Eriksson S, Persson A, et al. The metabolism and bioavailability of morphine in patients with severe liver cirrhosis. Br J Clin Pharmacol 1990;29:289–97.
7. Bernard SA, Bruera E. Drug interactions in palliative care. J Clin Oncol 2000;18:1780–99.
8. Swegle JM, Logemann C. Management of common opioid-induced adverse effects. Am Fam Physician 2006;74:1347–54.
9. Cherny N, Ripamonti C, Pereira J, et al. Strategies to manage the adverse effects of oral morphine: an evidence-based report. J Clin Oncol 2001;19:2542–54.
10. Cepeda MS, Farrar JT, Baumgarten M, et al. Side effects of opioids during short-term administration: effect of age, gender, and race. Clin Pharmacol Ther 2003;74:102–12.
11. Smith HS, Cox LR, Smith BR. Dopamine receptor antagonists. Ann Palliat Med 2012;1:137–42.
12. Smith HS, Laufer A. Opioid induced nausea and vomiting. Eur J Pharmacol 2014;722:67–78.
13. Brenner DM, Stern E, Cash BD. Opioid-related constipation in patients with noncancer pain syndromes: a review of evidence-based therapies and justification for a change in nomenclature. Curr Gastroenterol Rep 2017;19:12.
14. Pappagallo M. Incidence, prevalence, and management of opioid bowel dysfunction. Am J Surg 2001;182:11S–8S.
15. Tarumi Y, Wilson MP, Szafran O, et al. Randomized, double-blind, placebo-controlled trial of oral docusate in the management of constipation in hospice patients. J Pain Symptom Manage 2013;45:2–13.
16. Allan L, Hays H, Jensen NH, et al. Randomised crossover trial of transdermal fentanyl and sustained release oral morphine for treating chronic non-cancer pain. BMJ 2001;322:1154–8.
17. Ford AC, Brenner DM, Schoenfeld PS. Efficacy of pharmacological therapies for the treatment of opioid-induced constipation: systematic review and meta-analysis. Am J Gastroenterol 2013;108:1566–74 [quiz: 1575].
18. Thomas J, Karver S, Cooney GA, et al. Methylnaltrexone for opioid-induced constipation in advanced illness. N Engl J Med 2008;358:2332–43.
19. FDA approves methylnaltrexone bromide for oral use, 2016. Available at: https://www.accessdata.fda.gov/drugsatfda_docs/label/2016/208271s000lbl.pdf. Accessed February 27, 2018.
20. NDA 21-775 ENTEREG (alvimopan) REMS October 6, 2008. Risk Evaluation and Mitigation Strategy (REMS). Available at https://www.accessdata.fda.gov/drugsatfda_docs/label/2009/021775s001REMS.pdf. Accessed February 27, 2018.
21. McNicol E, Horowicz-Mehler N, Fisk RA, et al. Management of opioid side effects in cancer-related and chronic noncancer pain: a systematic review. J Pain 2003;4:231–56.

22. Lawlor PG. The panorama of opioid-related cognitive dysfunction in patients with cancer: a critical literature appraisal. Cancer 2002;94:1836–53.
23. Bruera E, Miller MJ, Macmillan K, et al. Neuropsychological effects of methylphenidate in patients receiving a continuous infusion of narcotics for cancer pain. Pain 1992;48:163–6.
24. Reissig JE, Rybarczyk AM. Pharmacologic treatment of opioid-induced sedation in chronic pain. Ann Pharmacother 2005;39:727–31.
25. Mercadante S, Portenoy RK. Opioid poorly-responsive cancer pain. Part 1: clinical considerations. J Pain Symptom Manage 2001;21:144–50.
26. Cherny NI. The management of cancer pain. CA Cancer J Clin 2000;50:70–116 [quiz: 117–20].
27. O'Mahony S, Coyle N, Payne R. Current management of opioid-related side effects. Oncology (Williston Park) 2001;15:61–73 [77; discussion 77–8, 80–2].
28. Chaney MA. Side effects of intrathecal and epidural opioids. Can J Anaesth 1995; 42:891–903.
29. Bonnet MP, Mignon A, Mazoit JX, et al. Analgesic efficacy and adverse effects of epidural morphine compared to parenteral opioids after elective caesarean section: a systematic review. Eur J Pain 2010;14:894.e1-9.
30. Liu XY, Liu ZC, Sun YG, et al. Unidirectional cross-activation of GRPR by MOR1D uncouples itch and analgesia induced by opioids. Cell 2011;147:447–58.
31. Ganesh A, Maxwell LG. Pathophysiology and management of opioid-induced pruritus. Drugs 2007;67:2323–33.
32. Jannuzzi RG. Nalbuphine for treatment of opioid-induced pruritus: a systematic review of literature. Clin J Pain 2016;32:87–93.
33. Volkow ND, McLellan AT. Opioid abuse in chronic pain–misconceptions and mitigation strategies. N Engl J Med 2016;374:1253–63.
34. Passik SD, Weinreb HJ. Managing chronic nonmalignant pain: overcoming obstacles to the use of opioids. Adv Ther 2000;17:70–83.
35. World Health Organization. Cancer pain relief with a guide to opioid availability. 2nd edition. Geneva (Switzerland): World Health Organization; 1996. p. 19.
36. Derogatis LR, Morrow GR, Fetting J, et al. The prevalence of psychiatric disorders among cancer patients. JAMA 1983;249:751–7.
37. Dowell D, Haegerich TM, Chou R. CDC guideline for prescribing opioids for chronic pain-United States, 2016. JAMA 2016;315(15):1624–45.
38. Kwon JH, Tanco K, Park JC, et al. Frequency, predictors, and medical record documentation of chemical coping among advanced cancer patients. Oncologist 2015;20:692–7.
39. Starr TD, Rogak LJ, Passik SD. Substance abuse in cancer pain. Curr Pain Headache Rep 2010;14:268–75.
40. Wasan AD, Butler SF, Budman SH, et al. Psychiatric history and psychologic adjustment as risk factors for aberrant drug-related behavior among patients with chronic pain. Clin J Pain 2007;23:307–15.
41. Edlund MJ, Martin BC, Fan MY, et al. Risks for opioid abuse and dependence among recipients of chronic opioid therapy: results from the TROUP study. Drug Alcohol Depend 2010;112:90–8.
42. de la Cruz M, Reddy A, Balankari V, et al. The impact of an educational program on patient practices for safe use, storage, and disposal of opioids at a comprehensive cancer center. Oncologist 2017;22:115–21.
43. Chou R. 2009 clinical guidelines from the American Pain Society and the American Academy of Pain Medicine on the use of chronic opioid therapy in chronic

noncancer pain: what are the key messages for clinical practice? Pol Arch Med Wewn 2009;119:469–77.
44. Arthur JA, Edwards T, Lu Z, et al. Frequency, predictors, and outcomes of urine drug testing among patients with advanced cancer on chronic opioid therapy at an outpatient supportive care clinic. Cancer 2016;122:3732–9.
45. Anghelescu DL, Ehrentraut JH, Faughnan LG. Opioid misuse and abuse: risk assessment and management in patients with cancer pain. J Natl Compr Canc Netw 2013;11:1023–31.
46. Moore TM, Jones T, Browder JH, et al. A comparison of common screening methods for predicting aberrant drug-related behavior among patients receiving opioids for chronic pain management. Pain Med 2009;10:1426–33.
47. Williams N. The CAGE questionnaire. Occup Med (Lond) 2014;64:473–4.
48. Bernadt MW, Mumford J, Taylor C, et al. Comparison of questionnaire and laboratory tests in the detection of excessive drinking and alcoholism. Lancet 1982;1:325–8.
49. Dyson V, Appleby L, Altman E, et al. Efficiency and validity of commonly used substance abuse screening instruments in public psychiatric patients. J Addict Dis 1998;17:57–76.
50. Butler SF, Budman SH, Fernandez K, et al. Validation of a screener and opioid assessment measure for patients with chronic pain. Pain 2004;112:65–75.
51. Webster LR, Webster RM. Predicting aberrant behaviors in opioid-treated patients: preliminary validation of the Opioid Risk Tool. Pain Med 2005;6:432–42.
52. Barclay JS, Owens JE, Blackhall LJ. Screening for substance abuse risk in cancer patients using the Opioid Risk Tool and urine drug screen. Support Care Cancer 2014;22:1883–8.
53. Butler SF, Budman SH, Fanciullo GJ, et al. Cross validation of the current opioid misuse measure to monitor chronic pain patients on opioid therapy. Clin J Pain 2010;26:770–6.
54. Wu SM, Compton P, Bolus R, et al. The addiction behaviors checklist: validation of a new clinician-based measure of inappropriate opioid use in chronic pain. J Pain Symptom Manage 2006;32:342–51.
55. Wang J, Christo PJ. The influence of prescription monitoring programs on chronic pain management. Pain Physician 2009;12:507–15.
56. Prescription drug monitoring program training and technical assistance center. Available at: http://www.pdmpassist.org/content/state-pdmp-websites. Accessed February 27, 2018.
57. Feldman L, Skeel Williams K, Knox M, et al. Influencing controlled substance prescribing: attending and resident physician use of a state prescription monitoring program. Pain Med 2012;13:908–14.
58. Magnani B, Kwong T. Urine drug testing for pain management. Clin Lab Med 2012;32:379–90.
59. Lock it up: medicine safety in your home. US Food and Drug Administration Web site. Available at: www.fda.gov/forconsumers/consumerupdates/ucm272905.htm. Accessed February 27, 2018.
60. Kalso E, Edwards JE, Moore RA, et al. Opioids in chronic non-cancer pain: systematic review of efficacy and safety. Pain 2004;112:372–80.
61. Khantzian EJ, Treece C. DSM-III psychiatric diagnosis of narcotic addicts. Recent findings. Arch Gen Psychiatry 1985;42:1067–71.
62. Jamison RN, Ross EL, Michna E, et al. Substance misuse treatment for high-risk chronic pain patients on opioid therapy: a randomized trial. Pain 2010;150:390–400.

63. Passik SD, Portenoy RK, Ricketts PL. Substance abuse issues in cancer patients. Part 1: Prevalence and diagnosis. Oncology (Williston Park) 1998;12: 517–21, 524.
64. Arthur J, Edwards T, Reddy S, et al. Outcomes of a specialized interdisciplinary approach for patients with cancer with aberrant opioid-related behavior. Oncologist 2018;23(2):263–70.
65. Coffin PO, Behar E, Rowe C, et al. NOnrandomized intervention study of naloxone coprescription for primary care patients receiving long-term opioid therapy for pain. Ann Intern Med 2016;165:245–52.
66. Kwon JH, Hui D, Bruera E. A pilot study to define chemical coping in cancer patients using the Delphi method. J Palliat Med 2015;18:703–6.
67. Del Fabbro E. Assessment and management of chemical coping in patients with cancer. J Clin Oncol 2014;32:1734–8.
68. Rinaldi RC, Steindler EM, Wilford BB, et al. Clarification and standardization of substance abuse terminology. JAMA 1988;259:555–7.
69. Weissman DE, Haddox JD. Opioid pseudoaddiction–an iatrogenic syndrome. Pain 1989;36:363–6.

Smoking Cessation for Those Pursuing Recovery from Substance Use Disorders

Karen J. Derefinko, PhD[a],*, Francisco I. Salgado García, PhD[a],
Daniel D. Sumrok, MD[b],[1]

KEYWORDS

- Tobacco • Cessation • Alcohol use disorder • Substance use disorder
- Concomitant treatment

KEY POINTS

- Tobacco addiction risk is profound in substance users.
- Many alcohol and substance use disorder treatment providers do not prioritize tobacco use cessation in treatment.
- Smoking cessation actually improves alcohol and substance use disorder outcomes.
- Behavioral treatment strategies are similar across substance classes.

Individuals in treatment for alcohol use disorder (AUD) or substance use disorder (SUD) face a multitude of risks that need to be addressed by their service providers. Among the many comorbid issues of AUD/SUD is concomitant tobacco use, most commonly in the form of cigarette smoking. Tobacco use, smoking, nicotine dependence, and tobacco addiction risk are terms used interchangeably in the literature. Even though dependence on nicotine is important in the area of tobacco use, there is evidence that people who smoke intermittently (ie, weekly but not daily) and consistently score low on nicotine dependence measures[1] still face the health risks associated with cigarette smoking.[2,3] As such, the aim of this article was to attend to the broadest issue by reviewing the literature on tobacco use and nicotine dependence.

This article originally appeared in *Medical Clinics*, Volume 102, Issue 4, July 2018.
Conflict of Interest Statement: The authors report no commercial or financial conflicts of interest.
[a] University of Tennessee Health Science Center, 66 North Pauline Street, Suite 305, Memphis, TN 38163-2181, USA; [b] University of Tennessee Health Science Center, Department of Addiction Medicine, 6401 Popular Avenue, Suite 500, Memphis, TN 38119, USA
[1] Present address: 1894 Cedar Street, McKenzie, TN 38201.
* Corresponding author.
E-mail address: kderefin@uthsc.edu

Clinics Collections 9 (2020) 167–182
https://doi.org/10.1016/j.ccol.2020.07.032

According to the US Department of Health and Human Services, cigarette smoking is the leading cause of preventable death in the United States, accounting for approximately 1 in 5 deaths.[4] Although the rates of smoking have been steadily declining for the past 10 years, 15.1% of those over age 18 report current cigarette use, with the highest rates among adults age 25 to 44 years (17.7%).[5] Results from the National Epidemiologic Survey on Alcohol and Related Conditions suggest that prevalence rates of nicotine dependence based on criteria in the fourth edition of the *Diagnostic and Statistical Manual of Mental Disorders* (eg, the use of nicotine to relieve withdrawal symptoms, use of nicotine more than intended) are extraordinarily high in those with an AUD (45.4%) or nonalcohol SUD (69.3%).[6] Other studies have found similar,[7,8] or even higher rates.[9] In addition to high prevalence, research has indicated that the degree of dependence using diagnostic criteria and dependence measures is stronger in those with AUD/SUD than those without,[10–13] indicating that risk for nicotine dependence is profound in substance users.

Although often overlooked, the long-term impact of tobacco use among those with AUD/SUD is undeniable. Smoking quit rates among those with AUD/SUD are significantly lower than those without comorbid substance use; Lasser and colleagues[8] found that those with a history of AUD had a quit rate of 16.9%, compared with those who have no history of AUD (42.5%). Although often treated as a secondary outcome, smoking has dire consequences among those with AUD/SUD. Results from a large study of individuals in treatment for AUD/SUD (n = 845) indicated that, among documented deaths in the sample, a significantly greater proportion were caused by tobacco use than the alcohol use that brought them into treatment (50.9% vs 34.1%, respectively).[14]

Despite known comorbidity rates and clear adverse outcomes, it is estimated that only 42% of SUD treatment centers provide tobacco cessation services.[15] With the known risk factors associated with smoking, this statistic suggests a crucial need for tobacco cessation services. This article presents a summary of the literature regarding the similar biopsychosocial mechanisms of tobacco use and AUD/SUD. This article also includes a description of the commonly held beliefs regarding smoking in those with AUD/SUD, and the argument of "harm reduction" in the broad context of addiction. Although there are clear reasons why physicians and other addiction treatment providers do not prioritize or promote smoking cessation among those with AUD/SUD, the risks to optimal outcomes should eclipse this apathy. The practicality of treatment, focusing on the methods, timing, and innovations of intervention strategies, are also presented. Finally, the common methodologies that may be used across tobacco use and AUD/SUD to prevent long-term lapse and relapse are discussed. Physicians can and should adhere to the policy that tobacco use is a common and dangerous comorbid condition that demands concomitant treatment for those with AUD/SUD and should follow the guidelines for treating tobacco use.[16]

COMMON ETIOLOGY OF TOBACCO, ALCOHOL, AND ILLICIT SUBSTANCE USE

It is critical to consider the basis for the cooccurrence of tobacco use and AUD/SUD to understand their concomitant use. Many hypotheses about the cooccurrence of these disorders exist and are generally based on biological predispositions and psychosocial/environmental factors. In addition to a possible joint genetic predisposition,[17] neurobiological models indicate that nicotine modulates neurotransmitter systems directly implicated in other SUDs, including dopamine,[18,19] serotonin,[20,21] acetylcholine,[22] endogenous opioid peptides,[23,24] gamma-aminobutyric acid, glutamate,[25–27] and norepinephrine.[28] Research has also demonstrated that nicotine increases the effects of other substances, may serve as a gateway drug, and may contribute to increased risk of drug use.[29]

Further, developmental research suggests that specific mechanisms of dysfunction underlie both tobacco and AUD/SUD, including executive cognitive function. As noted by Tarter,[30] executive cognitive function is believed to be modulated by the dorsolateral prefrontal cortex, and involves planned behavior (vs impulsivity), self-monitoring, attention, memory, and mental flexibility.[31] These mechanisms of function have been validated as reliable predictors of both tobacco and AUD/SUD in numerous empirical studies,[32–38] and cognitive tasks such as delay discounting have provided a strong link between mechanisms of dysfunction and related therapeutic techniques.[39–41]

Still other research points to the shared psychosocial or environmental mechanisms of both tobacco use and SUDs.[7] Independent but related theories[30,42,43] have been posited to explain the interactions between, and the importance of, proximal (peer and family use, access, stressors, psychopathology, novelty seeking) and distal (media and cultural influences regarding tobacco and substance use) interpersonal and environmental influences. Although each of these mechanisms have been found to be important contributors to the development of tobacco and substance use, several deserve specific mention. First, early environmental experiences have been found to have a significant effect on later substance use. The Adverse Childhood Events (ACEs) study, a collaborative effort between Kaiser and the Centers for Disease Control and Prevention, identified 10 categories of negative childhood events that predict tobacco,[44] alcohol,[45] and substance use[46] well into adulthood. These events included a household member who uses alcohol or illicit drugs. Parental substance use as a risk factor has been demonstrated repeatedly in individual studies of tobacco, alcohol, and other substance use,[47–49] as has peer substance use,[50–52] suggesting that modeling plays a large role in the etiology of all forms of substance use. Further, different forms of psychopathology have been shown to predict or cooccur with multiple forms of substance use, particularly depression,[53–55] anxiety,[55,56] posttraumatic stress disorder,[57,58] and bipolar disorder.[59,60] Results from the Epidemiologic Catchment Area study suggest that among those with a mental disorder, 29% have a lifetime prevalence of a SUD.[53]

It is clear that these multiple environmental and individual factors do not exist in isolation, and often seem to work in tandem to increase substance use risk over the life course. Numerous individual studies have contributed to emergent work on the latent factor of SUD liability,[61] which identifies the many shared genotypic and phenotypic contributors to multiple forms of substance use. In support of a common liability concept, research has documented comorbidity between substances (even among those with opposite effects),[62] cross-tolerance and cross-dependence between substances,[63,64] and consistency across individuals in "staging," or the progression from tobacco and alcohol to illicit drugs over time.[65,66]

WHY ALCOHOL USE DISORDER/SUBSTANCE USE DISORDER TREATMENT PROVIDERS TURN A BLIND EYE TO TOBACCO USE

Although the risks for tobacco use are widely known, physicians and other addiction treatment providers do not prioritize combustible (ie, cigarettes) and noncombustible (ie, e-cigarettes) tobacco cessation in treatment.[15] There are several reasons why this would be the case. First, as noted by Romberger and Grant,[67] there exists a common belief among providers that it is simply too difficult for patients to address both smoking cessation and alcohol or other substance use abstinence at the same time, leading to failures in treatment.[68] As evidence of this belief, smoking is not addressed in one of the largest attended public support groups (Alcoholics Anonymous), and a large survey conducted in 1995 that included health professionals who provide AUD/SUD treatment, suggested that two-thirds of treatment providers did not support smoking cessation during active alcohol or other substance use treatment.[69] In addition, research has found that barriers to the provision of smoking cessation interventions in substance use treatment settings include a lack of skill in the area of tobacco use treatment and few resources.[70] Also, it is possible that a number of treatment facilities may make decisions to allow smoking to engage patient populations needed to meet financial goals. Facilities with smoking bans run the risk of alienating patients who smoke, which may result in patients choosing treatment facilities that allow smoking. Although the Joint Commission on Accreditation of Health Organizations introduced indoor restrictions on smoking as a quality indicator effective December 31, 1993,[71] many health care settings continue to allow smoking outdoors in designated areas to accommodate patients and staff who continue to smoke.

Second, owing to common effects on neurotransmitters of addiction, smoking has anecdotally been considered a replacement behavior for alcohol and other drugs, with no clear associations with relapse,[72] or even concerns that smoking cessation will result in a relapse of alcohol or other substances.[73] Owing to the neurophysiological mechanisms of nicotine, it is quite possible that those in recovery for AUD/SUD do indeed experience less craving for alcohol or other substances because AUD/SUD withdrawal symptoms may, in part, be avoided by tobacco use.[74] This reliance on tobacco during substance use treatment is reflected in research on readiness to change, and concerns over smoking cessation during treatment for AUD/SUD. For instance, studies have found that methadone patients recognize the health risks of smoking, but few plan on quitting in the next 30 days.[75] Also, most patients in treatment perceive smoking cessation to be as or more difficult than quitting drugs or alcohol.[68] Similarly, patients' perceived barriers to smoking cessation include fear of relapse and lack of emotional coping.[73]

Third, tobacco use is legal and does not cause marked inebriation. Impairment in the areas of attention, impulse control, working memory, executive functioning, motor coordination, and cognitive flexibility are some of the deficits related to acute and chronic drug use.[76,77] Unlike alcohol and illicit drugs, nicotine—the common substance across tobacco products—does not produce major cognitive or behavioral impairment.[78] In fact, research has found that nicotine improves memory and attention in clinical and nonclinical populations.[78,79] Other studies have found that nicotine may increase response accuracy and speed relative to a placebo.[80] The lack of acute and visible signs of cognitive and behavioral impairment may influence the perception that tobacco products are less harmful and not a focus of substance use treatment.

Fourth, e-cigarettes and other noncombustible tobacco products have become popular,[81] are perceived to aid in cigarette smoking cessation,[82] and have received support as a harm reduction strategy for tobacco use.[83] Nevertheless, reviews on this topic[81] and a recent report of the surgeon general[84] have strongly warned against the use of e-cigarettes as a harm reduction strategy owing to the lack of evidence for its safety and efficacy in reducing or quitting smoking. Thus, physician endorsement of e-cigarettes and similar devices as a way to reduce harm is not recommended and cessation of e-cigarette should be encouraged.

There are indeed counterpoints to all of these issues, but it is important to note that these beliefs against the treatment of tobacco use exist, and are commonly held by patients and treatment providers alike. It is often the case that treatment providers are former alcohol or substance users,[85] and former (or current) tobacco users themselves.[69,86,87] These providers in recovery are likely to have personal experiences that limit their motivation to urge those in treatment for AUD/SUD to stop smoking. Owing to these arguments, it is necessary to address each of these issues, as well as others, and provide compelling evidence for the provision of tobacco cessation services to those in treatment for AUD/SUD.

WHY ALCOHOL USE DISORDER/SUBSTANCE USE DISORDER TREATMENT PROVIDERS SHOULD ENCOURAGE TOBACCO CESSATION

Although it is indeed the case that tobacco use is both legal and does not cause marked inebriation, it remains a very harmful behavior to those with AUD/SUD, especially considering that 50% of concurrent users die from tobacco use.[14] Other issues raised with evidence-based supportive research are addressed herein.

Quitting Smoking Will Not Cause a Relapse in Alcohol or Substance Use

Concerns that smoking cessation will result in a relapse of alcohol or other substances[73] have been directly challenged by research. A number of studies have found either no association between smoking cessation and alcohol or substance use relapse,[72,88,89] or that smoking cessation actually improves AUD/SUD outcomes.[90–93] For instance, Stuyt[94] reported on the 1-year outcomes of a group of alcohol or substance users that received inpatient addiction treatment. No significant effect on the duration of sobriety after treatment was observed regarding primary drug of use of participants, but the duration of sobriety between tobacco users and nontobacco users was significantly different; nontobacco users (including nonsmokers at time of entry and those who engaged in cessation during treatment) had nearly twice the duration of sobriety time compared with tobacco users (6.9 vs 3.9 months of sobriety, respectively). Prochaska[95] has provided an extensive overview of this literature, and Prochaska and colleagues[96] completed a metaanalysis of 19 randomized, controlled trials evaluating tobacco treatment interventions for individuals with substance use problems. This metaanalysis indicated that smoking cessation interventions were associated with a 25% increased likelihood of long-term abstinence from alcohol and illicit drugs. Further, other work suggests that these benefits exist for the longer term; De Soto and colleagues[97] found that 10-year abstention from alcohol and smoking are highly correlated. Taken together, these findings suggest that smoking cessation dramatically improves treatment success for AUD/SUD.

Concurrent versus Successive Treatment Could Affect Outcomes

Regarding the timing of AUD/SUD and smoking cessation, study results are mixed. Some research has demonstrated that concurrent treatment for tobacco and AUD/SUD improves the outcomes of tobacco alone (with no detriment to AUD/SUD outcomes) or of both substances,[91,96,98–100] but studies in this area suffer from notable methodologic limitations, including nonrandomized designs.[101]

In contrast, recent work has suggested that concurrent treatment may have adverse effects on the outcomes for primary drug treatment.[102] Joseph and colleagues[102] randomized 499 smokers with AUD to a concurrent (during alcohol treatment) or delayed (6 months later) smoking cessation intervention. All individuals received the same cognitive–behavioral treatment that included nicotine replacement therapy. Results indicated that, although smoking cessation rates were similar at 18 months (12.4% vs 13.7%), abstinence and prolonged abstinence rates for alcohol were significantly worse in the concurrent (vs delayed) treatment group at the 6 (41% vs 56%), 12 (33% vs 42%), and 18 month (41% vs 48%) follow-ups.[102]

As noted by others,[103] it is difficult for individuals to make multiple health behavior changes, suggesting that the timing of intervention (concurrent vs delayed tobacco cessation provision) may be best decided in the collaborative relationship between the treatment provider and patient. Work in related areas has suggested that considerable economic savings are associated with the joint behavior change,[104] indicating that, regardless of the timing, tobacco cessation services for those with AUD/SUD provide benefits to both the individual and the community.

Smoking Bans Do Not Affect Admissions

There is evidence that those in AUD/SUD treatment are interested in tobacco cessation, even among military personnel, who smoke at higher rates than the general population.[105] One may argue that expectations for smoking cessation (eg, facility-wide bans) may decrease the engagement of patients in substance use programs. Nevertheless, patients in such programs have been shown to lower resistance to such expectations over time; Brown and colleagues[106] surveyed substance use treatment facility administrators in New York before and after tobacco-free regulation implementation. These regulations increased tobacco screening and cessation services (including pharmacotherapies) among settings, and increased support for policies was demonstrated. Importantly, although patient resistance was reported, patient admissions did not decrease.[106]

Alcohol Use Disorder/Substance Use Disorder Treatment Patients Actually Want to Quit Smoking

Despite potential concerns about adverse effects on craving and sobriety, evidence suggests that those in treatment for AUD/SUD know about the harms of smoking, are interested in quitting smoking, and are willing to consider to smoking cessation during their treatment.[68,107] McClure and colleagues[107] found that 80% of individuals in opioid use disorder treatment who were receiving opioid agonist treatment would consider trying the nicotine patch to stop smoking, and more than 40% would try nicotine gum. Kozlowski and colleagues[68] surveyed clients of the Addiction Research Foundation and found that 46% indicated that they were "moderately" to "very much" interested in receiving smoking cessation services, although there was a consistent preference for receipt of services after their alcohol or drug problem was treated.

TREATMENT

Smoking cessation for those in treatment for AUD/SUD should be multifaceted, with both behavioral therapy and medication. We describe recommended smoking cessation medications and their potential positive effects on alcohol or other substance use. Then, describe traditional psychological smoking cessation techniques are described, and emergent techniques that can be used with success across different substance use treatment settings are presented.

Pharmacotherapies for Smoking Cessation

The most widely used pharmacotherapies for smoking cessation include nicotine replacement therapy and nonnicotine products such as bupropion hydrochloride (Zyban) and varenicline (Chantix). Each is approved by the Food and Drug Administration for smoking cessation,[108] and each may be used in conjunction with pharmacotherapies for other addictions. Treatment is based on the individual case.

Bupropion is an antidepressant with simulant properties that inhibits the reuptake of norepinephrine and dopamine, and has shown to be an effective pharmacologic aid in smoking cessation. Little work exists regarding the additional benefits of bupropion for alcohol or other drug craving or use. Although 1 study has indicated that bupropion may reduce the craving and effect of methamphetamine,[109] bupropion has not demonstrated efficacy for the treatment of AUD.[110] Nicotine replacement therapy is one of the most well-studied pharmacotherapies for smoking, and is available over the counter in the form of a transdermal patch, gum, or lozenge. Nicotine replacement therapy inhalers and nasal mist are available by prescription. Although there are few known benefits of nicotine replacement therapy for the reduction of alcohol or other substance use, some work has suggested that nicotine replacement therapy administration reduces positive subjective alcohol response and urges to drink.[111,112]

Varenicline is a selective $\alpha4$ $\beta2$ partial nicotinic receptor agonist that diminishes nicotine's reinforcing effects. Currently, varenicline is the most effective medication for smoking cessation.[113–115] The benefits of varenicline include few side effects, and a lack of pharmacologic interaction with other medications owing to the fact that varenicline is not metabolized. Recent randomized trials with varenicline suggest that it may be effective at reducing alcohol use and craving.[116–119] However, warnings and precautions issued by the Food and Drug Administration indicate that patients may experience adverse effects when taking varenicline and drinking alcohol, including decreased tolerance to alcohol, increased drunkenness, unusual or aggressive behavior, or no memory of things that happened.[120] Thus, it is recommended that providers use varenicline with caution in patients with AUD.

Interestingly, recent work has also tested the possibility of using varenicline for opioid withdrawal. Based on work that found a relation between nicotinic acetylcholine receptor and opioid dependence, a placebo-controlled pilot study by Hooten and Warner[121] sought to test whether varenicline could decrease opioid withdrawal symptoms in patients with chronic pain during detoxification. In this small sample (only 7 patients remained in the varenicline group through completion of the study), results demonstrated that opioid withdrawal in patients receiving varenicline decreased over time whereas opioid withdrawal in patients receiving placebo increased, although results were not significant (regression coefficients were -0.116 and 0.086, respectively; $P = .26$).[121] Relatedly, in another study, varenicline was not effective for smoking cessation in smokers who were opiate dependent and undergoing methadone treatment.[122] Because this work is preliminary, further investigation of varenicline as a pharmacotherapy for concomitant smoking and AUD/SUD is warranted.

Psychological Treatments

The US Department of Health and Human Services recommended that pharmacologic treatments for smoking be accompanied by cognitive–behavioral therapy.[90] Cognitive–behavioral therapy helps individuals to learn to identify and correct maladaptive cognitions and behaviors. Accepted cognitive behavioral treatments for smoking cessation in medical settings include the "5 A's" model (ie, ask about use, advise to quit, assess willingness to make a quit attempt, assist in the quit attempt, and arrange follow-up) and motivational enhancement via discussion of the "5 R's (eg, relevance, risks, rewards, roadblocks, and repetition). These skills can be directly applied to those with AUD/SUD in the course of treatment. Other recommended cognitive–behavioral therapy skills include goal setting/making a commitment, self-monitoring of behavior, avoidance of triggers, management of cravings through alternative activities, problem-solving skills, and augmenting social support. Importantly, all of these techniques are common across treatment for different forms of substance use.[123,124]

There are also emergent areas of treatment provision that may be applicable to both tobacco use and other forms of substance use. One emergent treatment approach is behavioral economics, a model developed through psychology and economics that seeks to explain and ultimately treat the lapses in decision making commonly seen in substance users.[125] These lapses in judgment are notable in moments of extreme craving, where short-term reinforcement seems to be more valuable than the long-term goal of sobriety, thereby leading to lapse and relapse behavior.

Complementary to behavioral economics, specific forms of problem solving and mindfulness-based therapy targeting emotion regulation and the reduction of impulsive action are believed to directly address impulsivity and delay discounting deficits. Evidence demonstrates that mindfulness-based substance use treatment is effective in decreasing impulsivity, improving emotion regulation, and increasing perceived drug risk.[126,127] Moreover, a recent metaanalysis investigating the efficacy of mindfulness for smoking cessation on long-term follow-up (6 months) found that mindfulness may be as effective as other smoking cessation treatments (odds ratio, 2.52; 95% confidence interval, 0.76–8.29),[128] and individual studies have supported the efficacy of mindfulness-based approaches in relapse prevention (effect size d = 0.88, indicating a large effect size).[129] Other randomized controlled studies that have addressed potential mechanisms of mindfulness-based substance use treatment have found no significant differences with cognitive–behavioral therapy, but significant differences compared with usual care (eg, decreased anxiety, cravings, and dependence).[130]

Aside from cognitive–behavioral therapy-based methods, a related area of substance use treatment is contingency management, or reinforcing abstinence through external rewards.[131] Several clinical trials have supported the efficacy of contingency management for smoking,[92,132] alcohol,[133] cocaine,[134] and opioid use.[135] Metaanalytic reviews indicate that contingency management generates moderate effect sizes (Cohen's ds between 0.31 and 0.65, indicating small to medium effect sizes) in reducing multiple forms of substance use and other externalizing behaviors,[131,136] indicating impressive efficacy, but long-term financial feasibility has remained a significant limitation to its long-term use in most treatment settings.

Notably, combined treatment methods for smoking and AUD/SUD are lacking in this literature, despite the many common ingredients of successful treatment across these substances. Given the economic barriers to treatment (reduced duration of approved treatment and few resources available to physicians and other addiction treatment providers), the development of combined treatment methods may be of considerable individual and economic value. Although some mixed findings regarding concurrent treatment success likely dampen enthusiasm, it is clear that this work is in its infancy, and more sophisticated methods for evaluation of treatment components are becoming available. For instance, adaptive intervention methods can be developed to construct individualized treatment that varies in sequencing and intensity according to patient response, risk, burden, adherence, and preference.[137] Such modeling would be of considerable value in those with comorbid tobacco and AUD/SUD.

Relapse Prevention

It is notable that all forms of substance use come with a high risk of relapse. Smoking, for instance, is estimated to have a relapse rate of 10% per year after 1 year of abstinence.[138] Relapse prevention focuses on identifying high-risk relapse situations and problem solving possible urges to use. In addition, other skills include emotion regulation, goal adherence, and social support. Although relapse prevention is often used as a part of smoking cessation (and other substance use treatment), results from empirical work are not entirely encouraging. A metaanalysis reviewing the efficacy of 26 different relapse prevention programs for smoking, AUD, and SUD found only a small effect (r = 0.14).[139] Thus, although relapse prevention is intuitively a good practice, research does not suggest that patients are successful at using preventative skills long after treatment has ended.

It should be noted that relapse prevention in those with tobacco use and AUD/SUD may also include psychoeducation regarding the comorbidity of these behaviors, as well as the potential increases in relapse of AUD/SUD with smoking relapse. Other studies have indicated that smokers with AUD/SUD who are not ready to quit benefit from psychoeducation practices[140]; it is likely that this kind information can help former smokers with AUD/SUD to resist temptations to smoke after cessation in light of the considerable consequences to their sobriety.

SUMMARY

Many reviews of the comorbidity of smoking and AUD/SUD exist, and a number of studies have been directed at understanding concomitant risk, barriers to treatment, and the need for smoking cessation in AUD/SUD populations. These efforts have only indirectly impacted the field of practice, as evidenced by alarmingly low rates of available smoking cessation programs in AUD/SUD treatment settings, despite interest and need. Dissemination of empirically validated methods to reduce dangerous comorbid behaviors is important. It is also imperative for physicians and other addiction treatment providers to promote smoking cessation across all treatment foci to increase healthy behavior and challenge the misconception of incompatibility between smoking cessation and AUD/SUD treatment.

ACKNOWLEDGMENTS

The editors thank Hilary A. Tindle, Vanderbilt Center for Tobacco, Addiction and Lifestyle, Vanderbilt University Medical Center, for providing a critical review of this article.

REFERENCES

1. Salgado-Garcia FI, Cooper TV, Taylor T. Craving effect of smoking cues in smoking and antismoking stimuli in light smokers. Addict Behav 2013;38(10):2492–9.
2. Tverdal A, Bjartveit K. Health consequences of pipe versus cigarette smoking. Tob Control 2011;20(2):123–30.
3. Franceschini N, Deng Y, Flessner MF, et al. Smoking patterns and chronic kidney disease in US Hispanics: Hispanic Community Health Study/Study of Latinos. Nephrol Dial Transplant 2016;31(10):1670–6.
4. U.S. Department of Health and Human Services. The health consequences of smoking—50 years of progress: a report of the surgeon general. Atlanta (GA): U.S. Department of Health and Human Services; 2014.
5. Centers for Disease Control and Prevention. Cigarette smoking among adults—United States, 2005–2015. Morb Mortal Wkly Rep 2016;65(44):1205–11.
6. Grant BF, Hasin DS, Chou S, et al. Nicotine dependence and psychiatric disorders in the united states: results from the National Epidemiologic Survey on Alcohol and Related Conditions. Arch Gen Psychiatry 2004;61(11):1107–15.
7. Kalman D, Morissette SB, George TP. Co-morbidity of smoking in patients with psychiatric and substance use disorders. Am J Addict 2005;14(2):106–23.

8. Lasser K, Boyd JW, Woolhandler S, et al. Smoking and mental illness: a population-based prevalence study. Jama 2000;284(20):2606–10.

9. Gulliver SB, Kalman D, Rohsenow DJ, et al. Smoking and drinking among alcoholics in treatment: cross-sectional and longitudinal relationships. J Stud Alcohol 2000;61(1):157–63.

10. Hughes JR. Treating smokers with current or past alcohol dependence. American Journal of Health Behavior 1996;20:286–90.

11. Hughes J. Do smokers with current or past alcoholism need different or more intensive treatment? Alcohol Clin Exp Res 2002;26(12):1934–5.

12. Sobell MB. Alcohol and tobacco: clinical and treatment issues. Alcohol Clin Exp Res 2002;26(12):1954–5.

13. Marks JL, Hill EM, Pomerleau CS, et al. Nicotine dependence and withdrawal in alcoholic and nonalcoholic ever-smokers. J Subst Abuse Treat 1997;14(6): 521–7.

14. Hurt RD, Offord KP, Croghan IT, et al. Mortality following inpatient addictions treatment. Role of tobacco use in a community-based cohort. Jama 1996; 275(14):1097–103.

15. Substance Abuse and Mental Health Services Administration. Center for Behavioral Health Statistics and Quality. The N-SSATS report: tobacco cessation services. Rockville (MD): MD Substance Abuse and Mental Health Services Administration,; 2013. p. 2013.

16. 2008 PHS Guideline Update Panel, Liaisons, and Staff. Treating tobacco use and dependence: 2008 update U.S. Public health service clinical practice guideline executive summary. Respir Care 2008;53(9):1217–22.

17. Swan GE, Carmelli D, Cardon LR. The consumption of tobacco, alcohol, and coffee in Caucasian male twins: a multivariate genetic analysis. J Subst Abuse 1996;8(1):19–31.

18. Schilström B, Nomikos G, Nisell M, et al. N-methyl-D-aspartate receptor antagonism in the ventral tegmental area diminishes the systemic nicotine-induced dopamine release in the nucleus accumbens. Neuroscience 1997;82(3):781–9.

19. Clarke PB. Mesolimbic Dopamine Activation—The Key to Nicotine Reinforcement?. Bock J, Marsh J, editors. In Ciba Foundation Symposium 152- The Biology of Nicotine Dependence.

20. Awtry TL, Werling LL. Acute and chronic effects of nicotine on serotonin uptake in prefrontal cortex and hippocampus of rats. Synapse 2003;50(3):206–11.

21. Bang SJ, Commons KG. Age-dependent effects of initial exposure to nicotine on serotonin neurons. Neuroscience 2011;179:1–8.

22. Picciotto MR, Zoli M, Rimondini R, et al. Acetylcholine receptors containing the beta2 subunit are involved in the reinforcing properties of nicotine. Nature 1998; 391(6663):173.

23. Kishioka S, Kiguchi N, Kobayashi Y, et al. Nicotine effects and the endogenous opioid system. J Pharmacol Sci 2014;125(2):117–24.

24. Xue Y, Domino EF. Tobacco/nicotine and endogenous brain opioids. Prog Neuropsychopharmacol Biol Psychiatry 2008;32(5):1131–8.

25. Markou A, Paterson NE, Semenova S. Role of gamma-aminobutyric acid (GABA) and metabotropic glutamate receptors in nicotine reinforcement: potential pharmacotherapies for smoking cessation. Ann N Y Acad Sci 2004;1025: 491–503.

26. D'Souza MS, Markou A. The "Stop" and "Go" of nicotine dependence: role of GABA and glutamate. Cold Spring Harb Perspect Med 2013;3(6) [pii:a012146].

27. Perez de la Mora M, Mendez-Franco J, Salceda R, et al. Neurochemical effects of nicotine on glutamate and GABA mechanisms in the rat brain. Acta Physiol Scand 1991;141(2):241–50.
28. Picciotto M. Nicotine as a modulator of behavior: beyond the inverted U. Trends Pharmacol Sci 2003;23:494–9.
29. Kandel DB, Kandel ER. A molecular basis for nicotine as a gateway drug. N Engl J Med 2014;371(21):2038–9.
30. Tarter RE. Etiology of adolescent substance abuse: a developmental perspective. Am J Addict 2002;11(3):171–91.
31. Martin C, Earlywine M, Blackson TC, et al. Aggressivity, inattention, hyperactivity, and impulsivity in boys at high and low risk for substance abuse. J Abnorm Psychol 1994;22:177–203.
32. Doran N, Trim RS. The prospective effects of impulsivity on alcohol and tobacco use in a college sample. J Psychoactive Drugs 2013;45(5):379–85.
33. Balevich EC, Wein ND, Flory JD. Cigarette smoking and measures of impulsivity in a college sample. Subst Abuse 2013;34(3):256–62.
34. Mitchell MR, Potenza MN. Addictions and personality traits: impulsivity and related constructs. Curr Behav Neurosci Rep 2014;1(1):1–12.
35. Chase HW, Hogarth L. Impulsivity and symptoms of nicotine dependence in a young adult population. Nicotine Tob Res 2011;13(12):1321–5.
36. Holmes AJ, Hollinshead MO, Roffman JL, et al. Individual differences in cognitive control circuit anatomy link sensation seeking, impulsivity, and substance use. J Neurosci 2016;36(14):4038–49.
37. National Institute on Drug Abuse. Sensation seeking promotes initiation, impulsivity promotes escalation of substance use. 2016. Available at: https://www.drugabuse.gov/news-events/nida-notes/2016/05/sensation-seeking-promotes-initiation-impulsivity-promotes-escalation-substance-use. Accessed August 1, 2017.
38. Verdejo-García A, Lawrence AJ, Clark L. Impulsivity as a vulnerability marker for substance-use disorders: review of findings from high-risk research, problem gamblers and genetic association studies. Neurosci Biobehav Rev 2008;32(4):777–810.
39. Bickel WK, Marsch LA. Toward a behavioral economic understanding of drug dependence: delay discounting processes. Addiction 2001;96(1):73–86.
40. Sheffer C, MacKillop J, McGeary J, et al. Delay discounting, locus of control, and cognitive impulsiveness independently predict tobacco dependence treatment outcomes in a highly dependent, lower socioeconomic group of smokers. Am J Addict 2012;21(3):221–32.
41. Ashe ML, Newman MG, Wilson SJ. Delay discounting and the use of mindful attention versus distraction in the treatment of drug addiction: a conceptual review. J Exp Anal Behav 2015;103(1):234–48.
42. Bandura A. Social foundations of thought and action: a social cognitive theory. Englewood Cliffs (NJ): Prentice-Hall; 1986.
43. Petraitis J, Flay BR, Miller TQ. Reviewing theories of adolescent substance use: organizing pieces in the puzzle. Psychol Bull 1995;117(1):67–86.
44. Anda RF, Croft JB, Felitti VJ, et al. Adverse childhood experiences and smoking during adolescence and adulthood. Jama 1999;282(17):1652–8.
45. Dube SR, Anda RF, Felitti VJ, et al. Adverse childhood experiences and personal alcohol abuse as an adult. Addict behaviors 2002;27(5):713–25.

46. Dube SR, Felitti VJ, Dong M, et al. Childhood abuse, neglect, and household dysfunction and the risk of illicit drug use: the adverse childhood experiences study. Pediatrics 2003;111(3):564–72.

47. Chassin L, Curran PJ, Hussong AM, et al. The relation of parent alcoholism to adolescent substance use: a longitudinal follow-up study. J Abnorm Psychol 1996;105(1):70.

48. Patton GC, Carlin JB, Coffey C, et al. The course of early smoking: a population-based cohort study over three years. Addiction 1998;93(8):1251–60.

49. Webster RA, Hunter M, Keats JA. Peer and parental influences on adolescents' substance use: a path analysis. Int J Addict 1994;29(5):647–57.

50. West P, Sweeting H, Ecob R. Family and friends' influences on the uptake of regular smoking from mid-adolescence to early adulthood. Addiction 1999;94(9):1397–411.

51. Li C, Pentz MA, Chou C-P. Parental substance use as a modifier of adolescent substance use risk. Addiction 2002;97(12):1537–50.

52. Hu FB, Flay BR, Hedeker D, et al. The influences of friends' and parental smoking on adolescent smoking behavior: the effects of time and prior smoking1. J Appl Soc Psychol 1995;25(22):2018–47.

53. Regier DA, Farmer ME, Rae DS, et al. Comorbidity of mental disorders with alcohol and other drug abuse: results from the Epidemiologic Catchment Area (ECA) study. Jama 1990;264(19):2511–8.

54. Kessler RC, Crum RM, Warner LA, et al. Lifetime co-occurrence of DSM-III-R alcohol abuse and dependence with other psychiatric disorders in the National Comorbidity Survey. Arch Gen Psychiatry 1997;54(4):313–21.

55. Patton GC, Carlin JB, Coffey C, et al. Depression, anxiety, and smoking initiation: a prospective study over 3 years. Am J Public Health 1998;88(10):1518–22.

56. Grant BF, Stinson FS, Dawson DA, et al. Prevalence and co-occurrence of substance use disorders and independent mood and anxiety disorders: results from the national epidemiologic survey on alcohol and related conditions. Arch Gen Psychiatry 2004;61(8):807–16.

57. Acierno R, Kilpatrick DG, Resnick H, et al. Assault, PTSD, family substance use, and depression as risk factors for cigarette use in youth: findings from the National Survey of Adolescents. J Trauma Stress 2000;13(3):381–96.

58. Brown PJ, Stout RL, Mueller T. Substance use disorder and posttraumatic stress disorder comorbidity: addiction and psychiatric treatment rates. Psychol Addict Behav 1999;13(2):115.

59. Strakowski SM, DelBello MP. The co-occurrence of bipolar and substance use disorders. Clin Psychol Rev 2000;20(2):191–206.

60. Swann AC. The strong relationship between bipolar and substance-use disorder. Ann N Y Acad Sci 2010;1187(1):276–93.

61. Vanyukov MM, Tarter RE, Kirisci L, et al. Liability to substance use disorders: 1. Common mechanisms and manifestations. Neurosci Biobehavioral Rev 2003;27(6):507–15.

62. Helzer JE, Burnam A, McEvoy LT. Alcohol abuse and dependence. In: Robins LN, Regier DA, editors. Psychiatric disorders in America. The epidemiologic catchment area study. New York: The Free Press; 1991. p. 81–115.

63. Coper H. Cross-tolerance and cross-dependence between different types of addictive drugs. In: Fishman J, editor. The bases of addiction. Berlin: Abakon; 1978. p. 235–56.

64. Funk D, Marinelli PW, Le AD. Biological processes underlying co-use of alcohol and nicotine: neuronal mechanisms, cross-tolerance, and genetic factors. Alcohol Res Health 2006;29(3):186.
65. Kandel D, Yamaguchi K. From beer to crack: developmental patterns of drug involvement. Am J Public Health 1993;83(6):851–5.
66. Kirby T, Barry AE. Alcohol as a gateway drug: a study of US 12th graders. J Sch Health 2012;82(8):371–9.
67. Romberger DJ, Grant K. Alcohol consumption and smoking status: the role of smoking cessation. Biomed Pharmacother 2004;58(2):77–83.
68. Kozlowski LT, Skinner W, Kent C, et al. Prospects for smoking treatment in individuals seeking treatment for alcohol and other drug problems. Addict behaviors 1989;14(3):273–8.
69. Bobo JK, Slade J, Hoffman AL. Nicotine addiction counseling for chemically dependent patients. Psychiatr Serv 1995;46(9):945–7.
70. Daws C, Egan SJ, Allsop S. Brief intervention training for smoking cessation in substance use treatment. Aust Psychol 2013;48(5):353–9.
71. Joint Commission on the Accreditation of Healthcare Organizations. Accreditation manual for hospitals. Oakbrook Terrace (IL): Joint Commission on the Accreditation of Healthcare Organizations; 1992.
72. Hughes JR. Treatment of smoking cessation in smokers with past alcohol/drug problems. J Subst Abuse Treat 1993;10(2):181–7.
73. Asher MK, Martin RA, Rohsenow DJ, et al. Perceived barriers to quitting smoking among alcohol dependent patients in treatment. J Subst Abuse Treat 2003; 24(2):169–74.
74. Palfai TP, Monti PM, Ostafin B, et al. Effects of nicotine deprivation on alcohol-related information processing and drinking behavior. J Abnorm Psychol 2000;109:96–105.
75. Clemmey P, Brooner R, Chutuape MA, et al. Smoking habits and attitudes in a methadone maintenance treatment population. Drug Alcohol Depend 1997; 44(2–3):123–32.
76. Gould TJ. Addiction and cognition. Addict Sci Clin Pract 2010;5(2):4–14.
77. Crean RD, Crane NA, Mason BJ. An evidence based review of acute and long-term effects of cannabis use on executive cognitive functions. J Addict Med 2011;5(1):1–8.
78. Rezvani AH, Levin ED. Cognitive effects of nicotine. Biol Psychiatry 2001;49(3): 258–67.
79. Newhouse P, Kellar K, Aisen P, et al. Nicotine treatment of mild cognitive impairment: a 6-month double-blind pilot clinical trial. Neurology 2012;78(2):91–101.
80. Kumari V, Gray JA, Ffytche DH, et al. Cognitive effects of nicotine in humans: an fMRI study. Neuroimage 2003;19(3):1002–13.
81. Das S, Prochaska JJ. E-cigarettes, vaping, and other electronic nicotine products: harm reduction pathways or new avenues for addiction? Psychiatr Times 2017;34(8):24–5.
82. Sutfin EL, McCoy TP, Morrell HE, et al. Electronic cigarette use by college students. Drug Alcohol Depend 2013;131(3):214–21.
83. Nitzkin JL. The case in favor of E-cigarettes for tobacco harm reduction. Int J Environ Res Public Health 2014;11(6):6459–71.
84. U.S. Department of Health and Human Services. E-cigarette use among youth and young adults. A report of the surgeon general. Atlanta (GA): U.S. Department of Health and Human Services, Centers for Disease Control and Prevention; 2016.

85. Hecksher D. Former substance users working as counselors. A dual relationship. Subst Use Misuse 2007;42(8):1253–68.
86. Fuller BE, Guydish J, Tsoh J, et al. Attitudes toward the integration of smoking cessation treatment into drug abuse clinics. J Subst Abuse Treat 2007;32(1): 53–60.
87. Guydish J, Passalacqua E, Tajima B, et al. Staff smoking and other barriers to nicotine dependence intervention in addiction treatment settings: a review. J Psychoactive Drugs 2007;39(4):423–33.
88. Martin JE, Calfas KJ, Patten CA, et al. Prospective evaluation of three smoking interventions in 205 recovering alcoholics: one-year results of Project SCRAP-Tobacco. J Consult Clin Psychol 1997;65(1):190–4.
89. Reid MS, Fallon B, Sonne S, et al. Smoking cessation treatment in community-based substance abuse rehabilitation programs. J Subst Abuse Treat 2008; 35(1):68–77.
90. Frosch DL, Shoptaw S, Nahom D, et al. Associations between tobacco smoking and illicit drug use among methadone-maintained opiate-dependent individuals. Exp Clin Psychopharmacol 2000;8(1):97–103.
91. Bobo JK, McIlvain HE, Lando HA, et al. Effect of smoking cessation counseling on recovery from alcoholism: findings from a randomized community intervention trial. Addiction 1998;93:877–87.
92. Shoptaw S, Jarvik ME, Ling W, et al. Contingency management for tobacco smoking in methadone-maintained opiate addicts. Addict Behav 1996;21: 409–12.
93. Kohn CS, Tsoh JY, Weisner CM. Changes in smoking status among substance abusers: baseline characteristics and abstinence from alcohol and drugs at 12-month follow-up. Drug Alcohol Depend 2003;69(1):61–71.
94. Stuyt EB. Recovery rates after treatment for alcohol/drug dependence. Tobacco users vs. non-tobacco users. Am J Addict 1997;6(2):159–67.
95. Prochaska JJ. Failure to treat tobacco use in mental health and addiction treatment settings: a form of harm reduction? Drug Alcohol Depend 2010;110(3): 177–82.
96. Prochaska JJ, Delucchi K, Hall SM. A meta-analysis of smoking cessation interventions with individuals in substance abuse treatment or recovery. J Consult Clin Psychol 2004;72(6):1144–56.
97. De Soto CB, O'Donnell WE, De Soto JL. Long-term recovery in alcoholics. Alcohol Clin Exp Res 1989;13(5):693–7.
98. Cooney NL, Litt MD, Sevarino KA, et al. Concurrent alcohol and tobacco treatment: effect on daily process measures of alcohol relapse risk. J Consult Clin Psychol 2015;83(2):346–58.
99. Hurt RD, Eberman KM, Croghan IT, et al. Nicotine dependence treatment during inpatient treatment for other addictions: a prospective intervention trial. Alcohol Clin Exp Res 1994;18(4):867–72.
100. Joseph AM, Nichol KL, Anderson H. Effect of treatment for nicotine dependence on alcohol and drug treatment outcomes. Addict Behav 1993;18(6):635–44.
101. Kodl M, Fu SS, Joseph AM. Tobacco cessation treatment for alcohol-dependent smokers: when is the best time? Alcohol Res Health 2006;29(3):203–7.
102. Joseph AM, Willenbring ML, Nugent SM, et al. A randomized trial of concurrent versus delayed smoking intervention for patients in alcohol dependence treatment. J Stud Alcohol 2004;65(6):681–91.
103. Prochaska JJ, Spring B, Nigg CR. Multiple health behavior change research: an introduction and overview. Prev Med 2008;46(3):181–8.

104. Edington DW. Emerging research: a view from one research center. Am J Health Promot 2001;15(5):341–9.
105. Shealy SE, Winn JL. Integrating smoking cessation into substance use disorder treatment for military veterans: measurement and treatment engagement efforts. Addict Behav 2014;39(2):439–44.
106. Brown E, Nonnemaker J, Federman EB, et al. Implementation of a tobacco-free regulation in substance use disorder treatment facilities. J Subst Abuse Treat 2012;42(3):319–27.
107. McClure EA, Acquavita SP, Dunn KE, et al. Characterizing smoking, cessation services, and quit interest across outpatient substance abuse treatment modalities. J Subst Abuse Treat 2014;46(2):194–201.
108. U.S. Food and Drug Administration. FDA 101: smoking cessation products. 2016. Available at: https://www.fda.gov/ForConsumers/ConsumerUpdates/ucm198176.htm. Accessed August 7, 2017.
109. Newton TF, Roache JD, De La Garza R, et al. Bupropion reduces methamphetamine-induced subjective effects and cue-induced craving. Neuropsychopharmacology 2006;31(7):1537.
110. Ait-Daoud N, Lynch WJ, Penberthy JK, et al. Treating smoking dependence in depressed alcoholics. Alcohol Res Health 2007;29(3):213–20.
111. McKee SA, O'Malley SS, Shi J, et al. Effect of transdermal nicotine replacement on alcohol responses and alcohol self-administration. Psychopharmacology 2008;196(2):189–200.
112. Udo T, Harrison ELR, Shi J, et al. A preliminary study on the effect of combined nicotine replacement therapy on alcohol responses and alcohol self-administration. Am J Addict 2013;22(6):590–7.
113. Fagerström K, Hughes J. Varenicline in the treatment of tobacco dependence. Neuropsychiatr Dis Treat 2008;4(2):353–63.
114. Ebbert JO, Hughes JR, West RJ, et al. Effect of varenicline on smoking cessation through smoking reduction: a randomized clinical trial. Jama 2015;313(7):687–94.
115. Anthenelli RM, Benowitz NL, West R, et al. Neuropsychiatric safety and efficacy of varenicline, bupropion, and nicotine patch in smokers with and without psychiatric disorders (EAGLES): a double-blind, randomised, placebo-controlled clinical trial. Lancet 2016;387(10037):2507–20.
116. Mitchell JM, Teague CH, Kayser AS, et al. Varenicline decreases alcohol consumption in heavy-drinking smokers. Psychopharmacology 2012;223(3):299–306.
117. Erwin BL, Slaton RM. Varenicline in the treatment of alcohol use disorders. Ann Pharmacother 2014;48(11):1445–55.
118. Verplaetse TL, Pittman BP, Shi JM, et al. Effect of lowering the dose of varenicline on alcohol self-administration in drinkers with alcohol use disorders. J Addict Med 2016;10(3):166–73.
119. Litten RZ, Ryan ML, Fertig JB, et al. A double-blind, placebo-controlled trial assessing the efficacy of varenicline tartrate for alcohol dependence. J Addict Med 2013;7(4):277–86.
120. U.S. Food and Drug Administration. FDA drug safety communication: FDA updates label for stop smoking drug Chantix (varenicline) to include potential alcohol interaction, rare risk of seizures, and studies of side effects on mood, behavior, or thinking. 2015. Available at: https://www.fda.gov/Drugs/DrugSafety/ucm436494.htm. Accessed August 1, 2017.

121. Hooten WM, Warner DO. Varenicline for opioid withdrawal in patients with chronic pain: a randomized, single-blinded, placebo controlled pilot trial. Addict behaviors 2015;42:69–72.

122. Stein MD, Caviness CM, Kurth ME, et al. Varenicline for smoking cessation among methadone-maintained smokers: a randomized clinical trial. Drug Alcohol Depend 2013;133(2):486–93.

123. McHugh RK, Hearon BA, Otto MW. Cognitive-behavioral therapy for substance use disorders. Psychiatr Clin North Am 2010;33(3):511–25.

124. Fiore MC. US public health service clinical practice guideline: treating tobacco use and dependence. Respiratory care 2000;45(10):1200–62.

125. Bickel WK, Johnson MW, Koffarnus MN, et al. The behavioral economics of substance use disorders: reinforcement pathologies and their repair. Annu Rev Clin Psychol 2014;10:641–77.

126. Himelstein S. Mindfulness-based substance abuse treatment for incarcerated youth: a mixed method pilot study. Int J Transpers Stud 2011;30(1):3.

127. Tang YY, Tang R, Posner MI. Mindfulness meditation improves emotion regulation and reduces drug abuse. Drug Alcohol Depend 2016;163(Suppl 1):S13–8.

128. Maglione MA, Maher AR, Ewing B, et al. Efficacy of mindfulness meditation for smoking cessation: a systematic review and meta-analysis. Addict Behav 2017;69:27–34.

129. Vidrine JI, Spears CA, Heppner WL, et al. Efficacy of Mindfulness Based Addiction Treatment (MBAT) for smoking cessation and lapse. J consulting Clin Psychol 2016;84(9):824–38.

130. Spears CA, Hedeker D, Li L, et al. Mechanisms underlying mindfulness-based addiction treatment versus cognitive behavioral therapy and usual care for smoking cessation. J Consult Clin Psychol 2017;85(11):1029–40.

131. Prendergast M, Podus D, Finney J, et al. Contingency management for treatment of substance use disorders: a meta-analysis. Addiction 2006;101(11):1546–60.

132. Alessi SM, Petry NM, Urso J. Contingency management promotes smoking reductions in residential substance abuse patients. J Appl Behav Anal 2008;41(4):617–22.

133. Petry NM, Martin B, Cooney JL, et al. Give them prizes, and they will come: contingency management for treatment of alcohol dependence. J consulting Clin Psychol 2000;68(2):250–7.

134. Higgins ST, Wong CJ, Badger GJ, et al. Contingent reinforcement increases cocaine abstinence during outpatient treatment and 1 year of follow-up. J consulting Clin Psychol 2000;68(1):64–72.

135. Petry NM, Martin B. Low-cost contingency management for treating cocaine- and opioid-abusing methadone patients. J consulting Clin Psychol 2002;70(2):398–405.

136. Petry NM, Alessi SM, Olmstead TA, et al. Contingency management treatment for substance use disorders: how far has it come, and where does it need to go? Psychol Addict Behav 2017;31(8):897–906.

137. Murphy SA. An experimental design for the development of adaptive treatment strategies. Stat Med 2005;24(10):1455–81.

138. Hughes JR, Peters EN, Naud S. Relapse to smoking after 1 year of abstinence: a meta-analysis. Addict behaviors 2008;33(12):1516–20.

139. Irvin JE, Bowers CA, Dunn ME, et al. Efficacy of relapse prevention: a meta-analytic review. J consulting Clin Psychol 1999;67(4):563–70.

140. Rohsenow DJ, Monti PM, Colby SM, et al. Brief interventions for smoking cessation in alcoholic smokers. Alcohol Clin Exp Res 2002;26(12):1950–1.

Weighing the Risks and Benefits of Electronic Cigarette Use in High-Risk Populations

Deepa R. Camenga, MD, MHS[a],*, Hilary A. Tindle, MD, MPH[b]

KEYWORDS

- E-cigarette • Tobacco • Smoking cessation
- Electronic nicotine delivery systems (ENDS)

KEY POINTS

- The evidence surrounding the efficacy of electronic (e)-cigarettes for smoking cessation is inconclusive.
- Early evidence suggests that e-cigarette use among adults with cardiovascular or pulmonary disease may have less risk than continued cigarette smoking; however, it also most likely has more adverse health outcome risk than tobacco abstinence. Long-term health effects of e-cigarettes are unknown.
- Among adults with serious mental illness, initial findings support the possibility that e-cigarettes may help some smokers with smoking reduction.
- Primary care providers should continue to screen all adults and adolescents for tobacco use, including e-cigarette use, and offer evidence-based smoking cessation therapies including medications approved by the US Food and Drug Administration to all cigarette smokers.

INTRODUCTION

Electronic cigarettes (e-cigarettes) are battery-operated devices typically designed to deliver nicotine and other additives via aerosol.[1] Since the introduction of e-cigarettes into the US market more than a decade ago, rates of current (ie, past month) and ever e-cigarette use among US adults have increased, especially among cigarette smokers.[2] A recent analysis of the nationally representative sample of US adults in the Population Assessment of Tobacco and Health Study found that 5.5% of US adults reported current e-cigarette use and many (44%) of persons who currently

This article originally appeared in *Medical Clinics*, Volume 102, Issue 4, July 2018.
Disclosure Statement: The authors report no disclosures.
[a] Yale School of Medicine, 464 Congress Avenue Suite 260, New Haven, CT 06519, USA;
[b] Vanderbilt University Medical Center, 2525 West End, Suite 370, Nashville, TN 37203, USA
* Corresponding author.
E-mail address: deepa.camenga@yale.edu

use e-cigarette reported regular use some or most days of the week.[2] Among adults and youth who use more than 1 tobacco product, dual use of cigarettes and e-cigarettes is the most common pattern.[2] Thus, e-cigarette use rates are higher among cigarette smokers than nonsmokers, with 12.7% of daily cigarette smokers reporting concomitant e-cigarette use in 2015.[3]

Recent studies have found that more than half of cigarette smokers in primary care and about 20% of hospitalized smokers have ever used e-cigarettes, with the most popular reasons for use being cigarette smoking reduction or cessation and perceptions of reduced harm.[4–6] As awareness of e-cigarettes continues to increase among US adults and youth,[2] clinical discussions about e-cigarettes are also becoming more common.[7] Among 1500 primary care and specialty physicians surveyed, most reported regularly fielding patient questions about e-cigarettes.[7] Given the abundant scientific evidence demonstrating the numerous short-term and long-term health consequences of cigarette smoking and other tobacco use,[8,9] provider-patient discussions about the safety and efficacy of e-cigarettes for smoking cessation or reduction are likely to increase.

Public Health England and the Royal College of Physicians have published expert opinions that e-cigarettes are likely to be about 95% safer than conventional cigarettes.[10] This estimate has been widely contested in the literature and was based on the speculation that e-cigarettes have 5% of the risk of cigarettes because the levels of carcinogens in e-cigarette vapor are 5% of that in cigarette smoke.[11] In contrast, US professional organizations have been more cautious in affirming the safety of e-cigarettes because there is little direct evidence to assess their long-term health impact.[12] Additionally, given emerging evidence that e-cigarette experimentation is associated with cigarette smoking initiation among youth, and concerns that e-cigarettes may promote dual use or renormalize smoking, there is an ongoing debate about whether these products will indeed improve the health of the population.[13–15] These concerns are particularly salient for the more than 16 million Americans at risk for or with an existing smoking-attributable illness, including those with cardiovascular disease (CVD) and pulmonary disease.[9] Other high risk populations include adults with serious mental illness (SMI) and adolescents because they may have unique vulnerabilities to the potential risks and benefits of e-cigarettes.

Thus, in an effort to inform clinical counseling around e-cigarette use in primary care, this article reviews the evidence about e-cigarette safety and efficacy for smoking cessation. Given the burden of tobacco-related morbidity among smokers with cardiac disease, pulmonary disease, or SMI, this article also reviews the current evidence assessing the potential health impact of e-cigarette use in these populations, as well as among adolescents who are uniquely vulnerable to developing nicotine dependence. In addition, current recommendations for managing e-cigarette use in primary care are reviewed.

WHAT ARE ELECTRONIC CIGARETTES OR ELECTRONIC NICOTINE DELIVERY SYSTEMS?

E-cigarettes have been recognized by the US Food and Drug Administration (FDA) as a type of electronic nicotine delivery system (ENDS) that is a tobacco product.[16] There are more than 400 different brands of e-cigarettes available for purchase via retail stores and online, and several different types of products, including disposable, cartridge, and tank-style e-cigarettes; and personal vaporizers (**Fig. 1**).[17] Of note, tobacco companies produce several popular brands of e-cigarettes.[18]

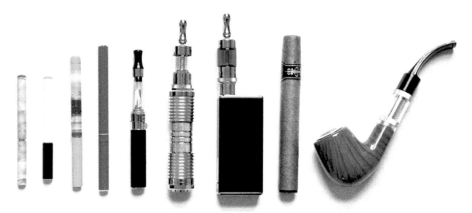

Fig. 1. There are several different types of e-cigarettes available, including disposable, cartridge and tank style, and personal vaporizers. (*From* US Department of Health and Human Services. US Food and Drug Administration (FDA). Tobacco products: vaporizers, e-cigarettes, and other Electronic Nicotine Delivery Systems (ENDS). Available at: https://www.fda.gov/TobaccoProducts/Labeling/ProductsIngredientsComponents/ucm456610.htm.   Accessed February 15, 2018.)

In general, an ENDS consists of a power source (ie, rechargeable lithium ion battery), heating element, and reservoir for e-liquid solution. The solution contains nicotine, propylene glycol and/or vegetable glycerin, flavorants, and other additives. Persons who use ENDSs can use prefilled cartridges of e-liquid or can pour the e-liquid directly into the device's chamber. When a person puffs on an e-cigarette, the e-liquid is heated and vaporized into a mist that is inhaled.[19] The act of inhaling is often called vaping rather than smoking because e-cigarettes do not burn tobacco and, therefore, do not produce smoke.

Patients may refer to e-cigarettes by a variety of names, including vape pens, e-pens, e-hookah, vape sticks, and mods.[20] ENDSs can resemble traditional cigarettes (cig-a-like models); however, newer products (also called advanced generation products) are especially popular among adult smokers and come in a variety of shapes, colors, and sizes.[21,22] Advanced generation products have been shown to deliver nicotine more efficiently than cig-a-like models,[23] and experienced adult who use them report that the ability to customize flavors and nicotine concentrations in advanced generation e-cigarettes helps promote traditional cigarette reduction or abstinence.[24,25]

SAFETY CONCERNS WITH ELECTRONIC NICOTINE DELIVERY SYSTEMS AND ELECTRONIC CIGARETTE LIQUIDS

Although the public may perceive that e-cigarettes contain only water vapor, the main ingredients in the e-cigarette (e)-liquid (e-juice) are nicotine, propylene glycol, vegetable glycerin, flavorants, and various additives.[1] E-liquid nicotine concentrations can vary from 0 to 24 or more mg per milliliter of e-liquid. The nicotine in many e-liquids has been shown to have vasoactive effects, although some studies suggest that the tobacco smoke compounds, rather than the nicotine, primarily contribute to increased cardiovascular risk.[9] Cardiovascular toxicants present in tobacco smoke, such as formaldehyde, acetaldehyde, acetone, acrolein, and butanol, have been found in e-cigarettes, although typically at lower concentrations than those found in combustible cigarettes.[26,27]

There are several safety concerns that have arisen in relation to e-liquids. First, studies have shown that the e-liquid nicotine content can be mislabeled, raising the concern that patients may unknowingly expose themselves to higher levels of nicotine than intended.[28,29] However, it is possible that mislabeling will become less of a problem as the FDA enacts regulations to standardize e-cigarette product labeling.[16] Second, although the e-liquids are intended to be consumed via inhalation, there are case reports of both e-liquid ingestion and transdermal poisonings. In fact, between 2012 and 2015 poison control centers reported a near 15-fold increase in the monthly number of exposures associated with e-cigarettes among children younger than 6 years (from 16 to 223 exposures).[30] Given that a 5-mL vial of an 18 mg per milliliter solution may contain up to 90 mg of nicotine, exposure to a vial of nicotine-containing e-liquid could result in intoxication or death.[16]

The potential for e-cigarette battery explosions has also risen as a safety concern.[31] Persons who use e-cigarette can inadvertently overheat the lithium ion battery, which results in explosion and fire due to the inherent flammability of the e-liquid.[32] Recent case series have reported burns and traumatic injuries of the oral or maxillofacial region (from explosions during e-cigarette use) and the extremities (from spontaneous explosions while the devices were stored in pockets).[33-38] Specific injuries to the oral cavity include intraoral burns, luxation injuries, and chipped and fractured teeth.[34] In addition, sight-threatening ocular injuries from ENDS explosions have been reported, including a penetrating corneoscleral laceration with iris prolapse, hyphema, and bilateral thermal and/or chemical corneal burns.[39,40] There is also a case report of ocular chemical injury due to inadvertent administration of the e-liquid (which was mistaken for antibiotic drops) to the eye.[41] To prevent the potential for explosion, some manufactured e-cigarettes have built-in timers to prevent battery overheating; however, these safety features are not regulated or standardized, and are not present in the modified devices.

ELECTRONIC CIGARETTES AND SMOKING CESSATION

In 2015, 68% of current smokers reported that they wanted to stop smoking completely; however, only 7% of adults reported success with smoking cessation in the past year.[42] Given well-documented obstacles to smoking cessation, many smokers are interested in trying e-cigarettes during efforts to quit or reduce smoking.[4-6] Hence, the role of e-cigarettes in smoking cessation is currently among the leading issues relevant to clinical and public health, and tobacco regulatory practice and policy.

Less than one-third of smokers use evidence-based medications during cigarette quit attempts.[43] Although not FDA-approved as a pharmacotherapy or device for smoking cessation, proponents of e-cigarettes argue that they help promote smoking cessation by providing a more attractive, and potentially effective, alternative to the 7 FDA-approved smoking cessation medications.[44,45] Both adolescents and adult smokers report that e-cigarettes are appealing because they are customizable, are available in a variety of flavors, can be used in traditionally smoke-free venues, and have fewer toxins than cigarettes.[46-50] Furthermore, unlike most FDA-approved smoking cessation therapies, persons who use e-cigarettes can mimic smoking behaviors (eg, via hand-to-mouth behaviors), which can provide a coping mechanism for conditioned smoking cues such as smoking when eating or consuming alcohol.[51]

To date, 2 randomized controlled clinical trials have examined the effectiveness of e-cigarettes for smoking cessation in adults. Bullen and colleagues[52] randomized 689 adult cigarette smokers in New Zealand who smoked more than 10 cigarettes per day to nicotine-containing (10–16 mg/mL) e-cigarettes, placebo (containing no nicotine) e-cigarettes, or nicotine patches (21 mg/24 h). At 6 months, the biochemically verified continuous abstinence rate was 7.3% in the e-cigarette group, 5.8% in the patch group, and 4.1% in the placebo e-cigarette group; however, the study was not statistically powered to detect a difference between the abstinence rates. Caponnetto and colleagues[19] randomized 300 smokers in Italy who were not intending to quit to placebo e-cigarettes, 7.2 mg nicotine-containing e-cigarettes, or e-cigarettes tapered from 7.2 to 5.4 mg nicotine. Twelve-month quit rates were statistically nonsignificant (13% for 7.2 mg nicotine e-cigarette, 9% for the e-cigarette tapered from 7.2 to 5.4 mg, and 4% for nonnicotine e-cigarettes).

A recent meta-analysis of 8 observational cohorts comparing e-cigarette use with no e-cigarette use failed to show a difference between the odds of cigarette abstinence between the 2 groups (odds ratio 0.74, $P = .051$, I^2 statistic $= 56\%$).[53] Of note, a variety of types and brands of e-cigarettes were provided or used by participants in both the randomized controlled trials and the observational studies, reducing the ability to determine if certain types of e-cigarette devices may be more helpful than others. Furthermore, the cohort studies are also limited because they generally did not report on other important predictors of successful smoking cessation, such as motivation to quit. By following a cohort of smokers, they may have underestimated the impact of e-cigarettes because they did not include smokers who had already successfully quit. Overall, given the small numbers of published clinical trials and the inherent limitations of observational studies, it is currently not possible for clinicians to determine whether e-cigarettes promote cessation from tobacco products among the general population of adult smokers.

SPECIAL POPULATIONS
Patients with Cardiovascular Disease

About 29% of the smoking-attributable deaths in the United States between 2005 and 2009 were due to CVD.[9] Among patients with established CVD, continued cigarette smoking is associated with poorer treatment outcomes; however, smoking cessation is a powerful secondary prevention technique and reduces mortality rates.[9,54] Data from the 2014 and 2015 National Interview Survey found that 21.9% of adult smokers ages 45 to 64 years with self-reported CVD and 14% of those with hypertension reported current e-cigarette use.[3] Adult smokers with CVD have a 1.54 increased likelihood of current e-cigarette use compared with smokers without any self-reported comorbidity.[3] These data indicate that it is especially important to understand how e-cigarette use affects overall cardiovascular health.

Currently, well-designed trials examining the efficacy of e-cigarettes for smoking cessation in adult smokers with CVD are lacking. Due to the vasoactive effects of nicotine and the presence of cardiovascular toxicants in e-liquids, there is ongoing concern in the field that long-term exposure to e-cigarette vapor may induce cardiac injury.[12,55] These toxicants can increase CVD risk by affecting blood pressure (BP) regulation, and promoting coagulation and atherosclerotic inflammation.[56–58] However, a recent longitudinal study showed that some persons who use e-cigarette have significantly lower levels of these carcinogens and toxins in their urine than cigarette smokers.[59]

Studies have yet to directly compare cardiovascular risk between cigarette smokers and persons who use e-cigarettes but early evidence suggests there is potential that e-cigarette use is associated with a range of cardiovascular effects. A recent study of 23 healthy adult volunteers who regularly use e-cigarette found that heart rate variability was shifted toward sympathetic predominance, a pattern associated with increased cardiovascular risk.[60] On the other hand, other small studies have reported positive effects on hypertension. For example, a medical record review of 43 patients with hypertension found that regular e-cigarette use reported on at least 2 occasions over a year was associated with a significant reduction in systolic and diastolic BP.[61] Another study of 52 adults with elevated systolic BP at baseline found that smoking reduction or abstinence via switching to e-cigarettes resulted in lower systolic BP at 1-year follow-up.[62] Furthermore, although the health effects of long-term exposure to nicotine among patients with CVD raises concern, studies have shown that patients with known CVD can tolerate short-term nicotine replacement therapy, raising the possibility that temporary e-cigarette use would be safe in this population.[63,64] These studies and others have led some experts to suggest that, although e-cigarette use may pose some heightened cardiovascular risk, especially among adults with existing CVD, the risk is likely to be less than that of cigarettes and, therefore, may result in reduced harm at the individual and population levels.[56]

Patients with Pulmonary Disease

E-cigarette use is also highly prevalent among adults with pulmonary disease such as asthma and chronic obstructive pulmonary disease (COPD), necessitating an understanding of the potential health effects in this group.[3] In 2015, about 12.5% of cigarette smokers with asthma and 15.8% of those with COPD reported past-month use of e-cigarettes.[3,65] Multiple studies demonstrate the relationship between cigarette smoking and worsened asthma symptoms, increased acute care utilization, missed days of school or work, and increased need for medications, which begs the question of whether e-cigarettes could result in harm reduction in this population if these individuals were able to completely stop using combustible tobacco.[66–68] Tobacco smoking is the leading cause of COPD globally. Cigarette smoking increases the risk of COPD exacerbations and lung function declines over time.[69,70]

There is emerging evidence that certain e-liquid flavorants have toxic pulmonary effects.[71] Cinnamon-flavored (ie, cinnamaldehyde) e-liquids and aerosols have been shown to be cytotoxic at low concentrations in human lung cells.[72] Recent studies have demonstrated that several flavorings induce expression of inflammatory cytokines in lung cell cultures.[73] One case report documented respiratory bronchiolitis interstitial lung disease, confirmed by open lung biopsy, in a person who uses e-cigarette who also smoked cigarettes.[74] Diacetyl is present in many e-cigarette liquids (found in caramel, butterscotch, watermelon, piña colada, and strawberry) and has been shown to be a cause of bronchiolitis obliterans (popcorn lung) in the occupational setting.[72,75]

There are few studies that tested the effect of e-cigarettes on human pulmonary function. Among healthy volunteers, several studies have shown short-term increases in airway hyperreactivity and airway resistance after using nicotine-containing e-cigarettes.[76,77] Studies have also shown that smokers with COPD who completely switched to e-cigarettes had a reduction in symptoms and an improved quality of life.[78] A small group of asthmatic smokers (18) who switched to e-cigarettes were followed prospectively and found to have improvements in spirometry and Asthma Control Questionnaire scores up to 2 years later.[79,80] Overall, the evidence regarding pulmonary outcomes is scant and future research is needed to understand the long-term impact of e-cigarettes on pulmonary health.

Patients with Serious Mental Illness

Primary care providers have an important role in improving health and care coordination of patients with SMI. Although smoking rates have declined significantly in the general population, they remain disproportionately high in individuals with mental health conditions.[81] Adults with SMI are those who have a current or past-year behavioral, mental, or emotional disorder that seriously impairs participation in major life activities.[82] Schizophrenia, schizoaffective disorder, bipolar disorder, or major depressive disorder, as well as other disorders, have the potential to produce impairment to a degree that a person would have SMI.[82] People with SMI generally have poorer physical health and life expectancy, which is partially attributed to the high prevalence of tobacco use in this population.[83] Smokers with SMI have greater difficulty quitting tobacco than those without SMI, which has been attributed to variety of factors, including higher levels of nicotine dependence, comorbid substance use, and psychosocial stress.[84]

The prevalence of e-cigarette use among adults with SMI varies, and studies have reported prevalence rates of current e-cigarette use from 11% to greater than 30%.[14,85,86] Prevalence rates are higher among adults with multiple mental health diagnoses compared with those with a single diagnosis.[87] A 2015 examination of a large representative sample of US adults found that 1 in 5 adults with SMI reported current e-cigarette use, and adults with mental health conditions were almost 2 times more likely to report past-month use of e-cigarettes than those without mental health conditions.[87]

Initial findings support the possibility that e-cigarettes may help with smoking reduction, whereas it is unknown how e-cigarette use will affect smoking cessation.[14] Thus, there is growing concern that e-cigarette use in this population may encourage dual e-cigarette and cigarette use. A 2015 study of a national representative sample of more than 6000 adult smokers found that adults with SMI were more likely than those without SMI to substitute some cigarettes with e-cigarettes during a quit attempt; however, they were also more likely to have completely switched to e-cigarettes during a smoking quit attempt.[87] However, a secondary analysis of the Bullen and colleagues[52] trial, which randomized 657 smokers to 16 mg nicotine e-cigarettes, 21 mg nicotine patches, or 0 mg nicotine e-cigarettes, with minimal behavioral support, found no differences in cessation rates (patches 14%, 16 mg e-cigarettes 5%, 0 mg e-cigarettes 0%, $P = .245$) among the subsample of 86 smokers with mental illness.[88]

More specific to SMI, a feasibility study of 14 smokers with schizophrenia not intending to quit found that 50% of the sample reported smoking 50% fewer cigarettes per day after 52 weeks, 14% had quit smoking, and schizophrenia symptoms did not increase with smoking.[19] Another pilot study provided e-cigarettes to 19 daily smokers with SMI for 4 weeks and found that self-reported use of combustible tobacco declined from 192 to 67 cigarettes per week ($P = .005$), confirmed by a reduction in breath carbon monoxide.[89] This initial evidence suggests that e-cigarette use is associated with reductions in cigarette smoking; however, future studies are needed in larger populations to validate these findings.

Considerations in Adolescents

When weighing the potential benefits of e-cigarette use in adult smokers, public health advocates and clinicians must also consider the potential risks if widespread use in adults facilitates youth exposure to nicotine through e-cigarettes and other tobacco products. Adolescents have heighted neurodevelopmental vulnerability to the development of nicotine addiction. A recognition of this enhanced vulnerability has led the United States to develop and implement multifaceted and comprehensive tobacco control efforts aimed at reducing youth access to tobacco.[90] As a result, rates of cigarette smoking among US adolescents have fallen in the last decade. In 2016, only

8.6% of high school students reported past-month cigarette smoking, whereas 19.6% reported this in 2006.[90–92] However, during this same period, rates of e-cigarette use have increased from less than 2% in 2011 to 11.3% of high school and 4.3% of middle school students reported current e-cigarette use in 2016.[91] Thus, whereas cigarettes are the most popular tobacco product used by US adults, e-cigarettes have surpassed cigarettes as the most common tobacco product used by youth.[20,91]

A recent meta-analysis of 9 longitudinal studies of 17,389 adolescents and young adults ages 14 to 30 years found that pooled probabilities of cigarette smoking initiation were 30.4% for baseline persons who ever used e-cigarette and 7.9% for baseline persons who never used e-cigarette.[13] The analysis reported that the baseline of ever using e-cigarettes (vs never using e-cigarettes) increased the odds of cigarette smoking initiation, with a pooled odds ratio of 3.62 (95% CI 2.42–5.41) when adjusting for known demographic, psychosocial, and behavioral risk factors for cigarette smoking. This raised the concern that e-cigarette use in youth may increase the burden of tobacco-related morbidity and mortality in future generations.[13] Several observational studies have found no association between e-cigarette use and smoking cessation in adolescents[93,94]; however, longitudinal studies in this area are lacking. Taken together, these findings led to the 2016 US Surgeon General's report, *E-cigarette Use Among Youth and Young Adults*, which recommended that "The use of products containing nicotine in any form among youth, including in e-cigarettes, is unsafe."[20]

ELECTRONIC CIGARETTES IN THE CONTEXT OF TOBACCO PRODUCT REGULATION AND PROPOSED POLICY CHANGES FOR TOBACCO CONTROL

In 2016, the FDA exercised its authority, as outlined in the 2009 Family Smoking Prevention and Tobacco Control Act, to regulate e-cigarettes as tobacco products with a goal of improving population health.[16,95] Building on this goal, the FDA has affirmed its commitment to encourage tobacco product innovations that offer smokers safer alternatives to cigarettes.[96] Additionally, the FDA has proposed a strategy that could reduce the nicotine content in cigarettes to levels that are low enough to be minimally addictive or even nonaddictive.[95] This strategy is aimed at encouraging millions of adult smokers to cease their use of combustible tobacco products but could also prompt the continued use or even initiation of less harmful, noncombustible nicotine delivery systems, such as e-cigarettes. For some populations, such as those with CVD, pulmonary disease, or SMI, this strategy offers both opportunities and challenges. Although harm reduction is expected with the complete cessation of combustible tobacco, chronic exposure to nicotine in e-cigarettes may not be totally benign due to the pharmacologic effects of nicotine on the cardiovascular system or the inflammatory effects of e-liquids on the lung. Furthermore, there could be unintended consequences for adolescents and young adults, especially if this policy encourages young people to erroneously view e-cigarettes as harmless instead of less harmful than combustible tobacco. Overall, the proposed US policy change will be considered successful if it achieves a similar outcome to that seen in the United Kingdom, where widespread use of e-cigarettes has been credited with reducing prevalence of cigarette smoking.[97]

SYNTHESIS OF THE EVIDENCE TO INFORM CLINICAL MANAGEMENT OF ELECTRONIC CIGARETTE USE IN PRIMARY CARE

Several professional organizations have put forth clinical policy statements that include e-cigarettes (**Box 1**). Of note, the US Preventative Services Task Force states

---

Box 1
Resources for current recommendations from US professional organizations

US Preventive Services Task Force (2015)[98]
  https://www.uspreventiveservicestaskforce.org/

American Heart Association (2015)[12]
  http://www.heart.org/HEARTORG/

The Forum of International Respiratory Society Position Statement (2014)[101]
  https://www.firsnet.org/

American Academy of Pediatrics (2015)[99]
  https://www.aap.org/en-us/Pages/Default.aspx

American Society of Clinical Oncology (2015)[102]
  https://www.asco.org/

---

the evidence is insufficient to determine the efficacy of e-cigarettes for smoking cessation, and the American Academy of Pediatrics recommends against e-cigarette use for smoking cessation.[98,99] However, the American Heart Association does point out that it is reasonable to support patients who use e-cigarettes for smoking cessation in settings in which the patient has repeatedly failed or is intolerant of guideline-based treatment or refuses conventional, FDA-approved smoking cessation medications.[12] In these cases, the clinician should advise patients about the potential risks of e-cigarette exposure and the lack of evidence to support their efficacy for smoking cessation.

COUNSELING ADULTS WHO USE ELECTRONIC CIGARETTES

When discussing e-cigarettes, primary care providers should educate patients about potential risks and benefits of e-cigarettes and specific concerns relevant to adults with heightened vulnerability tobacco-induced illnesses. In general, primary care providers should listen openly to patients' views on e-cigarettes and convey that there is not enough medical evidence to recommend e-cigarettes as a safe or efficacious product for smoking cessation. Based on the data presented in this article, medical professionals may tailor advice based on the patient's comorbid conditions. For example, patients with CVD should be counseled about the potential adverse effects of nicotine on cardiovascular health, whereas patients with pulmonary disease should be aware there is some inconclusive evidence of symptom improvement, as well as increased pulmonary inflammation, with e-cigarettes. Patients with SMI should learn that the current evidence supports the possibility that e-cigarettes may help with smoking reduction, whereas it is unknown how e-cigarette use will affect smoking cessation.[14] Nonetheless, all patients should be counseled on the potentially superior health impact of tobacco abstinence compared with prolonged e-cigarette use.

Primary care providers should continue to screen all adults for tobacco use, including e-cigarette use, and offer evidence-based smoking cessation therapies, including FDA-approved medications, to all cigarette smokers.[100] Additionally, e-cigarette use in smokers should be viewed as a step toward cessation, and trigger a deeper discussion between the physician and patient about goals for smoking cessation and the use of evidence-based medications. Overall, there is a great ongoing need to understand the potential impact of e-cigarettes on both individual smoking cessation and population health.

FUTURE CONSIDERATIONS AND SUMMARY

Tobacco exposure continues to be the leading cause of preventable morbidity and mortality in the United States. As a result, clinicians, policy makers, and public health professionals continue to strive to reduce cigarette and tobacco smoking rates. E-cigarettes are used by smokers in efforts to quit smoking; however, to date, the evidence regarding their efficacy for smoking cessation is inconclusive and does not meet the standard for evidence-based practice recommendations.

ACKNOWLEDGMENTS

The editors wish to thank Sara Kalkhoran, Massachusetts General Hospital and Harvard Medical School, for providing a critical review of this article.

REFERENCES

1. Grana R, Benowitz N, Glantz SA. E-cigarettes: a scientific review. Circulation 2014;129(19):1972–86.
2. Kasza KA, Ambrose BK, Conway KP, et al. Tobacco-product use by adults and youths in the United States in 2013 and 2014. N Engl J Med 2017;376(4):342–53.
3. Kruse GR, Kalkhoran S, Rigotti NA. Use of electronic cigarettes among U.S. Adults with medical comorbidities. Am J Prev Med 2017;52(6):798–804.
4. De Genna NM, Ylioja T, Schulze AE, et al. Electronic cigarette use among counseled tobacco users hospitalized in 2015. J Addict Med 2017;11(6):449–53.
5. Kalkhoran S, Alvarado N, Vijayaraghavan M, et al. Patterns of and reasons for electronic cigarette use in primary care patients. J Gen Intern Med 2017;32(10):1122–9.
6. Coleman BN, Rostron B, Johnson SE, et al. Electronic cigarette use among US adults in the Population Assessment of Tobacco and Health (PATH) Study, 2013–2014. Tob Control 2017;26(e2):e117–26.
7. Nickels AS, Warner DO, Jenkins SM, et al. Beliefs, practices, and self-efficacy of us physicians regarding smoking cessation and electronic cigarettes: a national survey. Nicotine Tob Res 2017;19(2):197–207.
8. U.S Department of Health and Human Services. How tobacco smoke causes disease: the biology and behavioral basis for smoking-attributable disease: a report of the Surgeon General. Atlanta (GA): U.S Department of Health and Human Services, Centers for Disease Control and Prevention, National Center for Chronic Disease Prevention and Health Promotion, Office on Smoking and Health; 2010.
9. US Department of Health and Human Services. The health consequences of smoking–50 years of progress: a report of the surgeon general. Atlanta (GA): US Department of Health and Human Services, Centers for Disease Control and Prevention, National Center for Chronic Disease Prevention and Health Promotion, Office on Smoking and Health; 2014.
10. McNeill A, Brose L, Calder R, et al. E-cigarettes: an evidence update. Public Health Engl 2015;3:76–80.
11. Hajek P. Underpinning evidence for the estimate that e-cigarette use is around 95% safer than smoking: authors' note. 2015. Available at: https://www.gov.uk/government/uploads/system/uploads/attachment_data/file/456704/McNeill-Hajek_report_authors_note_on_evidence_for_95_estimate.pdf. Accessed October 1, 2017.

12. Bhatnagar A, Whitsel LP, Ribisl KM, et al. Electronic cigarettes. A policy statement from the American Heart Association 2014;129(1):28–41.
13. Soneji S, Barrington-Trimis JL, Wills TA, et al. Association between initial use of e-cigarettes and subsequent cigarette smoking among adolescents and young adults: a systematic review and meta-analysis. JAMA Pediatr 2017;171(8): 788–97.
14. Hefner K, Valentine G, Sofuoglu M. Electronic cigarettes and mental illness: Reviewing the evidence for help and harm among those with psychiatric and substance use disorders. Am J Addict 2017;26(4):306–15.
15. Choi K, Grana R, Bernat D. Electronic nicotine delivery systems and acceptability of adult cigarette smoking among Florida youth: renormalization of smoking? J Adolesc Health 2017;60(5):592–8.
16. Food and Drug Administration, Health and Human Services. Deeming Tobacco Products To Be Subject to the Federal Food, Drug, and Cosmetic Act, as Amended by the Family Smoking Prevention and Tobacco Control Act; Restrictions on the Sale and Distribution of Tobacco Products and Required Warning Statements for Tobacco Products. Final rule. Fed Regist 2016;81(90): 28973–9106.
17. Grana RA, Ling PM. "Smoking revolution": a content analysis of electronic cigarette retail websites. Am J Prev Med 2014;46(4):395–403.
18. Richtel M. A bolder effort by big tobacco on e-cigarettes. New York Times, June 17, 2014. p. A1.
19. Caponnetto P, Campagna D, Cibella F, et al. EffiCiency and safety of an eLectronic cigAreTte (ECLAT) as tobacco cigarettes substitute: a prospective 12-month randomized control design study. PLoS One 2013;8(6):e66317.
20. US Department of Health and Human Services. E-cigarette use among youth and young adults: a report of the surgeon general. Atlanta (GA): US Department of Health and Human Services, Centers for Disease Control and Prevention, National Center for Chronic Disease Prevention and Health Promotion, Office on Smoking and Health; 2016.
21. Chen C, Zhuang YL, Zhu SH. E-cigarette design preference and smoking cessation: a U.S. population study. Am J Prev Med 2016;51(3):356–63.
22. Yingst JM, Veldheer S, Hrabovsky S, et al. Factors associated with electronic cigarette users' device preferences and transition from first generation to advanced generation devices. Nicotine Tob Res 2015;17(10):1242–6.
23. Lechner WV, Meier E, Wiener JL, et al. The comparative efficacy of first- versus second-generation electronic cigarettes in reducing symptoms of nicotine withdrawal. Addiction 2015;110(5):862–7.
24. Etter JF. Characteristics of users and usage of different types of electronic cigarettes: findings from an online survey. Addiction 2016;111(4):724–33.
25. Farsalinos KE, Romagna G, Tsiapras D, et al. Impact of flavour variability on electronic cigarette use experience: an internet survey. Int J Environ Res Public Health 2013;10(12):7272–82.
26. Goniewicz ML, Knysak J, Gawron M, et al. Levels of selected carcinogens and toxicants in vapour from electronic cigarettes. Tob Control 2014;23(2):133–9.
27. Goniewicz ML, Gawron M, Smith DM, et al. Exposure to nicotine and selected toxicants in cigarette smokers who switched to electronic cigarettes: a longitudinal within-subjects observational study. Nicotine Tob Res 2017;19(2):160–7.
28. Buettner-Schmidt K, Miller DR, Balasubramanian N. Electronic cigarette refill liquids: child-resistant packaging, nicotine content, and sales to minors. J Pediatr Nurs 2016;31(4):373–9.

29. Goniewicz ML, Kuma T, Gawron M, et al. Nicotine levels in electronic cigarettes. Nicotine Tobac Res 2013;15(1):158–66.
30. Kamboj A, Spiller HA, Casavant MJ, et al. Pediatric exposure to e-cigarettes, nicotine, and tobacco products in the United States. Pediatrics 2016;137(6) [pii:e20160041].
31. Ramirez JI, Ridgway CA, Lee JG, et al. The unrecognized epidemic of electronic cigarette burns. J Burn Care Res 2017;38(4):220–4.
32. Treitl D, Solomon R, Davare DL, et al. Full and partial thickness burns from spontaneous combustion of e-cigarette lithium-ion batteries with review of literature. J Emerg Med 2017;53(1):121–5.
33. Archambeau BA, Young S, Lee C, et al. E-cigarette blast injury: complex facial fractures and pneumocephalus. West J Emerg Med 2016;17(6):805–7.
34. Harrison R, Hicklin D Jr. Electronic cigarette explosions involving the oral cavity. J Am Dent Assoc 2016;147(11):891–6.
35. Hassan S, Anwar MU, Muthayya P, et al. Burn injuries from exploding electronic cigarette batteries: an emerging public health hazard. J Plast Reconstr Aesthet Surg 2016;69(12):1716–8.
36. Meernik C, Williams FN, Cairns BA, et al. Burns from e-cigarettes and other electronic nicotine delivery systems. BMJ 2016;354:i5024.
37. Goverman J, Schulz JT. Thigh burns from exploding E-cigarette. Burns 2016; 42(7):1618.
38. Colaianni CA, Tapias LF, Cauley R, et al. Injuries caused by explosion of electronic cigarette devices. Eplasty 2016;16:ic9.
39. Paley GL, Echalier E, Eck TW, et al. Corneoscleral laceration and ocular burns caused by electronic cigarette explosions. Cornea 2016;35(7):1015–8.
40. Khairudin MN, Mohd Zahidin AZ, Bastion ML. Front to back ocular injury from a vaping-related explosion. BMJ Case Rep 2016;2016 [pii:bcr2016214964].
41. Jamison A, Lockington D. Ocular chemical injury secondary to electronic cigarette liquid misuse. JAMA Ophthalmol 2016;134(12):1443.
42. Quitting smoking among adults–United States, 2001-2010. MMWR Morb Mortal Wkly Rep 2011;60(44):1513–9.
43. Babb S, Malarcher A, Schauer G, et al. Quitting smoking among adults - United States, 2000-2015. MMWR Morb Mortal Wkly Rep 2017;65(52):1457–64.
44. Correa JB, Ariel I, Menzie NS, et al. Documenting the emergence of electronic nicotine delivery systems as a disruptive technology in nicotine and tobacco science. Addict Behav 2017;65:179–84.
45. Pechacek TF, Nayak P, Gregory KR, et al. The potential that electronic nicotine delivery systems can be a disruptive technology: results from a national survey. Nicotine Tob Res 2016;18(10):1989–97.
46. Patrick ME, Miech RA, Carlier C, et al. Self-reported reasons for vaping among 8th, 10th, and 12th graders in the US: Nationally-representative results. Drug Alcohol Depend 2016;165:275–8.
47. Bold KW, Kong G, Cavallo DA, et al. Reasons for trying E-cigarettes and risk of continued use. Pediatrics 2016;138(3) [pii:e20160895].
48. Patel D, Davis KC, Cox S, et al. Reasons for current E-cigarette use among U.S. adults. Prev Med 2016;93:14–20.
49. Berg CJ. Preferred flavors and reasons for e-cigarette use and discontinued use among never, current, and former smokers. Int J Public Health 2016;61(2): 225–36.

50. Kong G, Morean ME, Cavallo DA, et al. Reasons for electronic cigarette experimentation and discontinuation among adolescents and young adults [published online ahead of print Dec 6 2014]. Nicotine Tob Res 2015;17(7):847–54.
51. Caponnetto P, Russo C, Bruno CM, et al. Electronic cigarette: a possible substitute for cigarette dependence. Monaldi Arch Chest Dis 2013;79(1):12–9.
52. Bullen C, Howe C, Laugesen M, et al. Electronic cigarettes for smoking cessation: a randomised controlled trial. Lancet 2013;382(9905):1629–37.
53. El Dib R, Suzumura EA, Akl EA, et al. Electronic nicotine delivery systems and/or electronic non-nicotine delivery systems for tobacco smoking cessation or reduction: a systematic review and meta-analysis. BMJ Open 2017;7(2): e012680.
54. Rigotti NA, Clair C. Managing tobacco use: the neglected cardiovascular disease risk factor. Eur Heart J 2013;34(42):3259–67.
55. Bhatnagar A. Are electronic cigarette users at increased risk for cardiovascular disease? JAMA Cardiol 2017;2(3):237–8.
56. Benowitz NL, Fraiman JB. Cardiovascular effects of electronic cigarettes. Nat Rev Cardiol 2017;14(8):447–56.
57. Rigotti NA, Clair C. Managing tobacco use: the neglected cardiovascular disease risk factor. Eur Heart J 2013;34(42):3259–67.
58. Morris PB, Ference BA, Jahangir E, et al. Cardiovascular effects of exposure to cigarette smoke and electronic cigarettes. J Am Coll Cardiol 2015;66(12): 1378–91.
59. Shahab L, Goniewicz ML, Blount BC, et al. Nicotine, carcinogen, and toxin exposure in long-term e-cigarette and nicotine replacement therapy users: a cross-sectional study. Ann Intern Med 2017;166(6):390–400.
60. Moheimani RS, Bhetraratana M, Yin F, et al. Increased cardiac sympathetic activity and oxidative stress in habitual electronic cigarette users: Implications for cardiovascular risk. JAMA Cardiol 2017;2(3):278–84.
61. Polosa R, Morjaria JB, Caponnetto P, et al. Blood Pressure Control in Smokers with Arterial Hypertension Who Switched to Electronic Cigarettes. International Journal of Environmental Research and Public Health 2016;13(11):1123.
62. Farsalinos K, Cibella F, Caponnetto P, et al. Effect of continuous smoking reduction and abstinence on blood pressure and heart rate in smokers switching to electronic cigarettes. Intern Emerg Med 2016;11(1):85–94.
63. Meine TJ, Patel MR, Washam JB, et al. Safety and effectiveness of transdermal nicotine patch in smokers admitted with acute coronary syndromes. Am J Cardiol 2005;95(8):976–8.
64. Mills EJ, Thorlund K, Eapen S, et al. Cardiovascular events associated with smoking cessation pharmacotherapies a network meta-analysis. Circulation 2014;129(1):28–41.
65. Centers for Disease Control. National current asthma prevalence (2015). 2017. Available at: https://www.cdc.gov/asthma/most_recent_data.htm. Accessed April 6, 2017.
66. Thomson NC, Chaudhuri R, Heaney LG, et al. Clinical outcomes and inflammatory biomarkers in current smokers and exsmokers with severe asthma. J Allergy Clin Immunol 2013;131(4):1008–16.
67. Thomson NC, Chaudhuri R. Asthma in smokers: challenges and opportunities. Curr Opin Pulm Med 2009;15(1):39–45.
68. Chaudhuri R, McSharry C, McCoard A, et al. Role of symptoms and lung function in determining asthma control in smokers with asthma. Allergy 2008;63(1): 132–5.

69. Rabe KF, Watz H. Chronic obstructive pulmonary disease. Lancet 2017; 389(10082):1931–40.
70. Jimenez-Ruiz CA, Andreas S, Lewis KE, et al. Statement on smoking cessation in COPD and other pulmonary diseases and in smokers with comorbidities who find it difficult to quit. Eur Respir J 2015;46(1):61–79.
71. Shields PG, Berman M, Brasky TM, et al. A review of pulmonary toxicity of electronic cigarettes in the context of smoking: a focus on inflammation. Cancer Epidemiol Biomarkers Prev 2017;26(8):1175–91.
72. Behar RZ, Wang Y, Talbot P. Comparing the cytotoxicity of electronic cigarette fluids, aerosols and solvents. Tob Control 2017. [Epub ahead of print].
73. Chun LF, Moazed F, Calfee CS, et al. Pulmonary toxicity of E-cigarettes. Am J Physiol Lung Cell Mol Physiol 2017;313(2):L193–206.
74. Flower M, Nandakumar L, Singh M, et al. Respiratory bronchiolitis-associated interstitial lung disease secondary to electronic nicotine delivery system use confirmed with open lung biopsy. Respirol Case Rep 2017;5(3):e00230.
75. Allen JG, Flanigan SS, LeBlanc M, et al. Flavoring chemicals in E-cigarettes: diacetyl, 2,3-pentanedione, and acetoin in a sample of 51 products, including fruit-, candy-, and cocktail-flavored E-cigarettes. Environ Health Perspect 2016;124(6):733–9.
76. Palamidas A, Gennimata SA, Kaltsakas G, et al. Acute effect of an e-cigarette with and without nicotine on lung function. Tob Ind Dis 2014;12(1):A34.
77. Vardavas CI, Anagnostopoulos N, Kougias M, et al. Short-term pulmonary effects of using an electronic cigarette: impact on respiratory flow resistance, impedance, and exhaled nitric oxide. Chest 2012;141(6):1400–6.
78. Polosa R, Morjaria JB, Caponnetto P, et al. Evidence for harm reduction in COPD smokers who switch to electronic cigarettes. Respir Res 2016;17(1):166.
79. Campagna D, Cibella F, Caponnetto P, et al. Changes in breathomics from a 1-year randomized smoking cessation trial of electronic cigarettes. Eur J Clin Invest 2016;46(8):698–706.
80. Cibella F, Campagna D, Caponnetto P, et al. Lung function and respiratory symptoms in a randomized smoking cessation trial of electronic cigarettes. Clin Sci 2016;130(21):1929.
81. Cook BL, Wayne GF, Kafali EN, et al. Trends in smoking among adults with mental illness and association between mental health treatment and smoking cessation. JAMA 2014;311(2):172–82.
82. SAMSHA's registry of evidence based practices and programs. Behind the term: serious mental illness. 2016. Available at: http://www.nrepp.samhsa.gov/Docs/Literatures/Behind_the_Term_Serious%20%20Mental%20Illness.pdf. Accessed August 2, 2017.
83. Sharma R, Gartner CE, Castle DJ, et al. Should we encourage smokers with severe mental illness to switch to electronic cigarettes? Aust N Z J Psychiatry 2017;51(7):663–4.
84. Sharma R. The challenge of reducing smoking in people with serious mental illness. Lancet Respir Med 2016;4(10):835–44.
85. Chen LS, Baker T, Brownson RC, et al. Smoking cessation and electronic cigarettes in community mental health centers: patient and provider perspectives. Community Ment Health J 2017;53(6):695–702.
86. Prochaska JJ, Grana RA. E-cigarette use among smokers with serious mental illness. PLoS One 2014;9(11):e113013.

87. Spears CA, Jones DM, Weaver SR, et al. Use of electronic nicotine delivery systems among adults with mental health conditions, 2015. Int J Environ Res Public Health 2016;14(1) [pii:E10].
88. O'Brien B, Knight-West O, Walker N, et al. E-cigarettes versus NRT for smoking reduction or cessation in people with mental illness: secondary analysis of data from the ASCEND trial. Tob Induc Dis 2015;13(1):5.
89. Pratt SI, Sargent J, Daniels L, et al. Appeal of electronic cigarettes in smokers with serious mental illness. Addict Behav 2016;59:30–4.
90. US Department of Health and Human Services. Preventing tobacco use among youth and young adults: a report of the surgeon general. Atlanta (GA): US Department of Health and Human Services, Centers for Disease Control and Prevention, National Center for Chronic Disease Prevention and Health Promotion, Office on Smoking and Health; 2012.
91. Jamal A, Gentzke A, Hu SS, et al. Tobacco use among middle and high school students - United States, 2011-2016. MMWR Morb Mortal Wkly Rep 2017; 66(23):597–603.
92. Centers for Disease Control and Prevention (CDC). Tobacco use among middle and high school students -- United States, 2000-2009. MMWR Morb Mortal Wkly Rep 2010;59(33):1063–8.
93. Camenga DR, Kong G, Cavallo DA, et al. Current and former smokers' use of electronic cigarettes for quitting smoking: an exploratory study of adolescents and young adults. Nicotine Tob Res 2017;19(12):1531–5.
94. Dutra LM, Glantz SA. Electronic cigarettes and conventional cigarette use among U.S. adolescents: a cross-sectional study. JAMA Pediatr 2014;168(7): 610–7.
95. Gottlieb S, Zeller M. A nicotine-focused framework for public health. N Engl J Med 2017;377(12):1111–4.
96. Warner KE, Schroeder SA. FDA's innovative plan to address the enormous toll of smoking. JAMA 2017;318(18):1755–6.
97. Brown J, WR. Quit success rates in England 2007-2017. Smoking in Britian 2017;(5):5–8. Available at: http://www.smokinginbritain.co.uk/read. Accessed March 3, 2018.
98. Siu AL. Behavioral and pharmacotherapy interventions for tobacco smoking cessation in adults, including pregnant women: U.S. Preventive services task force recommendation statement. Ann Intern Med 2015;163(8):622–34.
99. Clinical practice policy to protect children from tobacco, nicotine, and tobacco smoke. Pediatrics 2015;136(8):1008–17.
100. Fiore MC, Jaen CR, Baker TB, et al. Treating tobacco use and dependence: 2008 update. Clinical practice guideline. Rockville (MD): US Department of Health and Human Services. Public Health Services; 2008.
101. Bam TS, Bellew W, Berezhnova I, et al. Position statement on electronic cigarettes or electronic nicotine delivery systems. Int J Tuberc Lung Dis 2014; 18(1):5–7.
102. Brandon TH, Goniewicz ML, Hanna NH, et al. Electronic nicotine delivery systems: a policy statement from the American Association for Cancer Research and the American Society of Clinical Oncology. Clin Cancer Res 2015;21(3): 514–25. https://doi.org/10.1158/1078-0432.ccr-14-2544.

When and How to Treat Possible Cannabis Use Disorder

Annie Lévesque, MD, MSc[a],*, Bernard Le Foll, MD, PhD[b,c,d,e,f]

KEYWORDS

- Cannabis use disorder • Treatment • Psychosocial • Pharmacologic
- Synthetic cannabinoid

KEY POINTS

- Psychosocial interventions are the first-line for the treatment of cannabis use disorder.
- The most effective available treatments are cognitive–behavioral therapy and motivational enhancement therapy, with greater benefits found when combining approaches.
- Adding contingency management to these interventions can provide further benefit.
- There is no pharmacotherapy approved for the treatment of cannabis use disorder.
- Cannabinoid analogues and gabapentin have been tested with preliminarily positive results. Further research is warranted to clarify the potential role of these medications.

INTRODUCTION

Cannabis is the most frequently used illicit drug worldwide.[1] The lifetime probability of developing cannabis use disorder after a first exposure to the substance is approximately 9%.[2,3] Moreover, the likelihood of developing cannabis use disorder increases significantly if an individual starts using cannabis during adolescence.[4] In the United States, 4 million individuals were estimated to fulfill criteria for cannabis use disorder in the past year, representing approximately 1.5% of the American population aged 12 or older in 2015.[5]

This article originally appeared in *Medical Clinics*, Volume 102, Issue 4, July 2018.

Disclosure Statement: The authors have no conflict of interest to declare.

[a] Department of Psychiatry, Mount Sinai West Hospital, 1000 10th Avenue, Suite 8C-02, New York, NY 10019, USA; [b] Translational Addiction Research Laboratory, Centre for Addiction and Mental Health (CAMH), 33 Russell Street, Toronto, Ontario M5S 2S1, Canada; [c] Addiction Division, Addiction Medicine Service, Centre for Addiction and Mental Health, Toronto, Ontario M6J 1H4, Canada; [d] Department of Pharmacology and Toxicology, Institute of Medical Sciences, University of Toronto, Toronto, Ontario M5S 1A8, Canada; [e] Department of Psychiatry, Institute of Medical Sciences, University of Toronto, Toronto, Ontario M5S 1A8, Canada; [f] Department of Family and Community Medicine, Institute of Medical Sciences, University of Toronto, Toronto, Ontario M5S 1A8, Canada

* Corresponding author.

E-mail address: annie.levesque@mountsinai.org

Clinics Collections 9 (2020) 199–213

https://doi.org/10.1016/j.ccol.2020.07.034

The plant *Cannabis sativa* contains approximately 60 identified cannabinoid compounds, some of which exert an effect in the human body via interaction with the CB_1 and CB_2 receptors, located predominantly in the central nervous system and in the immune system, respectively.[6,7] The main psychoactive properties of cannabis are attributed to the cannabinoid compound delta-9-tetrahydrocannabinol (THC), a partial agonist of the CB_1 and CB_2 receptors, that has been associated with the high produced by cannabis use and with its effects that lead to the development of addiction.[6,8,9] Recently, there has been a growing interest in cannabidiol, a nonpsychotropic component also present in different strains of cannabis. Cannabidiol has been shown to have antiepileptic properties in well-conducted clinical trials, and preclinical studies suggest it may have possible therapeutic properties, including its ability to decrease THC induced paranoia and euphoria, in addition to exerting a positive impact on anxiety and depression.[6,10–15] It should be noted that, so far, only the antiepileptic effect of cannabidiol has been tested properly in human subjects, and the other properties of cannabidiol remain to be evaluated in rigorous large-scale clinical trials.[15]

Cannabis is often used recreationally for its euphoria-producing effects. Other symptoms and signs of acute cannabis intoxication include increased appetite, tachycardia, tachypnea, high blood pressure, ocular erythema, dry mouth, and altered judgment. Cannabis use has been associated with a number of deleterious health outcomes, including worsening of respiratory problems, worsening of bipolar disorder-associated symptoms, short-term impairment of learning and memory, and higher risks of death from motor vehicle accidents.[16] There is also substantial evidence regarding the association between frequent cannabis use and psychosis, including schizophrenia, although the exact interplay remains controversial.[16] It is possible that exposure to cannabis may precipitate an earlier occurrence of psychotic symptoms in predisposed subjects, as suggested by the transient occurrence of symptoms that resemble those of a psychosis after THC administration in human laboratory studies.[17] However, the fact that the prevalence of schizophrenia has been stable over time while the use of cannabis and the potency of cannabis used has increased does not support a causal relationship between cannabis use and schizophrenia.

A diagnosis of cannabis use disorder as defined by the fifth edition of the *Diagnostic and Statistical Manual of Mental Disorders* (DSM-5) is made when there is a problematic pattern of use leading to significant impairment or distress, as manifested by at least 2 of the symptoms listed in the DSM-5, occurring within a 12-month period.[18] Discontinuation of cannabis use after regular, prolonged use is associated with a withdrawal syndrome that is recognized by the DSM-5, characterized by the emergence of symptoms such as anxiety, dysphoria, sleep disturbance, irritability, and anorexia.[18,19] Although cannabis withdrawal can be distressing, it is not life threatening. Nonetheless, the experience of withdrawal symptoms makes cannabis cessation more challenging and individuals experiencing a higher number of withdrawal symptoms have greater risks of rapid relapse to cannabis use compared with those experiencing fewer symptoms.[20]

Demand for cannabis-related health care services has been increasing in most regions of the world, including North America.[1] This finding may partly be explained by a significant increase over the past decades in the concentration of THC in cannabis as well as by the emergence of synthetic cannabinoid, a group of chemically synthesized highly potent cannabinoid analogues that are often associated with more severe use-related outcomes.[21] Moreover, the recent legalization of marijuana use in numerous US states has contributed to easier access to the substance. Hence, data from the states that have legalized marijuana for recreational use indicate an increase in cannabis use and in cannabis-related emergency room visits and hospitalizations.[22–24]

Despite the high prevalence of cannabis use disorder, awareness regarding effective treatment options remain limited within the medical community. Better knowledge by clinicians regarding the management of cannabis use disorder could likely improve patient outcomes. This article offers an overview of the different effective approaches for the treatment of cannabis use disorder.

GENERAL TREATMENT PRINCIPLES

The intensity of the treatment recommended for a patient using cannabis largely depends on the clinical presentation. Therefore, a proper assessment and screening needs to be performed before establishing an appropriate treatment plan. Although no consensus screening recommendations have been published, authors have suggested the following recommendations. Physicians should question every patient at least once regarding cannabis use. Adolescents, young adults, and patients at high risk for cannabis-related harm (eg, patients with comorbid psychiatric or substance use disorders) should be asked about cannabis use more frequently, for example, at every routine medical visit.[25] When a patient reports using cannabis, the physician should inquire about clinical indicators of problematic cannabis use, including daily or near daily use, poor social functioning, poor functioning at work or school, unsuccessful attempts to reduce use, and concerns from family or friends.[25] When problematic use is suspected, the DSM-5 criteria should be reviewed to establish a diagnosis of cannabis use disorder.

Differentiating between recreational cannabis use and cannabis use disorder is an important step to determine what type of treatment is appropriate. The type of treatment offered also depends on a patient's motivation and desire to quit, and is often related to the level of distress experienced in relation to substance use. For patients using cannabis without fulfilling the criteria for cannabis use disorder, and for patients with cannabis use disorder who have no desire to diminish or discontinue their use, offering counseling as a part of medical visits is appropriate. Counseling can be based on the Lower Risk Cannabis Use Guidelines, a guideline based on a systematic literature review conducted by a group of international experts to identify behaviors that could be modified to decrease adverse health consequences from cannabis use.[26] The main recommendations issued by the group are summarized in **Box 1**.

For patients with a diagnosis of cannabis use disorder who are interested in receiving treatment, it is generally recommended to provide a referral to an addiction physician or to an addiction treatment program. If these options are not available, psychiatrists, psychologists, or counselors with expertise in addiction can also provide valuable specialized care. The treatment of cannabis use disorder is generally performed in an outpatient setting. Inpatient or residential treatments are generally limited to patients with comorbid psychiatric or substance use disorder justifying a higher level of care. It is recommended to establish treatment goals early in the episode of care to inform the appropriate treatment approach. Treatment goals are based on a patient's individual objectives, and may vary greatly, ranging from total abstinence, reducing the amount of cannabis used, to avoiding hazardous use. The use of urine drug screening may be useful in the course of treatment to monitor abstinence in patients aiming to fully discontinue cannabis use, but is of little usefulness in patients aiming to decrease their use, because routine drug screening only provides qualitative

> **Box 1**
> **Main recommendations from the lower risk cannabis use guidelines**
>
> 1. Abstaining from using cannabis to fully prevent cannabis-related health problems.
> 2. Avoiding initiation of cannabis use before the age of 16 years.
> 3. Choosing cannabis products with low THC potency or balanced THC-cannabidiol ratio.
> 4. Abstaining from using synthetic cannabinoid.
> 5. Favoring nonsmoking methods of consumption.
> 6. Avoiding deep inhalation practices, which may increase risks of respiratory problems.
> 7. Avoiding daily or near-daily cannabis use.
> 8. Abstaining from driving while impaired from cannabis to prevent motor vehicle accidents.
> 9. Populations at higher risk of cannabis-related adverse effects should refrain from using cannabis, including pregnant women and individuals with a predisposition for, or with a first-degree family history of psychosis or substance use disorder.
> 10. Avoiding to combine the aforementioned risk behaviors (eg, combining early initiation and high-frequency use could magnify the likelihood of experiencing cannabis-related adverse outcomes).
> *Abbreviation:* THC, delta-9-tetrahydrocannabinol.
>
> *Adapted from* Fischer B, Russell C, Sabioni P, et al. Lower-risk cannabis use guidelines: a comprehensive update of evidence and recommendations. Am J Public Health 2017;107(8):e4; with permission.

results. In patients with regular, heavy cannabis use, the interpretation of cannabis toxicology results can be challenging because qualitative results may remain positive up to 4 weeks after cessation of use. Furthermore, urine drug screening is of little usefulness in patients using synthetic cannabinoid because many of these compounds are not captured by urine drug testing.

Currently, psychosocial interventions are the first line for the treatment of cannabis use disorder, with some specific forms of such interventions having shown effectiveness in reducing cannabis use. A number of pharmacologic approaches have been tested in regard to their impact on cannabis use and on the severity of withdrawal symptoms yielding limited positive outcomes. Although a few medications have shown some promising results warranting further research, no medication is currently approved by the US Food and Drug Administration for the treatment of cannabis use disorder.

PSYCHOSOCIAL INTERVENTIONS

Different psychosocial interventions have been shown to be effective in reducing the frequency of cannabis use and the severity of cannabis use disorder.[27] The most effective approaches are cognitive–behavioral therapy (CBT), motivational enhancement therapy (MET), and a combination of both. Contingency management (CM) is also efficacious when combined with either of these interventions.[27] As a general principle, greater effectiveness is achieved when psychosocial treatments are implemented with higher intensity over longer periods of time (>4 treatment sessions over a period of >1 month).[27] This section presents an overview of the different psychosocial interventions available for the treatment of cannabis use disorder (**Table 1**).

Table 1
Main psychosocial interventions recommended for the treatment of cannabis use and cannabis use disorder

Condition	Intervention	Setting	Outcomes
Cannabis use	Brief counseling Education on safer cannabis use practices based on the LRCUG	Individual; can be delivered by any physician during a regular medical visit	Decrease adverse health consequences from cannabis use
Cannabis use disorder	CBT Identification and modification of problematic thoughts and behaviors	Individual or group setting; generally delivered by a trained addiction professional	Decrease cannabis use[a] Decrease cannabis related-problems
	MET Enhancement of intrinsic motivation to change by exploring and resolving ambivalence	Individual or group setting; generally delivered by a trained addiction professional	Decrease cannabis use[b] Decrease cannabis-related problems Decrease the severity of cannabis use disorder
	CM Providing incentives (vouchers) contingent upon positive treatment outcomes	Used as an augmentation treatment combined with CBT or MET	Enhances the effectiveness of CBT and MET to decrease cannabis use

Abbreviations: CBT, cognitive–behavioral therapy; CM, contingency management; LRCUG, lower risk cannabis use guidelines; MET, motivation enhancement therapy.
[a] The intervention is effective to decrease the number of days of use, to decrease the number of joints per day and to increase past month abstinence.
[b] The intervention is effective to decrease the number of days of use and the number of joints per day.

Cognitive–Behavioral Therapy

CBT is a psychotherapeutic approach that focuses on the identification and modification of problematic thoughts and behaviors. It can be delivered in a group or individual setting. In the context of substance use disorder, this approach emphasizes coping strategies learning, problem solving, and promoting the substitution of cannabis use by alternative, better adapted behaviors.[28] CBT effectively reduced the frequency of cannabis use among patients with cannabis use disorder.[27,29,30] A 2016 metaanalysis evaluating the effectiveness of different psychosocial interventions for the treatment of cannabis use disorder found that individuals receiving CBT used cannabis on fewer days in the month before assessment compared with those assigned to the inactive control group (mean difference, 10.94; 95% confidence interval [CI], 7.44–14.44; n = 134).[27] Compared with inactive control, CBT was also found effective in increasing abstinence in the month before assessment (risk ratio; 4.81; 95% CI, 1.17–19.70; n = 171), in reducing the number of joints used per day (standardized mean difference [SMD], 4.60; 95% CI, 2.21–7.00; 2 studies [n = 306]) and in decreasing cannabis-related problems (SMD, 7.88; 95% CI, 6.86–8.90; n = 135).[27]

Motivational Enhancement Therapy

MET is a psychotherapeutic approach that promotes the importance of self-efficacy and positive changes. It can be delivered in an individual or group setting. The objective of MET intervention is to enhance intrinsic motivation to change by exploring and resolving ambivalence in a nonjudgmental and empathic environment.[31] The aforementioned 2016 metaanalysis found a significant impact of MET on most of the primary outcomes examined (with the exception of past month abstinence), overall supporting the effectiveness of this psychotherapeutic approach for the treatment of cannabis use disorder.[27] MET was found effective in reducing the number of days of cannabis use in the month before assessment among participants treated with MET compared with inactive control (mean difference, 4.45; 95% CI, 1.90–7.00; 4 studies [n = 612]).[27] MET was also found superior to inactive control in reducing cannabis-related problems (SMD, 3.29; 95% CI, 1.85–4.72; 4 studies [n = 612]) and in decreasing the number of joints smoked per day (SMD, 3.14; 95% CI, 2.66–3.61; 4 studies [n = 611]) and the severity of cannabis use disorder (SMD, 4.07; 95% CI, 1.97–6.17; 2 studies [n = 316]).[27] The impact of MET on abstinence from cannabis in the month before assessment was not statistically significant (risk ratio, 1.19; 95% CI, 0.43–3.28; n = 197).[27]

Contingency Management

CM is often combined with other interventions as an augmentation approach for the treatment of substance use disorder. In CM, incentives are provided, often in the form of vouchers contingent upon positive treatment outcomes such as attendance at treatment appointments and abstinence from substance use verified with urine toxicology. A number of studies conducted in different populations of individuals with substance use disorders support the effectiveness of CM in improving retention to treatment and in promoting abstinence.[32,33] Although studies exploring the effectiveness of CM as a standalone treatment for cannabis use disorder are lacking, a number of clinical trials found that augmenting MET, CBT, or the combination of MET and CBT with abstinence-based CM improves the number of abstinent days compared with each of these psychotherapeutic approaches without CM.[27,34]

Alternative Approaches

Although the majority of studies on psychosocial interventions for the treatment of cannabis use disorder examined MET, CBT, or CM, alternative psychosocial approaches have also been tested, yielding weak or negative results. More specifically, evidence on mindfulness-based meditation, drug counseling, social support, and relapse prevention remain insufficient to recommend any of these approaches.[27] Marijuana Anonymous, a mutual help group based on the 12-step principle of Alcohol Anonymous, is widely available; however, its effectiveness has not been rigorously studied.

Combination Therapy

Although CBT and MET approaches were found equally effective for reducing cannabis use when compared with each other, a recent metaanalysis found maximal effectiveness of these interventions when delivered in combination compared with each treatment alone being delivered alone.[27] Furthermore, adding CM to either MET, CBT, or their combination likely further improves effectiveness.[27]

PHARMACOTHERAPY

There is currently no US Food and Drug Administration–approved medication for the treatment of cannabis use disorder, although a few trials have shown promising results. Cannabinoid agonists may be of potential value to decrease symptoms of withdrawal and improve retention to treatment. Some evidence also suggests gabapentin may improve abstinence from cannabis. N-Acetylcysteine (NCA) was thought to be a promising approach based on data from an adolescent trial, but the initial positive findings have not been replicated in a recent clinical trial conducted in an adult population.[35,36] Further research is needed to confirm the effectiveness of these treatments. This section reviews the main pharmacotherapies that have shown preliminarily positive results for the treatment of cannabis use disorder.

Cannabinoid Agonists

Delta-9-tetrahydrocannabinol analogues
Dronabinol Dronabinol (Marinol) is a synthetic form of THC that is bioavailable orally. It is currently approved by the US Food and Drug Administration for the treatment of chemotherapy-related nausea and vomiting and for appetite stimulation in patients with advanced human immunodeficiency virus infection.

A few studies support the effectiveness of dronabinol alone or in combination with lofexidine to improve symptoms of cannabis withdrawal.[37-41] A 12-week trial of 156 adults with cannabis use disorder found that dronabinol 20 mg 2 times per day was effective in reducing symptoms of withdrawal and in improving retention to treatment but had no effect on marijuana use and on abstinence at the end of treatment.[39] Two studies also suggested a dose-dependent effect of dronabinol in suppressing withdrawal symptoms with tested doses up to 120 mg/d.[37,40]

Each study reported that the medication was well-tolerated with minimal side effects and an absence of adverse cognitive effects. Possible side effects from dronabinol include palpitations, tachycardia, flushing, vasodilation, euphoria, abnormality in thinking, dizziness, anxiety, and gastrointestinal symptoms.

Nabilone Nabilone (Cesamet) is a synthetic form of delta THC that acts as an agonist of the CB_1 and CB_2 receptors. It is approved for the treatment of nausea and vomiting induced by chemotherapy.

One small study of 11 non–treatment-seeking individuals who smoked cannabis daily found that nabilone significantly decreased relapse and improved withdrawal symptoms of irritability, insomnia, and disrupted food intake.[42] A dose of 8 mg/d was associated with a modest impact on psychomotor task performance. This adverse effect was not found at a dose of 6 mg/d. Adverse effects most frequently reported from nabilone include drowsiness, dizziness, vertigo, euphoria, ataxia, depression, lack of concentration, sleep disorder, xerostomia, and visual disturbance.

Combined delta-9-tetrahydrocannabinol/cannabidiol product
Nabiximols (Sativex) is a medication delivered as a buccal spray that contains THC and cannabidiol in approximately equal proportions. It acts as an agonist at the CB_1 and CB_2 receptors. Although it is not currently available in the United States, it is approved in different countries for the treatment of cancer pain as well as for spasticity and neuropathic pain associated with multiple sclerosis.

One Australian 28-day inpatient study of 51 adults with cannabis use disorder demonstrated the effectiveness of nabiximols administered at a dose up to 86.4 mg of THC and 80 mg of cannabidiol daily to reduce symptoms of withdrawal (including withdrawal- induced irritability, depression, and cravings) and to improve retention to treatment compared with placebo.[43] No symptoms of intoxication were experienced. A Canadian study of 9 patients with cannabis use disorder found that high doses of nabiximols ($\leq$108 mg of THC and $\leq$100 mg of cannabidiol daily) were effective in reducing symptoms of withdrawal during cannabis abstinence, but had no impact on cravings.[44] In both studies, there was no impact of the treatment on cannabis use outcome. More research studies are required to validate its use for cannabis use disorder treatment. It should be noted that, in those trials, the rate of adverse effects did not differ between the medication and placebo. Importantly, symptoms of intoxication were not noted in the groups treated with nabiximols. Side effects most frequently reported with nabiximols include dizziness, drowsiness, fatigue, and nausea.

Gabapentin

Gabapentin is approved for the treatment of seizures and neuralgia. It acts by blocking voltage-dependent calcium channels, which indirectly modulates the inhibitory central nervous system neurotransmitter GABA. A 12-week randomized controlled trial of 50 adults with cannabis use disorder found that 1200 mg of gabapentin daily was effective in reducing cannabis use assessed both via urine drug testing and self-report, as well as in decreasing withdrawal symptoms including craving and improving executive function compared with the placebo group.[45] In this trial, gabapentin was administered 300 mg twice per day and 600 mg at bedtime. Both groups received weekly individual drug counseling. Although these results are promising, more research is needed to support the effectiveness of this medication for the treatment of cannabis use disorder.

The medication was well-tolerated and there was no difference in the proportion of adverse reactions between groups. The most frequent adverse effects reported with gabapentin are dizziness, drowsiness, ataxia, and fatigue.

N-Acetylcysteine

NAC is a derivative of the amino acid cysteine that modulates glutamate transmission. The presumed mechanism underlying NAC's possible efficacy is through the modulation of glutamate in the nucleus acumbens, a part of the brain reward circuitry that plays a significant role in the development of substance use disorders.

A study of 116 adolescents with cannabis use disorder aged between 15 and 21 years old showed that 8 weeks of treatment with NAC at a dose of 2400 mg/d doubled the odds of negative urine drug testing compared with placebo.[35] However, this finding was not replicated in a subsequent study by the same group, where 12 weeks of treatment with NAC at a dose of 2400 mg/d showed no difference in cannabis abstinence compared with placebo amongst 302 adults with cannabis use disorder aged 18 to 50 years old.[36]

Other

Numerous other tested pharmacologic approaches are likely of little value for the treatment of cannabis use disorder. These medications include escitalopram, fluoxetine, bupropion, nefazodone, venlafaxine, valproate, baclofen, modafinil, atomoxetine, buspirone, and naltrexone, all of which failed to demonstrate a significant positive impact on withdrawal or cannabis use outcomes.[38,46–57] In a human laboratory study, mirtazapine was found to improve sleep and food intake during abstinence, but did not impact withdrawal symptoms and relapse.[55] Similarly, a human laboratory study showed that the antipsychotic quetiapine improved sleep quality and food intake, but also increased marijuana craving and self-administration.[58]

Recently, data have emerged on the potential role of cannabidiol as a treatment option for cannabis use disorder given its ability to decrease THC-induced euphoria.[13,14] Although cannabidiol in combination with THC was found to improve symptoms of cannabis withdrawal, one laboratory study of cannabidiol administered alone did not show effectiveness in decreasing cannabis use or the subjective reinforcing effect of cannabis use.[43,44,59] It is unclear whether the impact of combination THC and cannabidiol treatment on reducing withdrawal symptoms can be partly attributed to the cannabidiol component or is instead owing to the effect of THC alone.

Rimonabant, an inverse agonist/antagonist of the CB_1 receptor was found to decrease drug taking behavior and cue-induced reinstatement of drug-seeking behavior in abstinent monkeys and to attenuate the physiologic effect of cannabis intoxication in humans.[60,61] However, it was found to cause adverse psychiatric outcomes such as anxiety and depression and was removed from the market in 2008.[62,63]

AM4113, a CB_1 receptor neutral antagonist has been studied in animal models, showing positive impact on reducing the use of cannabis without the negative psychiatric side effects of rimonabant.[61,64] This may be a promising treatment and further studies would be of interest.

Finally, a number of clinical trials are currently exploring the impact of different medications for the treatment of cannabis use disorder, including clonazepam, quetiapine, lorcaserin, FAAH-inhibitor, nabilone, NAC, cannabidiol, dronabinol in combination with clonidine, dextroamphetamine/amphetamine, and varenicline.

SYNTHETIC CANNABINOIDS

Synthetic cannabinoids are chemically synthesized compounds that are analogues to naturally occurring cannabinoids. They were first developed in laboratories for medical research in the 1960s and started being sold for recreational use around 2008 in the United States, most frequently under the names of "spice" or "K2."[65] Over the past decade, they have gained popularity owing to their accessibility, the unclear legal status regarding their use, and the lack of detection in routine drug screening. An important feature of synthetic cannabinoid is the variability of their composition, with frequent occurrence of new derivative compounds, presumably with the objective of avoiding regulations.[66] The heterogeneity of the synthetic cannabinoid group of compounds makes intoxication symptoms variable and less predictable.

Synthetic cannabinoids and cannabis bind to the same receptors and, therefore, both substances share common features in terms of signs and symptoms of intoxication and withdrawal. However, a number of synthetic cannabinoid compounds can have greater potency and binding affinity to the receptors compared with cannabis.[67,68] Moreover, certain synthetic cannabinoids produce active metabolites that act as full receptor agonists as opposed to the partial agonist activity of THC.[67,68] These pharmacologic properties contribute to the greater severity of synthetic cannabinoids intoxication and withdrawal symptoms compared with regular cannabis.

The majority of cases of intoxication are not life threatening and may present with tachycardia, nausea, vomiting, behavioral perturbation, and anxiety, although some severe symptoms of intoxication have been reported, including new-onset psychosis, kidney injury, rhabdomyolysis, respiratory depression, and seizures.[69–71] A few cases of death have been attributed to direct toxicity from synthetic cannabinoids causing cardiac arrhythmia, seizure, and kidney failure, whereas other cases of death were indirectly due to synthetic cannabinoids, such as hypothermia owing to individuals remaining unconscious outdoor in the winter or suicide.[69]

Management of Acute Intoxication

Mild to moderate symptoms of intoxication are managed in the emergency department until resolution of symptoms (which typically last 4–6 hours), although more severe symptoms may warrant inpatient admission. In the majority of cases, acute intoxication is managed with supportive care and with intravenous fluid repletion.[72] Benzodiazepines are used as a first line to treat agitation, irritability, psychosis, and seizure.[72] Antipsychotics may also be used to treat agitation and psychotic symptoms.[72] Antiemetic medications can be used to treat hyperemesis, although they are not always effective.[73,74] Poison control centers are available at all times and should be consulted for patients who are critically ill or for whom presentation symptoms are unclear.

Management of Withdrawal

Abrupt discontinuation of synthetic cannabinoid after daily use has been associated with withdrawal symptoms ranging from mild symptoms such as headaches, anxiety, insomnia, nausea, vomiting, loss of appetite, diaphoresis, and craving to severe symptoms including seizure, chest pain, palpitations, and dyspnea.[72] In the absence of instruments designed to assess withdrawal symptoms from synthetic cannabinoids specifically, we suggest that clinicians use the DSM-5 diagnostic criteria for cannabis withdrawal. Similar to the management of acute intoxication, mild to moderate withdrawal symptoms can be managed in an outpatient setting, although severe cases may require inpatient care and continuous monitoring.

Benzodiazepines are used as a first-line treatment for the management of withdrawal symptoms including agitation, anxiety, and seizure.[75,76] Quetiapine has been used with effectiveness to treat withdrawal induced agitation and anxiety after failure of a benzodiazepine trial.[75,76]

Given the recent emergence of synthetic cannabinoids, knowledge regarding best treatment options remain limited and further research is needed to better guide clinical interventions.

FUTURE CONSIDERATIONS AND SUMMARY

Despite the high prevalence of cannabis use disorder, there are few effective treatment options available. MET and CBT are the most effective psychosocial interventions to reduce cannabis use in individuals with cannabis use disorder, with maximal results achieved when combining both approaches.[27] Adding CM in the form of vouchers for negative urine drug test results can provide further benefit in the short term, although little evidence is available regarding long-term benefits.[27] Treatment of greater intensity (>4 sessions over >1 month) is more effective than lower intensity interventions.[27]

Although no pharmacotherapy is approved for the treatment of cannabis use disorder, data suggest that some medications may be of potential value. In line with the concept of using agonist medications to treat other substance use disorders, such as buprenorphine and methadone for opioid use disorder and nicotine replacement and varenicline for nicotine use disorder, there has been a growing interest in the potential role of cannabinoid analogues for the treatment of cannabis use disorder. It has been hypothesized that cannabinoid analogues could improve abstinence by attenuating withdrawal symptoms and by decreasing the pleasurable effect of cannabis. Although studies have consistently demonstrated the ability of cannabinoid analogues to decrease acute cannabis withdrawal symptoms, no impact was found on cannabis use outcomes.[37–44] Hence, the role of cannabinoid medications in the long-term treatment of cannabis use disorder remains to be investigated.

Gabapentin may provide some benefit in decreasing cannabis use and cannabis withdrawal symptoms.[45] There are mixed results regarding the effect of NAC.[35,36] Further research is warranted to clarify the potential role of the aforementioned medications. A number of pharmacotherapies are currently under investigation for the treatment of cannabis use disorder and may lead to the emergence of novel therapeutic options in the future.

Finally, data suggest gender differences in cannabis use and cannabis use disorder. Although men are more likely to initiate cannabis use and to have a lifetime diagnosis of cannabis use disorder, women demonstrate a faster progression from cannabis use to cannabis use disorder.[77,78] Women with cannabis use disorder are also more likely than men to experience withdrawal symptoms, to have low scores on quality of life assessment scales, and to have comorbid mood or anxiety disorders.[2,78–80] These gender differences could potentially lead to the development of gender-specific treatment approaches, such as placing a greater emphasis on withdrawal symptoms and on the treatment of comorbid psychiatric disorders for women. Future studies exploring the impact of gender on response to treatments for cannabis use disorder would be of great interest.

ACKNOWLEDGMENTS

The editors thank Jeanette M. Tetrault, Yale University School of Medicine, for providing a critical review of this article.

REFERENCES

1. United Nations Office on Drugs and Crime. World drug report 2016. Vienna (Austria): 2016. Available at: http://www.unodc.org/wdr2016/. Accessed June, 2017.
2. Lev-Ran S, Le Strat Y, Imtiaz S, et al. Gender differences in prevalence of substance use disorders among individuals with lifetime exposure to substances: results from a large representative sample. Am J Addict 2013;22(1):7–13.
3. Lopez-Quintero C, Perez de los Cobos J, Hasin DS, et al. Probability and predictors of transition from first use to dependence on nicotine, alcohol, cannabis, and cocaine: results of the National Epidemiologic Survey on Alcohol and Related Conditions (NESARC). Drug Alcohol Depend 2011;115(1–2):120–30.
4. Le Strat Y, Dubertret C, Le Foll B. Impact of age at onset of cannabis use on cannabis dependence and driving under the influence in the United States. Accid Anal Prev 2015;76:1–5.
5. SAMHSA. Key substance use and mental health indicators in the United States: results from the 2015 National Survey on Drug Use and Health. 2017. Available at: https://www.samhsa.gov/data/sites/default/files/NSDUH-FFR1-2015/NSDUH-FFR1-2015/NSDUH-FFR1-2015.htm#sudyr04. Accessed June, 2017.
6. Pertwee RG. Ligands that target cannabinoid receptors in the brain: from THC to anandamide and beyond. Addict Biol 2008;13(2):147–59.
7. Mechoulam R, Parker LA. The endocannabinoid system and the brain. Annu Rev Psychol 2013;64:21–47.
8. Solinas M, Goldberg SR, Piomelli D. The endocannabinoid system in brain reward processes. Br J Pharmacol 2008;154(2):369–83.
9. Mechoulam R, Hanus L. A historical overview of chemical research on cannabinoids. Chem Phys Lipids 2000;108(1–2):1–13.
10. Leweke FM, Piomelli D, Pahlisch F, et al. Cannabidiol enhances anandamide signaling and alleviates psychotic symptoms of schizophrenia. Transl Psychiatry 2012;2:e94.

11. Schier AR, Ribeiro NP, Silva AC, et al. Cannabidiol, a Cannabis sativa constituent, as an anxiolytic drug. Rev Bras Psiquiatr 2012;34(Suppl 1):S104–10.
12. Campos AC, Moreira FA, Gomes FV, et al. Multiple mechanisms involved in the large-spectrum therapeutic potential of cannabidiol in psychiatric disorders. Philos Trans R Soc Lond B Biol Sci 2012;367(1607):3364–78.
13. Englund A, Morrison PD, Nottage J, et al. Cannabidiol inhibits THC-elicited paranoid symptoms and hippocampal-dependent memory impairment. J Psychopharmacol 2013;27(1):19–27.
14. Karniol IG, Shirakawa I, Kasinski N, et al. Cannabidiol interferes with the effects of delta 9-tetrahydrocannabinol in man. Eur J Pharmacol 1974;28(1):172–7.
15. Devinsky O, Cross JH, Laux L, et al. Trial of cannabidiol for drug-resistant seizures in the Dravet syndrome. N Engl J Med 2017;376(21):2011–20.
16. National Academies of Sciences, Engineering, and Medicine. The health effects of cannabis and cannabinoids: the current state of evidence and recommendations for research. Washington, DC: The National Academies Press; 2017. p. 486.
17. D'Souza DC, Perry E, MacDougall L, et al. The psychotomimetic effects of intravenous delta-9-tetrahydrocannabinol in healthy individuals: implications for psychosis. Neuropsychopharmacology 2004;29(8):1558–72.
18. American Psychiatric Association. Diagnostic and statistical manual of mental disorders, fifth edition (DSM-5). Arlington (VA): American Psychiatric Association; 2013.
19. Gorelick DA, Levin KH, Copersino ML, et al. Diagnostic criteria for cannabis withdrawal syndrome. Drug Alcohol Depend 2012;123(1–3):141–7.
20. Cornelius JR, Chung T, Martin C, et al. Cannabis withdrawal is common among treatment-seeking adolescents with cannabis dependence and major depression, and is associated with rapid relapse to dependence. Addict Behav 2008; 33(11):1500–5.
21. ElSohly MA, Mehmedic Z, Foster S, et al. Changes in cannabis potency over the last 2 decades (1995-2014): analysis of current data in the United States. Biol Psychiatry 2016;79(7):613–9.
22. Wang GS, Roosevelt G, Heard K. Pediatric marijuana exposures in a medical marijuana state. JAMA Pediatr 2013;167(7):630–3.
23. Kim HS, Anderson JD, Saghafi O, et al. Cyclic vomiting presentations following marijuana liberalization in Colorado. Acad Emerg Med 2015;22(6):694–9.
24. Wen H, Hockenberry JM, Cummings JR. The effect of medical marijuana laws on adolescent and adult use of marijuana, alcohol, and other substances. J Health Econ 2015;42:64–80.
25. Turner SD, Spithoff S, Kahan M. Approach to cannabis use disorder in primary care: focus on youth and other high-risk users. Can Fam Physician 2014;60(9): 801–8.
26. Fischer B, Russell C, Sabioni P, et al. Lower-risk cannabis use guidelines: a comprehensive update of evidence and recommendations. Am J Public Health 2017;107(8):e1–12.
27. Gates PJ, Sabioni P, Copeland J, et al. Psychosocial interventions for cannabis use disorder. Cochrane Database Syst Rev 2016;(5):CD005336.
28. Beck A, Wright F, Newman C, et al. Cognitive therapy of substance abuse. New York: Guilford Press; 1993.
29. Stephens RS, Roffman RA, Curtin L. Comparison of extended versus brief treatments for marijuana use. J Consult Clin Psychol 2000;68(5):898–908.

30. Copeland J, Swift W, Roffman R, et al. A randomized controlled trial of brief cognitive-behavioral interventions for cannabis use disorder. J Subst Abuse Treat 2001;21(2):55–64 [discussion: 5–6].
31. Miller WR, Rollnick S. Motivational interviewing: preparing people for change. New York: The Guilford Press; 2002.
32. Petry NM, Peirce JM, Stitzer ML, et al. Effect of prize-based incentives on outcomes in stimulant abusers in outpatient psychosocial treatment programs: a national drug abuse treatment clinical trials network study. Arch Gen Psychiatry 2005;62(10):1148–56.
33. Peirce JM, Petry NM, Stitzer ML, et al. Effects of lower-cost incentives on stimulant abstinence in methadone maintenance treatment: a National Drug Abuse Treatment Clinical Trials Network study. Arch Gen Psychiatry 2006;63(2):201–8.
34. Stanger C, Budney AJ, Kamon JL, et al. A randomized trial of contingency management for adolescent marijuana abuse and dependence. Drug Alcohol Depend 2009;105(3):240–7.
35. Gray KM, Carpenter MJ, Baker NL, et al. A double-blind randomized controlled trial of N-acetylcysteine in cannabis-dependent adolescents. Am J Psychiatry 2012;169(8):805–12.
36. Gray KM, Sonne SC, McClure EA, et al. A randomized placebo-controlled trial of N-acetylcysteine for cannabis use disorder in adults. Drug Alcohol Depend 2017;177:249–57.
37. Budney AJ, Vandrey RG, Hughes JR, et al. Oral delta-9-tetrahydrocannabinol suppresses cannabis withdrawal symptoms. Drug Alcohol Depend 2007;86(1):22–9.
38. Haney M, Hart CL, Vosburg SK, et al. Marijuana withdrawal in humans: effects of oral THC or divalproex. Neuropsychopharmacology 2004;29(1):158–70.
39. Levin FR, Mariani JJ, Brooks DJ, et al. Dronabinol for the treatment of cannabis dependence: a randomized, double-blind, placebo-controlled trial. Drug Alcohol Depend 2011;116(1–3):142–50.
40. Vandrey R, Stitzer ML, Mintzer MZ, et al. The dose effects of short-term dronabinol (oral THC) maintenance in daily cannabis users. Drug Alcohol Depend 2013;128(1–2):64–70.
41. Haney M, Hart CL, Vosburg SK, et al. Effects of THC and lofexidine in a human laboratory model of marijuana withdrawal and relapse. Psychopharmacology 2008;197(1):157–68.
42. Haney M, Cooper ZD, Bedi G, et al. Nabilone decreases marijuana withdrawal and a laboratory measure of marijuana relapse. Neuropsychopharmacology 2013;38(8):1557–65.
43. Allsop DJ, Copeland J, Lintzeris N, et al. Nabiximols as an agonist replacement therapy during cannabis withdrawal: a randomized clinical trial. JAMA Psychiatry 2014;71(3):281–91.
44. Trigo JM, Lagzdins D, Rehm J, et al. Effects of fixed or self-titrated dosages of Sativex on cannabis withdrawal and cravings. Drug Alcohol Depend 2016;161:298–306.
45. Mason BJ, Crean R, Goodell V, et al. A proof-of-concept randomized controlled study of gabapentin: effects on cannabis use, withdrawal and executive function deficits in cannabis-dependent adults. Neuropsychopharmacology 2012;37(7):1689–98.
46. Weinstein AM, Miller H, Bluvstein I, et al. Treatment of cannabis dependence using escitalopram in combination with cognitive-behavior therapy: a double-blind placebo-controlled study. Am J Drug Alcohol Abuse 2014;40(1):16–22.

47. Carpenter KM, McDowell D, Brooks DJ, et al. A preliminary trial: double-blind comparison of nefazodone, bupropion-SR, and placebo in the treatment of cannabis dependence. Am J Addict 2009;18(1):53–64.
48. Levin FR, Mariani J, Brooks DJ, et al. A randomized double-blind, placebo-controlled trial of venlafaxine-extended release for co-occurring cannabis dependence and depressive disorders. Addiction 2013;108(6):1084–94.
49. Cornelius JR, Bukstein OG, Douaihy AB, et al. Double-blind fluoxetine trial in co-morbid MDD-CUD youth and young adults. Drug Alcohol Depend 2010;112(1–2): 39–45.
50. Penetar DM, Looby AR, Ryan ET, et al. Bupropion reduces some of the symptoms of marihuana withdrawal in chronic marihuana users: a pilot study. Subst Abuse 2012;6:63–71.
51. Haney M, Ward AS, Comer SD, et al. Bupropion SR worsens mood during marijuana withdrawal in humans. Psychopharmacology 2001;155(2):171–9.
52. Levin FR, McDowell D, Evans SM, et al. Pharmacotherapy for marijuana dependence: a double-blind, placebo-controlled pilot study of divalproex sodium. Am J Addict 2004;13(1):21–32.
53. McRae-Clark AL, Carter RE, Killeen TK, et al. A placebo-controlled trial of buspirone for the treatment of marijuana dependence. Drug Alcohol Depend 2009; 105(1–2):132–8.
54. McRae-Clark AL, Carter RE, Killeen TK, et al. A placebo-controlled trial of atomoxetine in marijuana-dependent individuals with attention deficit hyperactivity disorder. Am J Addict 2010;19(6):481–9.
55. Haney M, Hart CL, Vosburg SK, et al. Effects of baclofen and mirtazapine on a laboratory model of marijuana withdrawal and relapse. Psychopharmacology 2010;211(2):233–44.
56. Sugarman DE, Poling J, Sofuoglu M. The safety of modafinil in combination with oral 9-tetrahydrocannabinol in humans. Pharmacol Biochem Behav 2011;98(1): 94–100.
57. Haney M, Bisaga A, Foltin RW. Interaction between naltrexone and oral THC in heavy marijuana smokers. Psychopharmacology 2003;166(1):77–85.
58. Cooper ZD, Foltin RW, Hart CL, et al. A human laboratory study investigating the effects of quetiapine on marijuana withdrawal and relapse in daily marijuana smokers. Addict Biol 2013;18(6):993–1002.
59. Haney M, Malcolm RJ, Babalonis S, et al. Oral cannabidiol does not alter the subjective, reinforcing or cardiovascular effects of smoked cannabis. Neuropsychopharmacology 2016;41(8):1974–82.
60. Huestis MA, Boyd SJ, Heishman SJ, et al. Single and multiple doses of rimonabant antagonize acute effects of smoked cannabis in male cannabis users. Psychopharmacology 2007;194(4):505–15.
61. Schindler CW, Redhi GH, Vemuri K, et al. Blockade of nicotine and cannabinoid reinforcement and relapse by a cannabinoid CB1-receptor neutral antagonist AM4113 and inverse agonist rimonabant in squirrel monkeys. Neuropsychopharmacology 2016;41(9):2283–93.
62. Despres JP, Golay A, Sjostrom L. Effects of rimonabant on metabolic risk factors in overweight patients with dyslipidemia. N Engl J Med 2005;353(20):2121–34.
63. Scheen AJ. CB1 receptor blockade and its impact on cardiometabolic risk factors: overview of the RIO programme with rimonabant. J Neuroendocrinol 2008; 20(Suppl 1):139–46.
64. Gueye AB, Pryslawsky Y, Trigo JM, et al. The CB1 neutral antagonist AM4113 retains the therapeutic efficacy of the inverse agonist rimonabant for nicotine

dependence and weight loss with better psychiatric tolerability. Int J Neuropsychopharmacol 2016;19(12) [pii:pyw068].

65. European Monitoring Centre for Drugs and Drug Addiction. Understanding the 'spice' phenomenon. Luxembourg: Office for Official Publications of the European Communities: EMCDDA; 2009. Available at: http://www.emcdda.europa.eu/system/files/publications/537/Spice-Thematic-paper-final-version.pdf_en.

66. Seely KA, Lapoint J, Moran JH, et al. Spice drugs are more than harmless herbal blends: a review of the pharmacology and toxicology of synthetic cannabinoids. Prog Neuropsychopharmacol Biol Psychiatry 2012;39(2):234–43.

67. Huffman JW, Padgett LW. Recent developments in the medicinal chemistry of cannabimimetic indoles, pyrroles and indenes. Curr Med Chem 2005;12(12): 1395–411.

68. Brents LK, Reichard EE, Zimmerman SM, et al. Phase I hydroxylated metabolites of the K2 synthetic cannabinoid JWH-018 retain in vitro and in vivo cannabinoid 1 receptor affinity and activity. PLoS One 2011;6(7):e21917.

69. Tait RJ, Caldicott D, Mountain D, et al. A systematic review of adverse events arising from the use of synthetic cannabinoids and their associated treatment. Clin Toxicol (Phila) 2016;54(1):1–13.

70. Riederer AM, Campleman SL, Carlson RG, et al. Acute poisonings from synthetic cannabinoids - 50 U.S. toxicology investigators consortium registry sites, 2010-2015. MMWR Morb Mortal Wkly Rep 2016;65(27):692–5.

71. Hoyte CO, Jacob J, Monte AA, et al. A characterization of synthetic cannabinoid exposures reported to the National Poison Data System in 2010. Ann Emerg Med 2012;60(4):435–8.

72. Cooper ZD. Adverse effects of synthetic cannabinoids: management of acute toxicity and withdrawal. Curr Psychiatry Rep 2016;18(5):52.

73. Hermanns-Clausen M, Kneisel S, Szabo B, et al. Acute toxicity due to the confirmed consumption of synthetic cannabinoids: clinical and laboratory findings. Addiction 2013;108(3):534–44.

74. Ukaigwe A, Karmacharya P, Donato A. A gut gone to pot: a case of cannabinoid hyperemesis syndrome due to K2, a synthetic cannabinoid. Case Rep Emerg Med 2014;2014:3.

75. Nacca N, Vatti D, Sullivan R, et al. The synthetic cannabinoid withdrawal syndrome. J Addict Med 2013;7(4):296–8.

76. Macfarlane V, Christie G. Synthetic cannabinoid withdrawal: a new demand on detoxification services. Drug Alcohol Rev 2015;34(2):147–53.

77. Hernandez-Avila CA, Rounsaville BJ, Kranzler HR. Opioid-, cannabis- and alcohol-dependent women show more rapid progression to substance abuse treatment. Drug Alcohol Depend 2004;74(3):265–72.

78. Khan SS, Secades-Villa R, Okuda M, et al. Gender differences in cannabis use disorders: results from the National Epidemiologic Survey of Alcohol and Related Conditions. Drug Alcohol Depend 2013;130(1–3):101–8.

79. Copersino ML, Boyd SJ, Tashkin DP, et al. Sociodemographic characteristics of cannabis smokers and the experience of cannabis withdrawal. Am J Drug Alcohol Abuse 2010;36(6):311–9.

80. Herrmann ES, Weerts EM, Vandrey R. Sex differences in cannabis withdrawal symptoms among treatment-seeking cannabis users. Exp Clin Psychopharmacol 2015;23(6):415–21.

Epidemiology of Alcohol Consumption and Societal Burden of Alcoholism and Alcoholic Liver Disease

Page D. Axley, MD[a], Crit Taylor Richardson, MD[b],
Ashwani K. Singal, MD, MS[c],*

KEYWORDS

- Alcoholic cirrhosis • Alcoholic hepatitis • Liver cirrhosis • Prevalence of disease
- Burden of disease • Epidemiology

KEY POINTS

- Alcohol consumption is a significant cause of mortality, morbidity, and social problems, accounting for approximately 5% of deaths worldwide.
- The World Health Organization's 2010 goal was at least a 10% reduction in the harmful use of alcohol. Instead, the burden of alcohol consumption has continued to increase.
- Abstinence remains the cornerstone of treatment, with an additional need for public awareness on the toxic effects of alcohol use and the implementation of policies to restrict availability of alcohol.
- There is an unmet need for the development of more effective treatment options for patients with alcoholic liver disease.

INTRODUCTION

Alcohol consumption is the third most important preventable cause of any disease after smoking and hypertension.[1] About 38% of adults worldwide and 60% to 70% in the United States report alcohol consumption within the past 12 months.[2] According to the World Health Organization (WHO), alcohol consumption is linked to more than 200 diseases and injury-related health conditions.[2] Alcohol consumption accounts for

This article originally appeared in *Clinics in Liver Disease*, Volume 23, Issue 1, February 2019.
Disclosure Statement: There are no conflicts of interest. This work was supported by a faculty development grant from the American College of Gastroenterology to A.K. Singal.
[a] Department of Medicine, University of Alabama at Birmingham, 1720 2nd Avenue South, BDB 327, Birmingham, AL 35294, USA; [b] Division of Gastroenterology and Hepatology, University of Alabama at Birmingham, 1720 2nd Avenue South, BDB 380, Birmingham, AL 35294, USA; [c] Division of Gastroenterology and Hepatology, Porphyria Center, University of Alabama at Birmingham, 1720 2nd Avenue South, BDB 380, Birmingham, AL 35294, USA
* Corresponding author.
E-mail address: ashwanisingal.com@gmail.com

https://doi.org/10.1016/j.ccol.2020.07.035
2352-7986/20/© 2020 Elsevier Inc. All rights reserved.

4.2% of the global burden of disease measured in disability-adjusted life years (DALYs), especially among individuals in their most productive years, between the ages of 15 and 59 years.[3] DALYs attributed to alcohol consumption have increased by more than 25% among men and women since 1990.[3]

To understand the impact of alcohol consumption, it is important to have an accurate estimation of alcohol exposure and the burden of alcohol-related disease.[4] In the United States, 1 drink contains 14 g of alcohol. This amount is contained in 12 ounces of beer (5% weight/volume), 5 ounces of wine (8%–10% weight/volume), or 1.5 ounces of hard liquor (40%–45% weight/volume).[5] Approximately 1 in 12 adults report heavy alcohol consumption, defined as consumption of greater than 3 drinks per day in men and greater than 2 drinks per day in women, or engagement in binge drinking (>5 drinks in men and >4 drinks in women over 2 hours).[6] Chronic heavy use of alcohol can lead to hepatic steatosis, alcoholic hepatitis, alcoholic cirrhosis, and liver cancer.[7] Whereas hepatic steatosis and, possibly, fibrosis are potentially reversible on cessation of alcohol use, alcoholic cirrhosis can progress to decompensation and liver cancer despite abstinence.[8] Of the various factors responsible for liver disease, duration and amount of alcohol consumed are the most important factors.[9] Mortality rates from alcoholic cirrhosis closely parallel alcohol consumption prevalence rates worldwide.[10] With the growing burden of alcohol-related disease, there is increased need to develop and implement population-based approaches to reduce the health and social burdens caused by alcohol consumption.

WORLD-WIDE DISTRIBUTION AND HOT SPOTS OF ALCOHOL CONSUMPTION

For epidemiologic purposes, alcohol consumption is traditionally reported per capita, or the amount of alcohol consumed in liters per person.[11] Several limitations in the reporting of per capita alcohol consumption contribute to inaccurate estimates of alcohol use. For example, data on alcohol exposure are often derived from surveys of self-reported consumption that might underestimate true alcohol use.[12] Further, global studies of disease burden frequently use *International Statistical Classification of Diseases and Related Health Problems* (ICD) codes, which are inconsistently used across the world. Use of ICD codes may fail to capture those who do not seek medical care and thus miss a large proportion of these individuals.[13,14] Another limitation relates to the reporting of national consumption figures that rely on calculations of legal sales of alcohol and do not account for illegally produced alcohol.[15] It is estimated that approximately a quarter of the total alcohol consumed globally is unrecorded (**Fig. 1**).[16]

According to the most recent WHO data, average alcohol consumption per person among individuals aged 15 years and older is about 6.2 L of pure alcohol per year or 13.5 g of pure alcohol per day. Given that only 38% of the world's population consumes alcohol, drinkers consume an average of 17 L of pure alcohol annually.[2] In 2015, the global estimated prevalence of heavy episodic alcohol use over the past 30 days was 18.3% among adults.[17]

The highest rates of alcohol consumption are in Eastern Europe and the former Soviet Union at greater than 10 L per capita. In contrast, the lowest drinking rates are reported from the Middle East and Southeast Asia at less than 2.5 L per capita, likely due to significant Islamic populations in these regions of the world (**Fig. 2**). The type of alcohol consumed also varies by geographic region. Globally, the most frequent alcohol consumed is spirits (50.1%), followed by beer (34.8%) and wine (8%).[2]

There are differences in trends of per capita alcohol consumption over time across the world (**Fig. 3**). For example, alcohol consumption in North America remains high

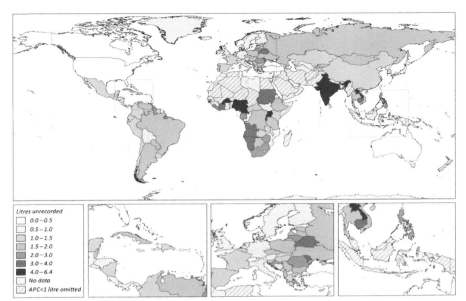

Fig. 1. Proportion of unrecorded alcohol consumption of the total alcohol consumption per capita (APC) in 2015. Countries with less than 1 L of recorded APC were omitted. (*From* Probst C, Manthey J, Merey A, et al. Unrecorded alcohol use: a global modelling study based on nominal group assessments and survey data. Addiction 2018;113(7):1231–41; with permission.)

but has been relatively stable over time.[18] Between 2000 and 2015, among persons older than 18 years of age, alcohol consumption increased by 3% (from 67% to 70%). This was associated with approximately 1% decrease in the prevalence of

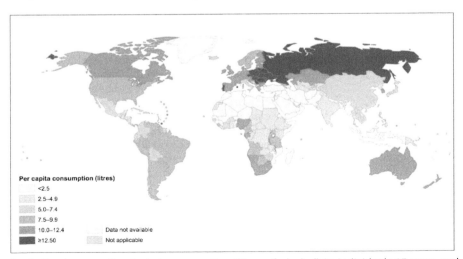

Fig. 2. Total per capita alcohol consumption (liters of alcohol) in individuals 15 years and older in 2010 in WHO member states. (*From* World Health Organization. Global status report on alcohol and health. Geneva (Switzerland): World Health Organization; 2014; with permission.)

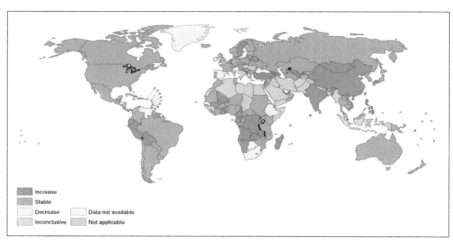

Fig. 3. Five-year change in recorded alcohol per capita among persons aged 15 years and older, 2006 to 2010. (*From* World Health Organization. Global status report on alcohol and health. Geneva (Switzerland): World Health Organization; 2014; with permission.)

alcohol use disorder in this population (from 7.4% to 6.2%).[18,19] Similarly, data from National Institute on Alcohol Abuse and Alcoholism demonstrated a decrease in alcohol consumption from the 1980s to mid-1990s, followed by a slight uptrend from 8.1 L per year in 1990 to 8.9 L per year in 2016.[20] Although consumption has remained relatively stable in the United States, binge drinking has significantly increased, particularly among women.[21]

On the other hand, many Asian countries, such as India and China, are experiencing a significant increase in per capita alcohol consumption, with more than 90% of their alcohol consumption in the form of spirits.[22] Per capita alcohol use by adults in India increased by 107% from 1970 to 1996.[23] This trend has continued into the twenty-first century with the per capita alcohol consumption increasing from 3.6 L to 4.4 L in 2010,[2] and a growing culture of heavy and binge drinking among younger adults.[24] Similarly, in China, per capita alcohol consumption increased from 4.9 L to 6.7 L between 2003 and 2010, with about 70% in the form of spirits.[2] Because greater than 50% of alcohol consumption per capita is unrecorded in Southeast Asia, these figures likely underestimate true alcohol consumption.[22] The trend in increased alcohol consumption in these countries is expected to continue on the background of increased disposable incomes, limited alcohol control policies, and aggressive alcohol marketing strategies.[2,25] Furthermore, demographic patterns in alcohol consumption are also expected to continue, with increased use among younger people and women.[26]

SOCIETAL COST OF ALCOHOLIC LIVER DISEASE

The burden of alcohol use and alcohol use disorders contributes significantly to the health care costs for alcohol-related diseases. For example, patients with alcoholic liver disease (ALD) incur direct costs to the health care system for medical care, and indirect costs to society due to a loss of workforce productivity, absenteeism, injury, early retirement, and mortality.[27] Costs related to alcohol consumption have been estimated at 125 billion Euros in the European Union in 2003[28] and 249 billion dollars in the United States in 2010[29] (these figures account for 1.3%–3.3% of gross domestic product, respectively).[27,30] With an estimated 223.5 billion dollars spent on alcohol abuse in 2006, the societal cost is estimated at $1.90 per individual alcoholic beverage consumed.[31]

Data from the Centers for Disease Control in the United States attributed an average annual number of 87,798 deaths to alcohol between 2006 and 2010, which accounts for 1 in 10 deaths among adults aged 18 to 65 years. This was associated with 2,560,290 years of potential life lost.[32] Age standardized death rates due to alcohol in the United States increased by 17.5% between 1990 and 2016, with 2.89 deaths per 100,000 persons in 2016.[33] Alcohol consumption has also had a significantly global impact on mortality. For example, 3.3 million deaths, or 5.9% of all deaths worldwide, were attributable to alcohol consumption in 2012.[2]

A large portion of the disease burden associated with alcohol use and mortality is due to ALD. For example, the US mortality rate from any cirrhosis increased by 8.2% between 2000 and 2013, from 9.7 to 10.5 deaths per 100,000. Based on the cause of the cirrhosis, the mortality increase over time was much higher for alcohol-related cirrhosis, with an 18.6% increase from 4.3 to 5.1 deaths per 100,000 people.[34] ALD contributed to 48% of all hospitalizations and cirrhosis-related deaths in the United States,[35] with 76% of these affecting individuals aged 25 to 34 years.[34] Transplantation for ALD is also increasing[36] and has now surpassed hepatitis C virus infection as the most common indication for liver transplantation in the United States.[37]

Alcoholic hepatitis, a unique presentation among individuals with chronic active heavy alcohol consumption, presents with acute-on-chronic liver failure and contributes significantly to the morbidity, health care burden, and mortality from ALD.[38,39] Analysis of the National Inpatient Sample database showed that average length of stay and hospital charges in 2010 per hospital admission for alcoholic hepatitis were 6.1 days and $46,264, respectively.[40] In another study on a cohort of 15,496 subjects hospitalized for alcoholic hepatitis, about $2 billion was spent in the 5-year follow-up from 2006 to 2010.[41]

The burden of ALD in Europe is considerably higher than in the United States and is estimated to be the highest in the world.[42,43] In the European Union, one-fifth of the population older than the age of 15 years reports binge drinking (5 or more drinks on an occasion) at least once a week.[44] Currently, it is estimated that 70% of the adults in the WHO European region drink alcohol, consuming an average of 10.7 L annually.[45] An analysis of mortality data from 14 European Union countries demonstrated that a 1 L increase in per capita consumption was associated with a 10% increase in cirrhosis diagnoses.[46]

In the United Kingdom, liver disease is the third leading cause of death before age 75 years, and alcohol contributes to 75% of liver disease mortality.[47] A recent report from the Lancet Standing Commission on liver disease in the United Kingdom projected that ALD will shortly overtake ischemic heart disease with regard to years of working life lost (before the age of 65 years).[48] The National Health Service spends approximately £21 billion annually related to alcohol misuse,[48] and £3.5 billion annually on complications related to ALD.[49] In 2015, there were 1.1 million alcohol-related hospital admissions, representing 7% of total hospital admissions.[48] Admissions for ALD to intensive care units tripled in the United Kingdom over the 10 years from 1996 to 2005.[50] In Portugal, 84% of hospital admissions for cirrhosis to all state hospitals from 1993 to 2008 were related to ALD, with a disproportionate increase in admissions for cirrhosis in men aged 40 to 54 years. Patients with ALD had longer length of stay and increased mortality.[51] Across Europe, prevalence and mortality data indicate that increasing rates of cirrhosis in Europe are linked to dramatic increases in harmful alcohol consumption, most notably in Northern European countries.[52]

China shares the worldwide burden of liver disease with an estimated 300 million people suffering from liver disease.[53] Although chronic viral hepatitis remains the largest cause of liver disease in China, alcohol use disorders are increasing on the background of increased screening and treatment programs for viral hepatitis.[54] Although nationwide large-scale epidemiologic data for ALD are unavailable, the prevalence as reported from specific regions of China ranges from 2.3% to 6.1% of the total population.[55] In a large tertiary referral hospital in Beijing, patients hospitalized with ALD continuously increased from 1.7% in 2002% to 4.6% in 2013, and hospitalizations for severe alcoholic hepatitis increased 2.43 times over the same period.[56] The annual incidence of hospitalizations related to ALD relative to other types of liver disease is growing steadily and an increased number of patients are undergoing liver transplantation for ALD.[55,57]

Of more than 1 million deaths (2% of all deaths) worldwide from cirrhosis,[58] 493,300 (47.9%) were due to ALD, which contributes to 1.2% of all deaths in men and 0.7% of deaths in women.[59] Proportion of cirrhosis deaths due to alcohol is highest in Central Europe at 72.3% and lowest in the Middle East and Northern Africa at 15.9% and 14%, respectively.[59]

POPULATION APPROACHES TO REDUCE ALCOHOLISM

Regional variations in the incidence and burden of ALD influence population-based strategies to reduce its burden. Taken together, these data underscore the current unmet need for strategies to reduce the disease burden from alcohol consumption. WHO-endorsed research has shown that the most economical public policy interventions to reduce alcohol-related mortality are taxation of alcoholic beverages, restricting the availability of alcoholic beverages, and imposing bans or restrictions on alcohol advertising.[60]

In most countries, the purchase of alcohol is limited by its availability and laws restricting sales to individuals below a certain minimum age.[61] Price is an important determinant of sales and, ultimately, consumption of alcohol.[62] There is strong evidence that affordability and availability of alcohol drive its consumption.[63–65] Examples of this association are demonstrated by areas of Europe with strong relationships in mortality rates from ALD tied to strategies to limit alcohol availability. For example, in Iceland, the deregulation of beer sales in 1989 was associated with a steady increase in rates of consumption and subsequent increase in mortality from ALD.[66] A study of alcohol consumption in Russia highlights a link between socioeconomic events that correlate with the availability and affordability of alcohol and overall mortality.[67] With the fall of the Soviet Union and the removal of state monopoly in 1992, alcohol consumption and alcohol-attributed disease burden increased significantly, contributing to 50% of all-cause mortality.[68] In 2006, policy changes in Russia, including restricting sale locations and regulations on licensing for producers and distributors, has led to a steady reduction in overall harms from excess alcohol consumption, including the risks of liver-related mortality.[69]

The use of taxation and minimum unit pricing to increase the cost of alcohol are effective approaches to curb excess alcohol consumption.[70,71] For example, in Taiwan the alcohol retail price increased by 7-fold after implementing significant increase in taxation of alcohol-related products in 2002. This resulted in an immediate decrease in alcoholic consumption and a significant reduction in hospital inpatient charges for alcohol-attributable diseases.[72] Regions in Canada have also implemented policies to increase the cost of alcohol, with an appreciable effect on alcohol-related mortality. In British Columbia, between 2002 and 2009, alcohol-related mortality decreased by 32% after the implementation of a 10% increase in the minimum unit price of all alcoholic beverages.[73] Minimum unit pricing has recently been passed into law in Scotland after ongoing legal challenges by the alcohol industry.[74] It is estimated that with a 50 pence minimum alcohol consumption will decrease by 3.5%, leading to 120 fewer alcohol attributable deaths, 1200 fewer hospital admissions, and a saving of £12.1 million each year.[75]

There are several other population-based approaches for limiting alcohol consumption, including use of a legal drinking age,[76] regulation in the number of alcohol selling outlets,[77] and restricting alcohol sales to certain hours of the day or days of the week.[78] Governments have also employed monopolies with licensing power to control the supply and availability of alcoholic beverages.[79] Laws against drinking and driving and public intoxication have also been implemented to curb the consumption of alcohol.[80] In many countries, advertisements on alcohol have been shown to drive increase in alcohol consumption, with an unhealthy pattern of drinking.[81,82] Exposure to alcohol marketing is associated with earlier drinking age, increased initiation of drinking, and heightened drinking intensity among current drinkers.[83,84] Data from the WHO in 2012 from 159 countries showed that nearly 40% of countries had no restrictions on alcohol marketing policies in place, with little change from 2002 to 2012.[2,85] On the other end of the spectrum, approximately 10% of countries located in the predominantly Islamic regions of northern Africa and the Middle East, reported a complete ban to reduce exposure to alcohol marketing.[2] Alcohol marketing restrictions have been successful in minimizing the allure of alcohol, particularly in vulnerable populations.[86] However, the most cost-effective policies and interventions to reduce alcohol consumption are limiting alcohol sale availability or increasing alcohol price.[87]

SUMMARY

Trends in the epidemiology of ALD reflect the current burden of disease and underscore the need for effective strategies to combat harmful alcohol use and management of ALD. The best current therapy remains complete abstinence of alcohol.[88-91] Alcohol consumption and the incidence of ALD are expected to continue to increase in the upcoming decades on the background of limited effective pharmacologic therapies for this disease.[92] Clearly, there remains an unmet need for the development of other effective treatment options for patients with ALD. With increased research efforts, there may be new treatment options, as well as strategies, to reduce alcohol consumption. Population-based approaches can affect the consumption of alcohol with direct health benefits and cost savings. Advances in medical therapies and worldwide reduction of harmful alcohol use are desperately needed to curtail the growing global burden of ALD and to achieve the WHO target of 3 to 4 alcohol-related deaths per 100,000 people.[1]

REFERENCES

1. Singal AK, Anand BS. Epidemiology of ALD. Clin Liv Dis 2013;2(2):53–6.
2. World Health Organization. Global status report on alcohol and health. Geneva (Switzerland): World Health Organization; 2014.
3. Gakidou E, Afshin A, Abajobir AA, et al. Global, regional, and national comparative risk assessment of 84 behavioural, environmental and occupational, and metabolic risks or clusters of risks, 1990–2016: a systematic analysis for the Global Burden of Disease Study 2016. Lancet 2017;390(10100):1345–422.
4. Immunological abnormalities in ALD. Lancet 1983;2(8350):605–6.

5. Mandayam S, Jamal MM, Morgan TR. Epidemiology of ALD. Semin Liver Dis 2004;24(3):217–32.

6. Rehm J, Gmel GE Sr, Gmel G, et al. The relationship between different dimensions of alcohol use and the burden of disease-an update. Addiction 2017; 112(6):968–1001.

7. Crawford JM. Histologic findings in ALD. Clin Liver Dis 2012;16(4):699–716.

8. Bataller R, Gao B. Liver fibrosis in ALD. Semin Liver Dis 2015;35(2):146–56.

9. Becker U, Deis A, Sorensen TI, et al. Prediction of risk of liver disease by alcohol intake, sex, and age: a prospective population study. Hepatology 1996;23(5): 1025–9.

10. Stein E, Cruz-Lemini M, Altamirano J, et al. Heavy daily alcohol intake at the population level predicts the weight of alcohol in cirrhosis burden worldwide. J Hepatol 2016;65(5):998–1005.

11. Bloomfield K, Stockwell T, Gmel G, et al. International comparisons of alcohol consumption. Alcohol Res Health 2003;27(1):95–109.

12. Ramstedt M. How much alcohol do you buy? A comparison of self-reported alcohol purchases with actual sales. Addiction 2010;105(4):649–54.

13. World Health Organization. Alcohol and Injuries. Emergency department studies in an international perspective. In: Cherpitel CJ, Borges G, Hungerford D, et al, editors. Room R. The relation between blood alcohol content and clinically assessed intoxication: lessons from applying the ICD-10 Y90 and Y91 codes in the emergency room. France: WHO; 2009. p. 135–46.

14. Faiad Y, Khoury B, Daouk S, et al. Frequency of use of the *International Classification of Diseases* ICD-10 diagnostic categories for mental and behavioural disorders across world regions. Epidemiol Psychiatr Sci 2017;1–9. https://doi.org/ 10.1017/S2045796017000683.

15. Greenfield TK, Kerr WC. Tracking alcohol consumption over time. Alcohol Res Health 2003;27(1):30–8.

16. Probst C, Manthey J, Merey A, et al. Unrecorded alcohol use: a global modelling study based on nominal group assessments and survey data. Addiction 2018; 113(7):1231–41.

17. Peacock A, Leung J, Larney S, et al. Global statistics on alcohol, tobacco and illicit drug use: 2017 status report. Addiction 2018;113(10):1905–26.

18. Kim W. Burden of liver disease in the United States: summary of a workshop. Hepatology 2002;36(1):227–42.

19. Liver transplantation for alcoholic liver disease. Proceedings of a meeting. Bethesda, Maryland, December 6-7, 1996. Liver Transpl Surg 1997;3(3):197–350.

20. Role of iron in alcoholic liver disease. Proceedings of a symposium. October, 2002. Bethesda, Maryland, USA. Alcohol 2003;30(2):91–158.

21. Dwyer-Lindgren L, Flaxman AD, Ng M, et al. Drinking patterns in US counties from 2002 to 2012. Am J Public Health 2015;105(6):1120–7.

22. Proceedings of the international symposium on alcoholic liver and pancreatic diseases and cirrhosis, 18-19 May 2006, Marina del Rey, California, USA. J Gastroenterol Hepatol 2006;21(Suppl 3):S1–110.

23. Das SK, Balakrishnan V, Vasudevan DM. Alcohol: its health and social impact in India. Natl Med J India 2006;19(2):94–9.

24. Bhattacharyya M, Barman NN, Goswami B. Survey of .alcohol-related cirrhosis at a tertiary care center in North East India. Indian J Gastroenterol 2016;35(3): 167–72.

25. Jiang H, Xiang X, Hao W, et al. Measuring and preventing alcohol use and related harm among young people in Asian countries: a thematic review. Glob Health Res Policy 2018;3:14.
26. Rehm J, Roerecke M. Patterns of drinking and liver cirrhosis – what do we know and where do we go? J Hepatol 2015;62(5):1000–1.
27. Laramée P, Kusel J, Leonard S, et al. The economic burden of alcohol dependence in Europe. Alcohol Alcohol 2013;48(3):259–69.
28. Anderson P, Baumberg B. Alcohol policy: who should sit at the table? Addiction 2007;102(2):335–6.
29. Sacks JJ, Gonzales KR, Bouchery EE, et al. 2010 National and State costs of excessive alcohol consumption. Am J Prev Med 2015;49(5):e73–9.
30. Rehm J, Mathers C, Popova S, et al. Global burden of disease and injury and economic cost attributable to alcohol use and alcohol-use disorders. Lancet 2009;373(9682):2223–33.
31. Bouchery EE, Harwood HJ, Sacks JJ, et al. Economic costs of excessive alcohol consumption in the U.S., 2006. Am J Prev Med 2011;41(5):516–24.
32. Stahre M, Roeber J, Kanny D, et al. Contribution of excessive alcohol consumption to deaths and years of potential life lost in the United States. Prev Chronic Dis 2014;11:E109.
33. Mokdad AH, Ballestros K, Echko M, et al. The state of US health, 1990-2016. JAMA 2018;319(14):1444.
34. Nemtsov AV. Alcohol-related human losses in Russia in the 1980s and 1990s. Addiction 2002;97(11):1413–25.
35. Singal AK, Salameh H, Kamath PS. Prevalence and in-hospital mortality trends of infections among patients with cirrhosis: a nationwide study of hospitalised patients in the United States. Aliment Pharmacol Ther 2014;40(1):105–12.
36. Kling CE, Perkins JD, Carithers RL, et al. Recent trends in liver transplantation for ALD in the United States. World J Hepatol 2017;9(36):1315–21.
37. Cholankeril G, Ahmed A. Alcoholic liver disease replaces hepatitis C virus infection as the leading indication for liver transplantation in the United States. Clin Gastroenterol Hepatol 2018;16:1356.
38. Singal AK, Kamath PS, Gores GJ, et al. Alcoholic hepatitis: current challenges and future directions. Clin Gastroenterol Hepatol 2014;12(4):555–64 [quiz: e31–2].
39. Lucey MR, Mathurin P, Morgan TR. Alcoholic hepatitis. N Engl J Med 2009; 360(26):2758–69.
40. Jinjuvadia R, Liangpunsakul S. Trends in alcoholic hepatitis related hospitalizations, financial burden, and mortality in the United States. J Clin Gastroenterol 2015;49(6):506–11.
41. Thompson JA, Martinson N, Martinson M. Mortality and costs associated with alcoholic hepatitis: a claims analysis of a commercially insured population. Alcohol 2018;71:57–63.
42. Abenavoli L, Milic N, Capasso F. Anti-oxidant therapy in non-alcoholic fatty liver disease: the role of silymarin. Endocrine 2012;42(3):754–5.
43. Abenavoli L, Milic N, De Lorenzo A, et al. A pathogenetic link between non-alcoholic fatty liver disease and celiac disease. Endocrine 2013;43(1):65–7.
44. Bräker AB, Soellner R. Alcohol drinking cultures of European adolescents. Eur J Public Health 2016;26(4):581–6.
45. Abenavoli L, Scarpellini E, Rouabhia S, et al. Probiotics in non-alcoholic fatty liver disease: which and when. Ann Hepatol 2013;12(3):357–63.

46. Ramstedt M. Per capita alcohol consumption and liver cirrhosis mortality in 14 European countries. Addiction 2002;96(1s1):19–33.
47. Williams R, Aspinall R, Bellis M, et al. Addressing liver disease in the UK: a blueprint for attaining excellence in health care and reducing premature mortality from lifestyle issues of excess consumption of alcohol, obesity, and viral hepatitis. Lancet 2014;384(9958):1953–97.
48. Williams R, Alexander G, Armstrong I, et al. Disease burden and costs from excess alcohol consumption, obesity, and viral hepatitis: fourth report of the lancet standing commission on liver disease in the UK. Lancet 2018;391(10125):1097–107.
49. Hazeldine S, Hydes T, Sheron N. ALD - the extent of the problem and what you can do about it. Clin Med 2015;15(2):179–85.
50. Welch C, Harrison D, Short A, et al. The increasing burden of ALD on United Kingdom critical care units: secondary analysis of a high quality clinical database. J Health Serv Res Policy 2008;13(Suppl 2):40–4.
51. Marinho RT, Duarte H, Gíria J, et al. The burden of alcoholism in fifteen years of cirrhosis hospital admissions in Portugal. Liver Int 2014;35(3):746–55.
52. Pimpin L, Cortez-Pinto H, Negro F, et al. Burden of liver disease in Europe: epidemiology and analysis of risk factors to identify prevention policies. J Hepatol 2018;69(3):718–35.
53. Fan JG. Epidemiology of alcoholic and nonalcoholic fatty liver disease in China. J Gastroenterol Hepatol 2013;28(Suppl 1):11–7.
54. Zheng X, Wang J, Yang D. Antiviral therapy for chronic hepatitis B in China. Med Microbiol Immunol 2015;204:115–20.
55. Wang F-S, Fan J-G, Zhang Z, et al. The global burden of liver disease: the major impact of China. Hepatology 2014;60(6):2099–108.
56. Huang A, Chang B, Sun Y, et al. Disease spectrum of ALD in Beijing 302 Hospital from 2002 to 2013: a large tertiary referral hospital experience from 7422 patients. Medicine 2017;96(7):e6163.
57. Wang W, Xu Y, Jiang C, et al. Advances in the treatment of severe alcoholic hepatitis. Curr Med Res Opin 2018;1–29. https://doi.org/10.1080/03007995.2018.
58. Rehm J, Samokhvalov AV, Shield KD. Global burden of ALDs. J Hepatol 2013;59(1):160–8.
59. Lozano R, Naghavi M, Foreman K, et al. Global and regional mortality from 235 causes of death for 20 age groups in 1990 and 2010: a systematic analysis for the Global Burden of Disease Study 2010. Lancet 2012;380(9859):2095–128.
60. Sornpaisarn BSK, Österberg E, Rehm J. Resource tool on alcohol taxation and pricing policies. Geneva (Switzerland): World Health Organization; 2017.
61. Babor TF, Caetano R, Casswell S, et al. Alcohol: no ordinary commodity. Oxford (UK): Oxford University Press; 2010.
62. Gallet CA. The demand for alcohol: a meta-analysis of elasticities. Aust J Agr Resource Econ 2007;51(2):121–35.
63. Sheron N. Alcohol and liver disease in Europe – simple measures have the potential to prevent tens of thousands of premature deaths. J Hepatol 2016;64(4):957–67.
64. Anderson P, Chisholm D, Fuhr DC. Effectiveness and cost-effectiveness of policies and programmes to reduce the harm caused by alcohol. Lancet 2009;373(9682):2234–46.
65. Elder RW, Lawrence B, Ferguson A, et al. The effectiveness of tax policy interventions for reducing excessive alcohol consumption and related harms. Am J Prev Med 2010;38(2):217–29.

66. Tyrfingsson T, Olafsson S, Bjornsson ES, et al. Alcohol consumption and liver cirrhosis mortality after lifting ban on beer sales in country with state alcohol monopoly: table 1. Eur J Public Health 2014;25(4):729–31.
67. Zaridze D, Lewington S, Boroda A, et al. Alcohol and mortality in Russia: prospective observational study of 151 000 adults. Lancet 2014;383(9927):1465–73.
68. Zaridze D, Brennan P, Boreham J, et al. Alcohol and cause-specific mortality in Russia: a retrospective case–control study of 48 557 adult deaths. Lancet 2009;373(9682):2201–14.
69. Neufeld M, Rehm J. Alcohol consumption and mortality in Russia since 2000: are there any changes following the alcohol policy changes starting in 2006? Alcohol Alcohol 2013;48(2):222–30.
70. Jiang H, Room R. Action on minimum unit pricing of alcohol: a broader need. Lancet 2018;391(10126):1157.
71. Meier PS, Holmes J, Angus C, et al. Estimated effects of different alcohol taxation and price policies on health inequalities: a mathematical modelling study. PLoS Med 2016;13(2):e1001963.
72. Lin CM, Liao CM. Inpatient expenditures on alcohol-attributed diseases and alcohol tax policy: a nationwide analysis in Taiwan from 1996 to 2010. Public Health 2014;128(11):977–84.
73. Zhao J, Stockwell T, Martin G, et al. The relationship between minimum alcohol prices, outlet densities and alcohol-attributable deaths in British Columbia, 2002-09. Addiction 2013;108(6):1059–69.
74. Gilmore W, Chikritzhs T, Stockwell T, et al. Alcohol: taking a population perspective. Nat Rev Gastroenterol Hepatol 2016;13(7):426–34.
75. Meier P, Brennan A, Angus C, et al. Minimum unit pricing for alcohol clears final legal hurdle in Scotland. BMJ 2017;359:j5372.
76. Plunk AD, Krauss MJ, Syed-Mohammed H, et al. The impact of the minimum legal drinking age on alcohol-related chronic disease mortality. Alcohol Clin Exp Res 2016;40(8):1761–8.
77. Gmel G, Holmes J, Studer J. Are alcohol outlet densities strongly associated with alcohol-related outcomes? A critical review of recent evidence. Drug Alcohol Rev 2016;35(1):40–54.
78. Holmes J, Guo Y, Maheswaran R, et al. The impact of spatial and temporal availability of alcohol on its consumption and related harms: a critical review in the context of UK licensing policies. Drug Alcohol Rev 2014;33(5):515–25.
79. Hahn RA, Middleton JC, Elder R, et al. Effects of alcohol retail privatization on excessive alcohol consumption and related harms: a community guide systematic review. Am J Prev Med 2012;42(4):418–27.
80. Esser MB, Bao J, Jernigan DH, et al. Evaluation of the evidence base for the alcohol industry's actions to reduce drink driving globally. Am J Public Health 2016;106(4):707–13.
81. Hollingworth W, Ebel BE, McCarty CA, et al. Prevention of deaths from harmful drinking in the United States: the potential effects of tax increases and advertising bans on young drinkers. J Stud Alcohol 2006;67(2):300–8.
82. Esser MB, Jernigan DH. Policy approaches for regulating alcohol marketing in a global context: a public health perspective. Annu Rev Public Health 2018;39(1):385–401.
83. Jernigan D, Noel J, Landon J, et al. Alcohol marketing and youth alcohol consumption: a systematic review of longitudinal studies published since 2008. Addiction 2017;112(Suppl 1):7–20.

84. Chang Fc, Lee Cm, Chen Ph, et al. Using media exposure to predict the initiation and persistence of youth alcohol use in Taiwan. Int J Drug Policy 2014;25(3): 386–92.
85. Esser MB, Jernigan DH. Assessing restrictiveness of national alcohol marketing policies. Alcohol Alcohol 2014;49(5):557–62.
86. Babor TF, Jernigan D, Brookes C, et al. Toward a public health approach to the protection of vulnerable populations from the harmful effects of alcohol marketing. Addiction 2017;112:125–7.
87. Martineau F, Tyner E, Lorenc T, et al. Population-level interventions to reduce alcohol-related harm: an overview of systematic reviews. Prev Med 2013;57(4): 278–96.
88. Guirguis J, Chhatwal J, Dasarathy J, et al. Clinical impact of alcohol-related cirrhosis in the next decade: estimates based on current epidemiological trends in the United States. Alcohol Clin Exp Res 2015;39(11):2085–94.
89. Singal AK, Kodali S, Vucovich LA, et al. Diagnosis and treatment of alcoholic hepatitis: a systematic review. Alcohol Clin Exp Res 2016;40(7):1390–402.
90. Louvet A, Labreuche J, Artru F, et al. Main drivers of outcome differ between short and long-term in severe alcoholic hepatitis: a prospective study. Hepatology 2017;66(5):1464–73.
91. Thursz MR, Forrest EH, Ryder S, et al. Prednisolone or pentoxifylline for alcoholic hepatitis. N Engl J Med 2015;373(3):282–3.
92. Singal AK, Bataller R, Ahn J, et al. ACG clinical guideline: ALD. Am J Gastroenterol 2018;113(2):175–94.

Behavioral Addictions
Excessive Gambling, Gaming, Internet, and Smartphone Use Among Children and Adolescents

Jeffrey L. Derevensky, PhD*, Victoria Hayman, BSc,
Lynette Gilbeau, BEd

KEYWORDS

- Behavioral disorders • Gambling • Gaming • Internet addiction • Smartphone use

KEY POINTS

- The introduction of behavioral addictions is a relatively new concept in psychiatry. Although many of the disorders subsumed under the term behavioral addictions have existed for decades, it was not until 2010 that the DSM workgroup, based on a growing body of literature, suggested adding the term *behavioral addictions* to their official classification of psychiatric diagnoses in the *Diagnostic and Statistical Manual of Mental Disorders, Fifth Edition*.
- Gambling, typically thought to be an adult behavior, has become commonplace among adolescents.
- Although technological advances have made accessing information and communication easier, excessive use of the Internet and smartphones can result in multiple mental and physical health issues.
- Gambling disorders, gaming disorders, Internet use disorder, and excessive smartphone use often begin during childhood and adolescence.

BEHAVIORAL ADDICTIONS

The introduction of behavioral addictions is a relatively new concept in psychiatry.[1] Although many of the disorders subsumed under the term behavioral addictions have existed for decades, it was not until 2010 that the DSM workgroup, based on a growing body of literature, suggested adding the term *behavioral addictions* to their official classification of psychiatric diagnoses in the *Diagnostic and Statistical Manual of Mental Disorders, Fifth Edition* (DSM-5).[2] There was strong empirical support

This article originally appeared in *Pediatric Clinics*, Volume 66, Issue 6, December 2019.
International Centre for Youth Gambling Problems and High-Risk Behaviors, McGill University, 3724 McTavish Street, Montreal, Quebec H3A 1Y2, Canada
* Corresponding author.
E-mail address: Jeffrey.derevensky@mcgill.ca

Clinics Collections 9 (2020) 227–246
https://doi.org/10.1016/j.ccol.2020.07.036
2352-7986/20/© 2020 Elsevier Inc. All rights reserved.

indicating that a number of potentially risky behaviors, besides psychoactive sub-stance ingestion, produce short-term rewards that may result in persistent behaviors despite the individual's understanding and awareness of adverse consequences.[3–6] The American Psychiatric Association (DSM-5),[2] World Health Organization (*Interna-tional Classification of Diseases, Eleventh Revision* [ICD-11])[7] and the American Soci-ety of Addiction Medicine[8] have all recognized that such disorders, characterized as *behavioral addictions*, to varying degrees and with different, but similar, clinical criteria should be recognized.

Our current conceptualization of behavioral addictions is that those disorders under the rubric of behavioral addictions share many similarities and commonalities with other forms of addictive behaviors.[3] The DSM workgroup concluded that the emerging neuroscientific data supported a unified neurobiological theory of addictions indepen-dent of the specific substances, substrates, or activities, which should allow for the inclusion of behavioral addictions as well as chemical addictions.[1] Although a number of behavioral addictions were suggested for inclusion, the workgroup concluded that there was sufficient evidence for inclusion of a gambling disorder and that further research was necessary before including a gaming disorder, Internet use disorder, smartphone disorder, sex addiction, exercise addiction, and shopping addiction. The World Health Organization has nevertheless elected to include gaming disorder in its ICD-11.[7]

Behavioral addictions may be best understood from a biopsychosocial model.[1,9] The essential feature of behavioral addictions lies in the individual's failure to resist im-pulses, drives, or temptations, which if engaged in excessively may result in harmful consequences. Griffiths,[9] early on, articulated 6 core elements found among individ-uals experiencing a behavioral addiction; these being salience (the activity becomes highly valued and takes precedence over other activities), mood modification (the emotional response to the behavior; this may be in the form of an adrenalin rush when engaged in the behavior or may lead to a reduction in a depressive state), toler-ance (the need for increasing amounts of the behavior to achieve the desired level of mood modification), withdrawal symptoms (unpleasant feelings or physiologic with-drawal symptoms when cutting down or stopping the activity), conflict (conflicts with other activities or persons due to the behavior), and relapse (a relatively high rate of returning back to the initial behavior). Each of these core elements can be found among all behavioral addictions.[10]

Although several behavioral addictions (eg, compulsive shopping, sexual addiction, smartphone addiction) seem to be more typical of middle age or even older adults, the onset of many of these behavioral disorders has been shown to occur during child-hood, adolescence, and/or early adulthood. It may well be that the consequences and problems associated with a behavioral addiction may be more severe during adulthood, but the resulting problems associated with a behavioral addiction for chil-dren and adolescents also can be pervasive.

CHILD AND ADOLESCENT RISKY BEHAVIORS

Over the past few decades, there has been a significant and remarkable invigoration of both theoretic and empirical research on child and adolescent risk behaviors (those behaviors that if engaged in excessively can, directly or indirectly, compromise the in-dividual's physical and mental health, and the life course trajectories of young peo-ple).[10–12] Today's conceptualizations of child and adolescent risky behaviors encompass a wide array of causal domains, including cultural, genetic, biological, so-cial, psychological, and environmental factors.[11] Much of the early work focused on adolescent problematic behaviors (substance and alcohol abuse, cigarette smoking, unprotected sexual activity, drinking and driving, and delinquency), all of which had potentially serious negative short-term and long-term consequences for the individual, the individual's family, and society. These risky behaviors often compromise one's "healthy development," and result in mental health, social, educational, and in some cases legal difficulties for adolescents.[13] Given the pervasiveness of the problems, researchers and clinicians have sought a better understanding as to the reasons why individuals engage in these behaviors, their risk factors, both proximal and distal, as well as the identification and assessment of protective factors.[11] This has further led to issues related to prevention programs focused on harm minimization or harm reduction.[14]

As previously noted, although there is much commonality among different behavioral addictions, there also remains increasing evidence that different problem behaviors are associated with distinct risk factors, which is reflected in differential diagnoses applicable to specific mental health disorders occurring during childhood or adolescence.[2,7] Derevensky[10] argued that although it is important to study individuals displaying a single form of problem behavior, understanding youth displaying problems in multiple domains can significantly add to our knowledge. He points to Jacobs'[15] *General Theory of Addictions* suggesting that an addiction is a dependent state acquired over time to relieve stress. Jacobs[15] postulated that 2 interrelated sets of factors predispose individuals to addictions: (1) an abnormal physiologic resting state, and (2) childhood experiences producing a deep sense of inadequacy. The unipolar physiologic resting state (over or under stimulation) is a key factor within this theoretic model, suggesting that an addiction may be in part inherited through a genetic disposition. In an attempt to reduce or minimize the effects of this physiologic state, individuals, through maladaptive coping strategies, turn to some addictive behavior as a form of stress reduction.[15]

Although a large number of behavioral addictions have been clinically reported, this review focuses on gambling disorders (recognized in the DSM-5),[2] gaming disorders (recognized in ICD-11),[7] as well Internet addiction and excessive smartphone use, given these disorders appear to have emerged as important clinical and social issues.

GAMBLING DISORDERS

Society has witnessed a dramatic expansion of all forms of gambling. Once thought to be an activity only for adults, gambling has become a popular mainstream activity in most parts of the world along with its concomitant associated problems.[10,12] Whether purchasing lottery scratch cards with familiar themes, playing poker or other card games among friends, or wagering on sports, international studies have consistently reported that gambling has become part of the life experiences for large numbers of adolescents.[12,16–21]

Despite prohibitions from engaging in government-regulated gambling activities (the age varies based on the type of gambling and jurisdiction), adolescents have been reported to have engaged in all forms of gambling, including online gambling.[12,16,17,21,22] There is abundant evidence suggesting that a pattern of gambling behavior often occurs early, with children as young as ages 9 and 10 engaging in some form of gambling,[12,16–18,22,23] yet few parents,[24] teachers,[25,26] and even mental health professionals[27,28] perceive gambling to be a serious issue for youth. Although most youth who gamble can be best described as social, recreational, occasional, or infrequent gamblers, a small but identifiable number of adolescents develop a serious gambling problem.

With almost 80% of adolescents reporting having gambled for money at least once during their lifetime,[12] there is a growing concern that problem and disordered gambling among adolescents is a significant issue. Calado and colleagues,[16] in reviewing the adolescent gambling literature, reported that between 0.2% and 12.3% of youth meet criteria for problem gambling, notwithstanding assessment differences, cutoff scores, timeframes, accessibility, and availability of different gambling activities. They also suggested that in addition to male individuals being more likely to report gambling and experiencing problems, individuals who belong to an ethnic minority may be at a higher risk for problem/disordered gambling. Their analyses further revealed that youth engaged in online Internet wagering are more prone to experience gambling and gambling-related problems, likely the result of its easy accessibility, affordability, convenience, and anonymity.[16,19,29,30] It is important to note that youth with gambling problems typically do not elect to seek treatment for gambling problems.[10,12]

The types of gambling activities in which youth are engaged is often related to the accessibility and availability of specific forms of gambling. School age children are much more prone to engage in gambling activities among peers (often related to skill-related games), lottery tickets (eg, scratch-instant win tickets) and sports gambling. As they get older and have greater access to money and credit cards, they may begin to get involved in video lottery terminals (where available), casinos, and online gambling.[12]

Risk Factors Associated with a Gambling Disorder

There is a growing list of risk and protective factors associated with youth experiencing gambling problems. The cumulative body of gambling research suggests male individuals are more likely to engage in gambling and experience gambling problems,[12,16,31] they begin gambling at an earlier age,[32] they may be members of an ethnic minority,[33,34] may have had disrupted familial and peer relationships,[35] and have a parent or close family member with a gambling disorder.[12,32] From a psychological perspective, many of these adolescents, like their adult counterparts, report significant mental health issues, including anxiety disorders,[36] depression,[37–39] and impulsivity.[37] These individuals score lower on measures of conformity and self-discipline, and they report high rates of suicide ideation and attempts.[39,40] Academically, adolescents with gambling problems experience a wide variety of school-related problems, including impaired academic performance, interpersonal difficulties, and conduct-related problems.[12,41] Other factors associated with youth gambling problems include having a "big win" (this being dependent on their socioeconomic level and age of the individual),[32] with peer influences being predictive of gambling problems.[42]

Adolescent problem gamblers, like their adult counterparts, exhibit erroneous beliefs, their cognitive thinking lacks a knowledge of the independence of events, and they report an exaggerated level of skill when gambling. As well, they typically have poor or maladaptive general coping skills,[40,43] have a high-risk propensity,[14] and have poor resiliency in light of adversity.[44,45] In addition, adolescent problem gamblers report more daily hassles and traumatic life events.[46]

Despite these well-established risk factors and their associations with youth gambling problems, many children and adolescents never develop significant problems, suggesting that there are protective factors that play an important role in minimizing and decreasing the likelihood of youth problem gambling.[45] Several early studies by Dickson and her colleagues[14] revealed that low-risk propensity, family cohesion, school connectedness, achievement motivation, and effective coping skills served as protective factors. Lussier and colleagues[45] further reported on the importance of resilience being an important protective factor. Those youth having high scores on resiliency measures were significantly less likely to experience gambling problems. These factors may serve to counteract risk factors through a cancellation process.[14,44,45]

Assessing Gambling Problems Among Adolescents and Young Adults

Due to the growing awareness of gambling problems among adolescents, a number of instruments have been adapted from adult scales for this age group. The South Oaks Gambling Screen-Revised for Adolescents,[47] DSM-IV-J[48] and its revision the DSM-IV-MR-J,[49] and the Massachusetts Gambling Screen[50] have been used in a large number of adolescent prevalence studies. Each of these instruments was modeled on adult screening instruments; however, more recently, the Canadian Adolescent Gambling Inventory[51] was specifically developed to assess gambling severity among adolescents.

Like adult scales, common constructs underlie all the instruments. The notion of deception (lying), stealing money to support gambling, preoccupation, and chasing losses are common to all of these instruments. Similarly, although the number of items and constructs differ, each criterion item has equal weighting, and a cut score is provided identifying pathologic gambling for each respective instrument (see Derevensky[12] for a more comprehensive discussion and description of these instruments).

The Changing Face of Gambling

Gambling has dramatically changed during the past decade. Not only has it become more socially acceptable, easily accessible, and readily available, but technological innovations have revolutionized the industry and the way we gamble. Online gambling, wagering through one's smartphone, fantasy sports wagering, in-play and micro sports betting, are just a few examples. In some jurisdictions, Video Lottery Terminals are available on almost every corner, and sports wagering is prevalent. There is little doubt that youth, in spite of prohibitions, have managed to access and engage in many of these forms of gambling.[12] Recently, Derevensky and Gainsbury[52] raised concerns about social casino gaming; simulated forms of gambling that individuals play for points or chips but that may have higher than average payout rates. In a series of studies by Kim and colleagues,[53–55] there seems to be a crossover and migration from gambling on online social casino games to actual online gambling among young adults. King,[56] in reviewing the available literature, pointed to the convergence between gaming and gambling and suggested some forms of gaming may be a "gateway" to actual gambling. He concluded, after a review of the available empirical evidence, that simulated gambling during adolescence increases risk of monetary gambling during adulthood. McBride and Derevensky[57] also reported that social casino game playing among adolescents was related to more problematic gambling behaviors. Other forms of gambling, such as fantasy sports wagering, appear to be popular among adolescent boys. Those individuals engaging in these behaviors frequently were reported to experience a number of gambling-related behaviors.[58]

GAMING DISORDERS

With the appearance of electronic games in the 1990s and technological advances associated with game consoles and smartphones, video games and online gaming continue to increase in popularity and accessibility. There is evidence that more than 90% of children and adolescents in the United States play video games, with a large percentage spending an increasingly substantial amount of time playing.[59,60] Király and colleagues[61] argued that online video games are currently one of the most widespread recreational activities irrespective of culture, age, and gender. Newzoo[62] suggested that in spite of some concerns, the gaming market continues to grow and is expected to become a $180 billion market by 2021 (more than doubling in size since 2014). It should not be interpreted that gaming in and of itself is harmful. On the contrary, video games may satisfy certain psychological needs of the users, including identity expression, a sense of mastery and achievement, and the desire to escape from reality.[63] Despite some positive attributions associated with gaming, if done excessively, individuals can experience a number of negative consequences (eg, financial losses, as online games often require money to continue play, psychological detachment, sleep deprivation, eating and nutritional problems, a lack of personal and social interaction, depression, and anxiety, among others). Given its attractiveness, widespread popularity, easy accessibility and availability, it is not surprising that an identifiable number of individuals appear to engage in this behavior excessively. Although the DSM-5[2] Work Group identified gaming disorder as a potential disorder worthy of further investigation, the World Health Organization decided there was sufficient clinical and experimental evidence to include it in the ICD-11[7] as a behavioral disorder requiring treatment for individuals meeting the clinical criteria. A gaming disorder is defined as a pattern of gaming behavior ("digital gaming" or "video gaming") characterized by impaired control over gaming, and increased priority given to gaming over other activities, interests, and daily activities. It is marked by a continuation or escalation of gaming despite the occurrence of negative consequences. As part of the clinical criteria, this behavior is not episodic and must be of sufficient severity (both intensity and frequency) to result in significant impairment in personal, familial, social, educational, occupational, or other important areas of functioning. The World Health Organization diagnostic criteria also indicate that this behavior must be present for at least 12 months; however, in exceptional cases of a severe gaming disorder, a shorter timeframe is used.[7]

A consensus concerning prevalence rates of a gaming disorder has been difficult to achieve given significant variability among studies in terms of definition, assessment criteria, geographic considerations, accessibility (related to income and Internet access), and different methodological approaches. Several reviews of the literature examining the prevalence rates of gaming disorders[61,64,65] suggest that approximately 1.5% to 9.9% of adolescents appear to have a gaming disorder, with some research reporting rates as high as 25% among US university students.[66] Although adults can also exhibit symptoms of a gaming disorder, Kuss and Griffiths[67–69] concluded that gaming disorders are more typical among children and adolescents (possibly because of more free time). A recent study revealed that excessive gaming time may not only be gender-dependent but also dependent on the individual's preference of game genre.[70] Role-playing games and shooter-type games may be related to higher time spent gaming.[70] Eichenbaum and colleagues[71] reported that Massively Multiplayers Online Role-Playing Games were highly related to Internet gaming disorders, whereas action and puzzle games were found to be minimally linked to a gaming disorder.[72] However, if done excessively, these games can lead to a gaming disorder. One's motivation for gaming has also been shown to be related to a gaming disorder. For example, if gaming is primarily used for social reasons versus psychological escape, it may be less problematic. Nevertheless, as gaming frequency and play time escalate, the likelihood of a gaming disorder increases. In addition, the more game genres engaged in, the greater the incidence of a gaming disorder.[73]

Although there are several studies that have found an association between Internet use and a gaming disorder, those with a severe gaming disorder have a variety of psychosocial problems and psychiatric conditions (eg, depressive symptomatology, attention-deficit hyperactivity, mood disorders, anxiety disorders, personality disorders, and obsessive-compulsive disorders).[61,74–78] However, it is important to note that there is very little research examining the temporal or causal relationships between psychiatric disorders and gaming disorders.[79–82] Further, disordered gaming significantly predicted poorer academic performance, even after controlling for sex, age, and weekly amounts of game playing.[59] Long-term effects of violent games also seem to be predictive of more aggressive behavior.[83] Kuss and colleagues[84] further suggested that understanding one's cultural context is important, as it embeds gamers into a community with shared beliefs and practices, endowing their gaming with a particular meaning.

Whether it is due to gaming's social features, the ability to manipulate and control aspects of the game itself, reward and punishment features (eg, earning or losing points), the aesthetic quality of the games, the ability to assume an alternate identity with the game characters, or the ability to interact with others, children and adolescents are particularly drawn to these games.[67–69,85] Online gaming has become a space of "virtual socialization" in which players experience social interactions as an integral part of the gaming process.[78] For some, the increased frequency of gaming represents a need for completion of more intricate, time-consuming, or difficult goals to achieve satisfaction and the need to rectify perceived gaming inadequacies.[81]

Gaming: Some Recent Developments

One evolution of the gaming movement has been what is referred to as e-Sports, whereby individuals watch teams of gamers compete against each other in real time. These competitions have attracted tens of thousands of spectators, and some players have developed a strong cultlike following. This has resulted in an increase in young people reporting a desire to become "professional gamers." Collegiate and professional e-Sports (competitive video gaming) have become more organized and popular.[86,87] Since their establishment in the early 2000s, professional and club e-Sports have seen a rapid growth in both participation and viewership,[88,89] with some colleges and universities now offering scholarships for top players.[87] The gambling industry has now capitalized on this emerging market, with some casinos now accepting wagers on the outcome of the matches.

Assessing Internet Gaming Disorders

The need for common diagnostic criteria has been repeatedly emphasized in the psychological literature.[90] The existence of multiple instruments reflects the divergence of opinions in the field regarding how best to diagnose this condition. This has not precluded researchers from developing several scales, some of which include the Internet Gaming Disorder Test-20[91] and its short form (IGDS-9)[92] (assesses severity of online and offline gaming behaviors), Internet Gaming Disorder Test-10[61] (a 10-item scale based on the DMS-5 criteria for a gambling disorder), and the Internet Gaming Disorders Scales (both 9-item and 27-item versions).[93,94] All of these scales are designed to assess negative consequences associated with a gaming disorder.

INTERNET ADDICTION DISORDER

Similar to a gaming disorder, the American Psychiatric Association[2] suggested that Internet use disorder as an addiction is in need of further study. Internet addiction follows a trajectory similar to substance-related addictions, as well as gambling and gaming disorders.[9,84] Although Griffiths[9] points to the symptoms traditionally associated with an Internet addiction (salience, mood modification, tolerance, withdrawal, conflict, and relapse), Kuss and Griffiths[67–69] also suggest there is an abundance of neurobiological evidence suggesting its addictive properties. Problematic Internet Use, Internet Addiction Disorder, or Internet Addiction (IA) is characterized by excessive preoccupation, urges, and/or behaviors that ultimately lead to significant impairment and negative consequences.[95]

Several researchers contend that rather than looking at IA per se, an emphasis and focus should be on the specific type of Internet activities in which the individual is engaged (eg, online gambling, gaming disorders, smartphone use) that may prompt them to become addicted.[84,96] For example, studies examining the use of social networking applications, including online chatting,[97,98] and social networking sites,[64,99] have been reported to be highly associated with IA.[84]

Prevalence of Internet Addiction

Although no current "gold standard" measure exists for identifying IA, international prevalence rates of IA have varied considerably, ranging from 1.5% to 8.2%.[100] These rates are dependent on the ages of individuals being assessed as well as geographic differences.[101–103] Given the popularity and widespread accessibility of the Internet, a large number of studies have been conducted among adolescents[104] and university students.[66,84,105] Kuss and colleagues[84] attribute high rates of Internet use among children and adolescents to their unlimited Internet access, flexible schedules, and expectations by teachers and peers that they make use of technology. Studies of youth appear to indicate extremely high prevalence rates of Facebook and Twitter use, with a large percentage of youth indicating an inability to stop using social networking sites and frequently spending excessive amounts of time on these sites.[106] Whether used for gaming or social networking sites, Internet use enables adolescents to stay "connected" with their peers and thus remains highly socially acceptable and desirable to youth.

The fact that IA has been associated with aggression,[107,108] introversion,[107] high sensation seeking,[108] social inhibition,[109] neuroticism,[110,111] lower scores on measures of extroversion,[112] depression and depressive mood disorders,[113,114] anxiety,[115] emotional stability,[116] conduct disorders,[117] general mental health disorders,[118] poor coping strategies, difficulties in school and at home,[119] and the need for psychological escape from their current reality,[120] all point to the potential seriousness of the problem.[10,84] There is a growing body of literature suggesting that Internet-addicted adolescents suffer loss of control, have a poor self-image, low self-esteem, experience social withdrawal, and report familial conflicts.[121] Studies have revealed that under extreme circumstances, a severe IA can lead to dysthymia; bipolar, affective social-anxiety disorders; and major depression.[121] Excessive Internet use has been associated with impaired sleep and eating disorders.[122]

Assessment of Internet Addiction

Diagnosing IA can be challenging.[122] As previously indicated, there are no "gold standard" assessment instruments. Many of the scales developed have been based on the DSM clinical criteria for substance dependence or a gambling disorder (assessing preoccupation, the need to increase the behavior, efforts to control the behavior, emotional responses when trying to reduce or stop Internet use, lying to family members about time spent on the Internet, the use of the Internet to reduce a dysphoric mood, the continuous need for increased use, and negative consequences associated with excessive Internet use). Examples of such scales include the Internet Addiction Diagnostic Questionnaire,[123] the Problematic Internet Use Questionnaire developed by Demetrovics and colleagues,[124] and the Compulsive Internet Use Scale.[125]

THE AGE OF SMARTPHONES

Today's smartphones are part mini-computer and part cell phone. Connected to the Internet, they allow individuals to communicate with anyone; search for information; check email or Facebook messages; play games; do banking; order goods; watch favorite movies, sports, or television shows; and easily find directions.[126] In addition, in recent years there has been an explosion in the number of applications (*apps*) developed for smartphones, enabling users to do anything from monitoring their health to controlling environmental conditions (eg, alarm, lights, heating/cooling schedules) in their homes.

The number of smartphone users is nearing 2.5 billion in 2019,[127] with analysts projecting more than 6 billion smartphones being in use by 2020.[128] Although user growth is expected to level off in developing markets (ie, North America and Europe), the exponential growth will be led by penetration in less mature markets (ie, Africa, the Middle East).[129]

Youth and Smartphones

In the United States, smartphone ownership has become a nearly ubiquitous element of teen life, with 95% of teens reporting they have a smartphone or access to one, representing a 22% increase from 2014.[130] Smartphone ownership is nearly universal in North America and parts of Europe and Asia, independent of gender, race, ethnicity, and socioeconomic background.[130] Although Internet and smartphone use is on the rise, geographic differences have been noted. A large-scale study in 2014 across Europe (Belgium, Denmark, Ireland, Italy, Portugal, Romania, United Kingdom) revealed that 46% of children ages 9 to 16 years reported owning a smartphone.[131] In South Korea, 84% of individuals older than 3 were found to use a smartphone, with approximately 96% of teenagers reporting smartphone usage,[132] in the United Kingdom, 46% of 9-year-olds own a smartphone and 93% of youth aged 15 own one,[133] and in Switzerland, nearly all adolescents aged 12 to 19 (98%) own a mobile phone (97% of which are smartphones).[134] Although these prevalence studies are not directly comparable given they were conducted over different time periods and use different-age populations, they clearly indicate a growing number of children and adolescents possess or have access to a smartphone. The most commonly reported reason for parents initially giving their children a smartphone is to facilitate contact (either from parent to child or child to parent).[135] In the United States and Japan, youth spend most of the time on their mobile device playing games, watching videos, accessing social networking sites, and messaging.[136,137] Interestingly, individuals (American) between 18 and 24 years old send and receive an average of 2022 texts per month,[138] with texting surpassing voice calls and emails as the most common means of transmitting information, particularly for adolescents and young adults.[139] Whether using one's smartphone for texting, tweeting, sexting, or using social media communications, the prevalence and appeal are overwhelming.

Smartphone Addiction

Similar to excessive gambling, gaming, and Internet use, excessive smartphone use can have adverse mental and physical health consequences. The Pew Research Center[130] reported that 45% of US teens indicate they are online "almost constantly," and this figure has nearly doubled from 24% in their 2014 to 2015 survey. Youth sleep with their smartphones, eat with their smartphones at their side, and repeatedly check for messages and texts. International research shows similar upward trends in usage. Among Korean youth (aged 11–12), research has revealed they spend, on average, 5.4 hours daily on their smartphones.[140] Although some studies reported a predominance of female individuals addicted to their smartphone, others have revealed greater use and problems among male individuals.[141] Internationally, smartphone addiction prevalence rates among youth have been reported to be 19.9% in Switzerland,[142] 30.9% in South Korea,[143] 10.0% in the United Kingdom,[144] and 6.4% in Turkey.[145] The wide variability in prevalence rates is attributable to the use of different scales and methodologies for measurement.[146,147]

Risks Associated with Excessive Smartphone Use

Despite the many advantages associated with smartphone use (eg, communication, ability to immediately access information, social networking), its increasing popularity and overuse by children and adolescents has resulted in multiple problems.[126] The consequences of excessive smartphone use include depression, anxiety, impulsivity, poor self-regulation, academic difficulties, reduced social interaction, and a lack of familial interaction.[145,148–158] Increased time spent on smartphones also has been shown to be related to lower physical activity and more sedentary behavior, sleep disturbances, and a number of physical problems (neck stiffness, blurred vision, wrist or back pain), and fewer leisure pursuits, such as reading or creating art or music.[126,142,154,159]

Assessing Smartphone Addiction

There are a limited number of instruments for assessing potential smartphone addiction among children and adolescents.[144] Several of the scales in current use include the Smartphone Addiction Scale,[160] Cellular Phone Dependence Questionnaire,[161] and Problematic Mobile Phone Use Questionnaire (PMPUQ)[153] and its short version (PMPUQ-SV).[153] The 27-item Mobile Phone Problem Use Scale (MPPUS) of Bianchi and Phillips[162] is among the most widely used with adults, and has been adapted for use with adolescents (MPPUSA, a 26-item scale).[144]

TREATING GAMBLING, INTERNET, GAMING, AND SMARTPHONE ADDICTIONS

Although it is beyond the scope of this article to go into depth concerning the treatment of behavioral disorders, it is important to note that few children and adolescents voluntarily seek treatment for any of the behavioral disorders discussed. Issues related to abstinence versus controlled use still remain. Although one could argue for abstinence in gambling (especially for children and adolescents), it is difficult to make this argument for Internet or smartphone use. In some jurisdictions, in-patient treatment is growing, especially for individuals with a gaming addiction. Some schools are now requiring children to place their smartphones in their locker at the beginning of the school day and retrieve them only at the end of the day[163]; and governments around the world are trying to develop more effective systems for prohibiting underage youth from gambling. Traditional forms of treatment for several behavioral disorders include cognitive/cognitive behavioral therapy, motivational interviewing, family therapy, and a growing number of online forums and support groups. Yau and colleagues[164] suggest that a comprehensive treatment program for behavioral addictions may want to use an integrated treatment approach, drawing on several different therapeutic approaches that focus on addressing symptoms, as well as the underlying dynamics that contribute to the addictive behavior. Although Yau and colleagues[164] were discussing treatment of a food addiction, this model would be beneficial in working with youth experiencing other forms of behavioral addictions.

Parents play an essential role in helping both prevent and modify their children's behavioral addictions. There is little doubt about the social acceptance of many of the behaviors discussed, and there is ample evidence that children are increasingly being exposed to gambling, gaming, the Internet, and use of mobile technologies earlier and earlier.[165] Gaming, the Internet, and smartphones are commonly used as forms of entertainment and communication. They are also used by parents as a way of keeping their children occupied. The issue remains as to when casual use or engagement becomes problematic. There is considerable evidence that parents remain unaware of the extent to which children engage in these behaviors until they become problematic. Much of this behavior is often modeled on parental behavior. Parents should be encouraged to set limits early on, model appropriate behavior, recognize the warning signs as to when a behavior becomes problematic, and to modify and/or curb excessive use. Time limitations for Internet use, gaming, and smartphone use are often dependent on the age of the individual, the free time available and whether the behavior is interfering with social interactions and school performance. There exists an enormous wealth of knowledge via the Internet concerning strategies to help curb excessive problematic behaviors. There are also a growing number of pediatricians, psychologists, and psychiatrists with clinical expertise to help children and parents.

SUMMARY

Today's youth face different stressors than any generation before them. Not only are they dealing with physiologic changes, increasing academic demands, social pressures, and a difficult employment market, they are doing this in front of an online audience. Youth are expected to be "on" 24 hours a day, 7 days a week. Although technology has made certain tasks easier, the social pressures placed on our teens has increased exponentially. Suicide rates have increased for children younger than 15, and dramatically jumped for youth between age 15 and 24.[166] Based on the 2017 Youth Risk Behaviors Survey, 7.4% of youth in grades 9 to 12 (ages 12–17) reported having made at least one suicide attempt during the past 12 months (2.4% of youth required medical treatment).[166] Although it is impossible to draw a causal link with many of the behavioral disorders discussed, the psychosocial stresses placed on youth resulting from any of the behaviors discussed certainly leads to a wide variety of mental health issues.

There is little doubt that the behavioral addictions discussed (gambling disorders, gaming disorders, IA disorders, and smartphone problems) often develop during childhood and adolescence. Today's youth are not only "connected," but fear they will miss something important when not connected. The excessive use of "screen time" has led to major confrontations with parents over their devices. Awareness of these disorders is essential. Setting limits by parents often results in more conflict. Tracking the amount of screen time children use can provide parents with a better picture of the severity of the problem. Other behavioral disorders, such as gambling, are often more difficult to observe.

Although, with time, some youth may outgrow these disorders as they become adults through a process of natural recovery or, in some cases, through psychological or psychiatric interventions (there is evidence that adult prevalence rates for many of these behavioral disorders are lower compared with adolescents), their consequences and harms may be severe. It is important to recognize that concomitant mental health, academic, social, familial, and interpersonal issues may have longstanding consequences. Although many of the treatment approaches have evolved from work in substance abuse, each disorder requires an understanding of the motivations underlying the behaviors to determine whether abstinence or controlled behavior may be feasible. Although abstinence from gambling and gaming behaviors might be possible, use of the Internet and smartphones is essential. Further understanding of the developmental trajectories and the risk and protective factors for each of these behavioral disorders will ultimately enable us to develop more effective prevention and treatment strategies.

REFERENCES

1. Rosenberg K, Feder L. An introduction to behavioral addictions. Behavioral addictions: criteria, evidence and treatment. New York: Elsevier; 2014. p. 1–17.
2. American Psychiatric Association. Diagnostic and statistical manual of mental disorders: DSM-5. Washington, DC: American Psychiatric Publishing; 2013.
3. Grant J, Potenza MN, Weinstein A, et al. Introduction to behavioral addictions. Am J Drug Alcohol Abuse 2010;36(5):233–41.
4. Rosenberg K, Feder L, editors. Behavioral addictions: criteria, evidence, and treatment. New York: Elsevier; 2014.
5. Petry NM, editor. Behavioral addictions: DSM-5 and beyond. New York: Oxford University Press; 2016.
6. Young K, De Abreu C. Internet addiction: a handbook and guide to evaluation and treatment. New York: John Wiley & Sons; 2010.
7. World Health Organization. International classification of diseases-eleventh revision (ICD-11). (Switzerland): World Health Organization; 2018.
8. American Society of Addiction Medicine. Public policy statement: definition of addiction. Chevy Chase (MD): American Society of Addiction Medicine; 2011.
9. Griffiths MD. A 'components' model of addiction within a biopsychosocial framework. J Subst Use 2005;10(4):191–7.
10. Derevensky J. Behavioral addictions: some developmental consideration. Curr Addict Rep 2019;6(3):313–22.
11. Jessor R, editor. New perspectives on adolescent risk behavior. New York: Cambridge University Press; 1998.
12. Derevensky J. Teen gambling: understanding a growing epidemic. New York: Rowman & Littlefield Publishers; 2012.
13. Jessor R, Van Den Bos J, Vaderryn J, et al. Protective factors in adolescent problem behavior: moderator effects and developmental change. Dev Psychol 1995;31(6):923–33.
14. Dickson L, Derevensky JL, Gupta R. Youth gambling problems: examining risk and protective factors. Int Gamb Stud 2008;8(1):25–47.
15. Jacobs DF. A general theory of addictions: a new theoretical model. J Gambl Behav 1986;2(1):15–31.
16. Calado F, Alexandre J, Griffiths MD. Prevalence of adolescent problem gambling: a systematic review of recent research. J Gambl Stud 2017;33(2): 397–424.
17. Volberg R, Gupta R, Griffiths MD, et al. An international perspective on youth gambling prevalence studies. Int J Adolesc Med Health 2010;22:3–38.
18. Gupta R, Derevensky J. Adolescents with gambling problems: from research to treatment. J Gambl Stud 2000;(16):315–42.

19. Andrie E, Tzavara C, Tzavela E, et al. Gambling involvement and problem gambling correlates among European adolescents: results from the EU NET ADB study. Soc Psychiatry Psychiatr Epidemiol 2019. [Epub ahead of print].
20. Hayer T, Griffiths MD. The prevention and treatment of problem gambling in adolescence. In: Gullotta T, Adams G, editors. Handbook of adolescent behavioural problems: evidence-based approaches to prevention and treatment. New York: Springer; 2014. p. 467–86.
21. Jacobs DF. Juvenile gambling in North America: an analysis of long-term trends and future prospects. J Gambl Stud 2000;(16):119–52.
22. Jacobs DF. Youth gambling in North America: long-term trends and future prospects. In: Derevensky J, Gupta R, editors. Gambling problems in youth: theoretical and applied perspectives. New York: Kluwer Academic/Plemun Publishers; 2004.
23. Derevensky J, Gupta R. Prevalence estimates of adolescent gambling: a comparison of the SOGS-RA, DSM-IV-J, and the GA 20 Questions. J Gambl Stud 2000;16:227–51.
24. Campbell C, Derevensky J, Meerkamper E, et al. Parents' perceptions of adolescent gambling: a Canadian national study. J Gamb Iss 2011;25:36–53.
25. Derevensky J, St-Pierre R, Temcheff C, et al. Teacher awareness and attitudes regarding adolescent risky behaviours: is adolescent gambling perceived to be a problem? J Gambl Stud 2014;30:435–51.
26. Sansanwal R, Derevensky J, Lupu I, et al. Knowledge and attitudes regarding adolescent problem gambling: a cross-cultural comparative analysis of Romanian and Canadian teachers. Int J Ment Health Addict 2015;13(1):33–48.
27. Sansanwal R, Derevensky J, Gavriel-Fried B. What mental health professionals in Israel know and think about adolescent problem gambling. Int Gamb Stud 2016;16:67–84.
28. Temcheff C, Derevensky J, St-Pierre R, et al. Beliefs and attitudes of mental health professionals with respect to gambling and other high risk behaviors in schools. Int J Ment Health Addict 2014;12:716–29.
29. Griffiths MD, Parke J. Adolescent gambling on the Internet: a review. Int J Adolesc Med Health 2010;22:59–75.
30. Delfabbro P, King D, Griffiths MD. From adolescent to adult gambling: an analysis of longitudinal gambling patterns in South Australia. J Gambl Stud 2014; 30(3):547–63.
31. Productivity Commission. Gambling productivity inquiry report. Melbourne (Australia): Australian Government; 2010.
32. Gupta R, Derevensky J. Familial and social influences on juvenile gambling. J Gambl Stud 1997;13:179–92.
33. Stinchfield R, Winters KC. Gambling and problem gambling among youth. Ann Am Acad Pol Soc Sci 1998;556:172–85.
34. Wallisch LS. Gambling in Texas: 1995 Surveys of adult and adolescent gambling behavior, Executive Summary. Austin (TX): Texas Commission on Alcohol & Drug Abuse; 1996.
35. Hardoon K, Derevensky J, Gutpa R. An examination of the influence of familial, emotional, conduct and cognitive problems, and hyperactivity upon youth risk-taking and adolescent gambling problems. Ontario (Canada): Ontario Problem Gambling Research Center; 2002.
36. Ste-Marie C, Gutpa R, Derevensky J. Anxiety and social stress related to adolescent gambling behavior and substance use. J Child Adolesc Subst Abuse 2006; 16(4):55–74.

37. Dussault F, Brendgen M, Vitaro F, et al. Longitudinal links between impulsivity, gambling problems and depressive symptoms: a transactional model from adolescence to early adulthood. J Child Psychol Psychiatry 2011;52(2):130–8.

38. Gupta R, Derevensky J. An empirical examination of Jacobs' General Theory of Addictions: do adolescent gamblers fit the theory? J Gambl Stud 1998;14: 17–49.

39. Gupta R, Derevensky J. Adolescent gambling behaviour: a prevalence study and examination of the correlates associated with problem gambling. J Gambl Stud 1998;14:319–45.

40. Nower L, Gupta R, Blaszczynski A, et al. Suicidality and depression among youth gamblers: a preliminary examination of three studies. Int Gamb Stud 2004;4(1):70–80.

41. Welte JW, Barnes GM, Tidwell MC, et al. Association between problem gambling and conduct disorder in a national survey of adolescents and young adults in the United States. J Adolesc Health 2009;45(4):396–401.

42. Derevensky J, Gupta R. Adolescents with gambling problems: a synopsis of our current knowledge. J Gamb Iss 2004;10.

43. Gupta R, Derevensky J, Marget N. Coping strategies employed by adolescents with gambling problems. J Child Adolesc Ment Health 2004;9(3):115–20.

44. Lussier I, Derevensky J, Gupta R, et al. Youth gambling behaviors: an examination of the role of resilience. Psychol Addict Behav 2007;21:165–73.

45. Lussier I, Derevensky J, Gupta R, et al. Risk, compensatory, protective, and vulnerability factors related to youth gambling problems. Psychol Addict Behav 2014;28(2):404–13.

46. Bergevin T, Derevensky J, Gupta R, et al. Adolescent gambling: understanding the role of stress and coping. J Gambl Stud 2006;22(2):195–208.

47. Winters KC, Stinchfield RD, Fulkerson J. Toward the development of an adolescent gambling problem severity scale. J Gambl Stud 1993;9:63–84.

48. Fisher S. Measuring pathological gambling in children: The case of fruit machines in the U. K. J Gambl Stud 1992;8:263–85.

49. Fisher S. Developing the DSM-IV-MR-J criteria to identify adolescent problem gambling in non-clinical populations. J Gambl Stud 2000;(16):253–73.

50. Shaffer HJ, LaBrie R, Scanlen KM, et al. Pathological gambling among adolescents: Massachusetts Gambling Screen (MAGS). J Gambl Stud 1994;10: 339–62.

51. Tremblay J, Wiebe J, Stinchfield R, et al. Canadian Adolescent Gambling Inventory (CAGI). Report to the Canadian Centre on Substance Abuse and the Interprovincial Consortium on Gambling Research; Toronto, Ontario, 2015.

52. Derevensky J, Gainsbury S. Social casino gaming and adolescents: should we be concerned and is regulation in sight? Int J Law Psychiatry 2016;44:1–6.

53. Kim H, Hollingshead S, Wohl M. Who spends money to play for free? Identifying who makes micro-transactions on social casino games (and why). J Gambl Stud 2017;33(2):525–38.

54. Kim H, Wohl M, Gupta R, et al. Why do young adults gamble online? A qualitative study of motivations to transition from social casino games to online gambling. Asian J Gambl Issues Public Health 2017;7(1):6.

55. Kim H. Social casino games: current evidence and future directions. Ottawa (Canada): Carleton University; 2017.

56. King D. Online gaming and gambling in children and adolescents—normalising gambling in cyber places: a review of the literature. Melbourne (Australia): University of Adelaide; 2018.

57. McBride J, Derevensky J. Internet gambling and risk-taking among students: an exploratory study. J Behav Addict 2012;1(2):50–8.
58. Marchica L, Derevensky J. Fantasy sports: a growing concern among college student-athletes. Int J Ment Health Addict 2016;14(5):635–45.
59. Gentile D. Pathological video-game use among youth ages 8 to 18: a national study. Psychol Sci 2009;20(5):594–602.
60. Anderson C, Gentile D, Buckley K. Violent video game effects on children and adolescents: theory, research, and public policy. New York: Oxford University Press; 2007.
61. Király O, Nagygyörgy K, Griffiths MD, et al. Problematic online gaming. In: Rosenberg KP, Feder L, editors. Behavioral addictions: criteria, evidence and treatment. New York: Elsevier; 2014. p. 61–97.
62. Newzoo. Newzoo's 2017 report: Insights into the $108.9 billion global games market. 2017. Available at: https://newzoo.com/insights/articles/newzoo-2017-report-insights-into-the-108-9-billion-global-games-market/. Accessed February 5, 2019.
63. Ryan RM, Rigby CS, Przybylski A. The motivational pull of video games: a self-determination theory approach. Motiv Emot 2006;30(4):347–63.
64. Kuss D, Griffiths MD. Online social networking and addiction: a review of the psychological literature. Int J Environ Res Public Health 2011;8(9):3528–52.
65. Rehbein F, Kuhn S, Rumpf H, et al. Internet gaming disorder: a new behavioral addiction. In: Petry NM, editor. Behavioral addictions: DSM-5 and beyond. New York: Oxford University Press; 2016. p. 43–70.
66. Fortson B, Scotti J, Chen Y, et al. Internet use, abuse, and dependence among students at a Southeastern regional university. J Am Coll Health 2007;56(2):137–44.
67. Kuss D, Griffiths MD. Internet and gaming addiction: a systematic literature review of neuroimaging studies. Brain Sci 2012;2(3):347–74.
68. Kuss D, Griffiths MD. Online gaming addiction in children and adolescents: a review of empirical research. J Behav Addict 2012;1(1):3–22.
69. Kuss D, Griffiths MD. Internet gaming addiction: a systematic review of empirical research. Int J Ment Health Addict 2012;10(2):278–96.
70. Rehbein F, Staudt A, Hanslmaier M, et al. Video game playing in the general adult population of Germany: can higher gaming time of males be explained by gender specific genre preferences? Comput Hum Behav 2016;55:729–35.
71. Eichenbaum A, Kattner F, Bradford D, et al. Role-playing and real-time strategy games associated with greater probability of Internet gaming disorder. Cyberpsychol Behav Soc Netw 2015;18(8):480–5.
72. Lemmens JS, Hendriks SJF. Addictive online games: examining the relationship between game genres and Internet gaming disorder. Cyberpsychol Behav Soc Netw 2016;19(4):270–6.
73. Donati MA, Chiesi F, Ammannato G, et al. Versatility and addiction in gaming: the number of video-game genres played is associated with pathological gaming in male adolescents. Cyberpsychol Behav Soc Netw 2015;18(2):129–32.
74. Mößle T, Rehbein F. Predictors of problematic video game usage in childhood and adolescence. Sucht 2013;59(3):153–64.
75. Gentile D, Choo H, Liau A, et al. Pathological video game use among youths: a two-year longitudinal study. Pediatrics 2011;127:319–29.

76. Rumpf H, Vermulst A, Kastirke N, et al. Occurence of Internet addiction in a general population sample: a latent class analysis. Eur Addict Res 2014;20(4): 159–66.
77. Mihara S, Higuchi S. Cross-sectional and longitudinal epidemiological studies of Internet gaming disorder: a systematic review of the literature. Psychiatry Clin Neurosci 2017;71(7):425–44.
78. Laconi S, Pirès S, Chabrol H. Internet gaming disorder, motives, game genres and psychopathology. Comput Hum Behav 2017;75:652–9.
79. Rehbein F, Kleimann M, Mößle T. Prevalence and risk factors of video game dependency in adolescence: results of a German nationwide survey. Cyberpsychol Behav Soc Netw 2010;13(3):269–77.
80. Krossbakken E, Torsheim T, Mentzoni RA, et al. The effectiveness of a parental guide for prevention of problematic video gaming in children: a public health randomized controlled intervention study. J Behav Addict 2018;7(1):52–61.
81. King DL, Herd MCE, Delfabbro PH. Motivational components of tolerance in Internet gaming disorder. Comput Hum Behav 2018;78:133–41.
82. King DL, Delfabbro PH, Zwaans T, et al. Clinical features and axis I comorbidity of Australian adolescent pathological Internet and video game users. Aust N Z J Psychiatry 2013;47(11):1058–67.
83. Gentile D, Li D, Khoo A, et al. Mediators and moderators of long-term effects of violent video games on aggressive behavior: practice, thinking, and action. JAMA Pediatr 2014;168(5):450–7.
84. Kuss D, Griffiths MD, Binder J. Internet addiction in students: prevalence and risk factors. Comput Hum Behav 2013;29(3):959–66.
85. King D, Delfabbro PH, Griffiths MD. Video game structural characteristics: a new psychological taxonomy. Int J Ment Health Addict 2010;8(1):90–106.
86. Flaherty C. Cutting academic programs, spending on esports. 2018. Available at: https://www.insidehighered.com/quicktakes/2018/08/20/cutting-academic-programs-spending-esports. Accessed February 3, 2019.
87. Bauer-Wolf J. Video games as a college sport. 2017. Available at: https://www.insidehighered.com/news/2017/06/09/esports-quickly-expanding-colleges. Accessed February 22, 2019.
88. Smith N. eSports catching fire at Ohio State. Washington Post 2018.
89. Igelman A. eSports and Casinos. Available at: https://ggbnews.com/article/esports-and-casinos/2018. Accessed February 12, 2019.
90. Petry NM, Rehbein F, Gentile D, et al. An international consensus for assessing Internet gaming disorder using the new DSM-5 approach. Addiction 2014; 109(9):1399–406.
91. Pontes HM, Kiraly O, Demetrovics Z, et al. The conceptualisation and measurement of DSM-5 Internet Gaming Disorder: the development of the IGD-20 Test. PLoS One 2014;9(10):e110137.
92. Pontes HM, Griffiths MD. Measuring DSM-5 Internet gaming disorder: development and validation of a short psychometric scale. Comput Hum Behav 2015; 45:137–43.
93. Lemmens J, Valkenburg P, Gentile D. The Internet gaming disorder scale. Psychol Assess 2015;27(2):567–82.
94. Lemmens J, Valkenburg P, Peter J. Development and validation of a game addiction scale for adolescents. Media Psychol 2009;12:77–95.
95. Weinstein A, Feder L, Rosenberg K, et al. Internet addiction disorder: overview and controversies. In: Rosenberg K, Feder L, editors. Behavioral addictions: criteria, evidence and treatment. New York: Elsevier; 2014. p. 99–117.

96. Widyanto L, Griffiths MD. Internet addiction: a critical review. Int J Ment Health Addict 2006;4(1):31–51.
97. Huang Y-R. Identity and intimacy crises and their relationship to Internet dependence among college students. Cyberpsychol Behav 2006;9(5):571–6.
98. Leung L. Net-generation attributes and seductive properties of the Internet as predictors of online activities and Internet addiction. Cyberpsychol Behav 2004;7(3):333–48.
99. Leung L, Lee P. The influences of information literacy, Internet addiction and parenting styles on Internet risks. New Media Soc 2012;14(1):117–36.
100. Petersen K, Weymann N, Schelb Y, et al. Pathological Internet use: epidemiology, diagnostics, co-occurring disorders and treatment. Fortschr Neurol Psychiatr 2009;77(5):263–71.
101. Christakis D, Moreno M, Jelenchick L, et al. Problematic Internet usage in US college students: a pilot study. BMC Med 2011;9(1):77.
102. Poli R, Agrimi E. Internet addiction disorder: prevalence in an Italian student population. Nord J Psychiatry 2012;66(1):55–9.
103. Niemz K, Griffiths MD, Banyard P. Prevalence of pathological Internet use among university students and correlations with self-esteem, the General Health Questionnaire (GHQ), and disinhibition. Cyberpsychol Behav 2005;8(6):562–70.
104. Lam L, Peng Z, Mai J, et al. Factors associated with Internet addiction among adolescents. Cyberpsychol Behav 2009;12(5):551–5.
105. Moreno M, Jelenchick L, Cox E, et al. Problematic Internet use among US youth: a systematic review. Arch Pediatr Adolesc Med 2011;165(9):797–805.
106. Cabral J. Is generation Y addicted to social media? Elon Journal of Undergraduate Research in Communications 2011;2(1):5–13.
107. Caplan S, Williams D, Yee N. Problematic Internet use and psychosocial well-being among MMO players. Comput Hum Behav 2009;25(6):1312–9.
108. Mehroof M, Griffiths MD. Online gaming addiction: the role of sensation seeking, self-control, neuroticism, aggression, state anxiety, and trait anxiety. Cyberpsychol Behav 2010;13(3):313–6.
109. Porter G, Starcevic V, Berle D, et al. Recognizing problem video game use. Aust N Z J Psychiatry 2010;44(2):120–8.
110. Dong G, Wang J, Yang X, et al. Risk personality traits of Internet addiction: a longitudinal study of Internet-addicted Chinese university students. Asia Pac Psychiatry 2013;5(4):316–21.
111. Tsai H, Cheng S, Yeh T, et al. The risk factors of Internet addiction—a survey of university freshmen. Psychiatry Res 2009;167(3):294–9.
112. Van der Aa N, Overbeek G, Engels R, et al. Daily and compulsive Internet use and well-being in adolescence: a diathesis-stress model based on big five personality traits. J Youth Adolesc 2009;38(6):765.
113. Morrison C, Gore H. The relationship between excessive Internet use and depression: a questionnaire-based study of 1,319 young people and adults. Psychopathology 2010;43(2):121–6.
114. Tsitsika A, Critselis E, Louizou A, et al. Determinants of Internet addiction among adolescents: a case-control study. ScientificWorldJournal 2011;11:866–74.
115. Kratzer S, Hegerl U. Is "Internet Addiction" a disorder of its own? A study on subjects with excessive Internet use. Psychiatr Prax 2008;35(2):80–3.
116. Bernardi S, Pallanti S. Internet addiction: a descriptive clinical study focusing on comorbidities and dissociative symptoms. Compr Psychiatry 2009;50(6):510–6.

117. Kormas GS, Critselis E, Janikian M, et al. Risk factors and psychosocial characteristics of potential problematic and problematic Internet use among adolescents: a cross-sectional study. BMC Public Health 2011;11(1):595.

118. Kawabe K, Horiuchi F, Ochi M, et al. Internet addiction: prevalence and relation with mental states in adolescents. Psychiatry Clin Neurosci 2016;70(9):405–12.

119. Milani L, Osualdella D, Di Blasio P. Quality of interpersonal relationships and problematic Internet use in adolescence. Cyberpsychol Behav 2009;12(6): 681–4.

120. Kwon J, Chung C, Lee J. The effects of escape from self and interpersonal relationship on the pathological use of Internet games. Community Ment Health J 2011;47(1):113–21.

121. Cerniglia L, Zoratto F, Cimino S, et al. Internet addiction in adolescence: neurobiological, psychosocial and clinical issues. Neurosci Biobehav Rev 2017;76(Pt A):174–84.

122. Young K. Clinical assessment of Internet-addicted clients. In: Young K, Nabuco de Abreu C, editors. Internet addiction. New Jersey: John Wiley & Sons; 2011. p. 19–34.

123. Young KS. Internet addiction: the emergence of a new clinical disorder. Cyber Psychology Behav 1998;1(3):237–44.

124. Demetrovics Z, Szeredi B, Rozsa S. The three-factor model of Internet addiction: the development of the Problematic Internet Use Questionnaire. Behav Res Methods 2008;40(2):563–74.

125. Meerkerk GJ, Van Den Eijnden RJJM, Vermulst AA, et al. The compulsive Internet use scale (CIUS): some psychometric properties. Cyberpsychol Behav 2009;12(1):1–6.

126. Choi SW, Kim DJ, Choi JS, et al. Comparison of risk and protective factors associated with smartphone addiction and Internet addiction. J Behav Addict 2015; 4(4):308–14.

127. Statista. Number of smartphone users worldwide from 2014 to 2020 (in billions). 2019. Available at: https://www.statista.com/statistics/330695/number-of-smartphone-users-worldwide/. Accessed February 28, 2019.

128. IHS Markit. More than six billion smartphones by 2020. 2017. Available at: https://news.ihsmarkit.com/press-release/technology/more-six-billion-smartphones-2020-ihs-markit-says. Accessed January 20, 2019.

129. Lunden I. 6.1B smartphone users globally by 2020, Overtaking basic fixed phone subscriptions. 2015. Available at: https://techcrunch.com/2015/06/02/6-1b-smartphone-users-globally-by-2020-overtaking-basic-fixed-phone-subscriptions/. Accessed February 3, 2019.

130. Pew Research Center. Teens, social media & technology 2018. 2018. Available at: http://www.pewinternet.org/2018/05/31/teens-social-media-technology-2018/. Accessed February 5, 2019.

131. Mascheroni G, Ólafsson K. The mobile Internet: access, use, opportunities and divides among European children. New Media Soc 2015;18(8):1657–79.

132. Korea Internet and Security Agency. 2016 survey on Internet usage. Available at: http://www.kisa.or.kr/eng/usefulreport/surveyReport_View.jsp?cPage=1&p_No=262&b_No=262&d_No=80&ST=&SV=; 2018.

133. Statista. Share of children owning tablets and smartphones in the United Kingdom (UK) from 2017, by age. 2017. Available at: https://www.statista.com/statistics/805397/children-ownership-of-tablets-smartphones-by-age-uk/.

134. Willemse I, Waller G, Genner S, et al. JAMES: Jugend, Aktivitäten, Medien – Erhebung Schweiz [JAMES: Youth, Activities, Media– Survey Switzerland]. Zürich (Switzerland): Zürcher Hochschule für angewandte Wissenschaften; 2014.
135. Nielsen. Mobile kids: the parent, the child and the smartphone. 2017. Available at: https://www.nielsen.com/us/en/insights/news/2017/mobile-kids–the-parent-the-child-and-the-smartphone.html.
136. Statista. Minutes spent daily on mobile devices among Japanese teenagers in 2017, by activity and gender. 2017. Available at: https://www.statista.com/statistics/758200/japan-daily-mobile-device-use-teens-by-activity-gender/.
137. Statista. Share of teenage smartphone users in the United States who spent more than 3 hours on selected mobile activities every day as of August 2016. 2016. Available at: https://www.statista.com/statistics/722531/us-teen-mobile-time-spent-activities/.
138. Experian. Young adults: texting is just as meaningful as a phone call. 2012. Available at: http://www.experian.com/blogs/marketing-forward/2012/12/03/young-adults-texting-is-just-as-meaningful-as-a-phone-call/.
139. Newport F. The new era of communication among Americans. Available at: http://www.gallup.com/poll/179288/new-era-communication-americans.aspx.
140. Jeong S-H, Kim H, Yum J-Y, et al. What type of content are smartphone users addicted to? SNS vs. games. Comput Hum Behav 2016;54:10–7.
141. Randler C, Wolfgang L, Matt K, et al. Smartphone addiction proneness in relation to sleep and morningness-eveningness in German adolescents. J Behav Addict 2016;5(3):465–73.
142. Haug S, Castro RP, Kwon M, et al. Smartphone use and smartphone addiction among young people in Switzerland. J Behav Addict 2015;4(4):299–307.
143. Cha SS, Seo BK. Smartphone use and smartphone addiction in middle school students in Korea: prevalence, social networking service, and game use. Health Psychol Open 2018;5(1):1–15.
144. Lopez-Fernandez O, Honrubia-Serrano L, Freixa-Blanxart M, et al. Prevalence of problematic mobile phone use in British adolescents. Cyberpsychol Behav Soc Netw 2014;17(2):91–8.
145. Aker S, Sahin MK, Sezgin S, et al. Psychosocial factors affecting smartphone addiction in university students. J Addict Nurs 2017;28(4):215–9.
146. Lopez-Fernandez O. Short version of the Smartphone Addiction Scale adapted to Spanish and French: towards a cross-cultural research in problematic mobile phone use. Addict Behav 2017;64:275–80.
147. Lopez-Fernandez O, Honrubia-Serrano ML, Freixa-Blanxart M. Spanish adaptation of the "Mobile Phone Problem Use Scale" for adolescent population. Adicciones 2012;24(2):123–30 [in Spanish].
148. Hawi NS, Samaha M. The relations among social media addiction, self-esteem, and life satisfaction in university students. Soc Sci Comput Rev 2016;35(5):576–86.
149. Junco R. In-class multitasking and academic performance. Comput Hum Behav 2012;28(6):2236–43.
150. Junco R, Cotten SR. No A 4 U: The relationship between multitasking and academic performance. Comput Educ 2012;59(2):505–14.
151. Lin Y-H, Chang L-R, Lee Y-H, et al. Development and validation of the Smartphone Addiction Inventory (SPAI). PLoS One 2014;9(6):e98312.
152. Lin Y-H, Chiang C-L, Lin P-H, et al. Proposed diagnostic criteria for smartphone addiction. PLoS One 2016;11(11):e0163010.

153. Billieux J, Van Der Linden M, Rochat L. The role of impulsivity in actual and problematic use of the mobile phone. Appl Cogn Psychol 2008;22(9):1195–210.
154. Lepp A, Li J, Barkley JE, et al. Exploring the relationships between college students' cell phone use, personality and leisure. Comput Hum Behav 2015;43: 210–9.
155. Demirci K, Akgonul M, Akpinar A. Relationship of smartphone use severity with sleep quality, depression, and anxiety in university students. J Behav Addict 2015;4(2):85–92.
156. Samaha M, Hawi N. Relationships among smartphone addiction, stress, academic performance, and satisfaction with life. Comput Hum Behav 2016;57: 321–5.
157. Panek E, Khang H, Liu Y, et al. Profiles of problematic smartphone users: a comparison of South Korean and US college students. Korea Obs 2018;49(3): 437–64.
158. Kim D, Lee Y, Lee J, et al. Development of Korean Smartphone Addiction Proneness Scale for Youth. PLoS One 2014;9(5):e97920.
159. Hwang K, Yoo Y, Cho O. Smartphone overuse and upper extremity pain, anxiety, depression and interpersonal relationships among college students. Journal of the Korea Contents Association 2012;12(10):365–75.
160. Kwon M, Lee J-Y, Won W-Y, et al. Development and validation of a Smartphone Addiction Scale (SAS). PLoS One 2013;8(2).
161. Toda M, Monden K, Kubo K, et al. Cellular phone dependence tendency of female university students. Nihon Eiseigaku Zasshi 2004;59(4):383–6.
162. Bianchi A, Phillips JG. Psychological predictors of problem mobile phone use. Cyberpsychol Behav 2005;8(1):39–51.
163. Smith R. France bans smartphones from schools. 2018. Available at: https://www.cnn.com/2018/07/31/europe/france-smartphones-school-ban-intl/index.html.
164. Yau YH, Gottleib C, Krasna L, et al. Food addiction: evidence, evaluation and treament. In: Rosenberg K, Feder L, editors. Behavioral addictions. New York: Elsevier; 2014. p. 143–84.
165. Chiong C, Shuler C, editors. Learning: is there an app for that. Investigations of young children's usage and learning with mobile devices and apps. New York: The Joan Ganz Cooney Center at Sesame Workshop; 2010.
166. American Foundation for Suicide Prevention. Suicide statistics. 2019. Available at: https://afsp.org/about-suicide/suicide-statistics/.

Contingency Management
Using Incentives to Improve Outcomes for Adolescent Substance Use Disorders

Catherine Stanger, PhD*, Alan J. Budney, PhD

KEYWORDS

- Incentives • Contingency management • Adolescent • Substance use • Treatment
- Review

KEY POINTS

- Contingency management (CM) interventions can increase abstinence among youth with substance use problems.
- In developing CM interventions, it is important to consider target outcomes; objective monitoring; and the timing, magnitude, and type of rewards and consequences.
- Parents can successfully implement CM at home with training and support.

In the past decades, multiple studies testing interventions for adolescent substance use problems have shown that youth in treatment of substance use problems have better outcomes than those not in treatment, and there are multiple interventions that have been identified as well established or probably efficacious.[1] Contingency management (CM) is one such intervention. The CM approach grew out of the disciplines of behavioral pharmacology and behavior analysis that demonstrated substance use can be conceptualized as a learned behavior that is maintained, in part, by pharmacological actions (reinforcing effects) of the substance in conjunction with social and other nonpharmacological reinforcements that occur in the context of substance use. As such, CM capitalizes on knowledge that drug seeking and drug use can be reduced by arranging relevant environmental contingencies, such that incompatible or competing prosocial reinforcing activities are made more available and drug abstinence is directly reinforced while drug use is punished. Typically, CM interventions are used as part of a comprehensive substance use treatment program, including some form of individual or family-based intervention.

This article originally appeared in *Pediatric Clinics*, Volume 66, Issue 6, December 2019.
This work was supported by NIH Grants DA15186 and P30DA029926. None of the authors has any conflict of interest or other disclosures.
Center for Technology and Behavioral Health, Geisel School of Medicine at Dartmouth, Dartmouth College, 46 Centerra Parkway, EverGreen Center Suite 300, HB 7255, Lebanon, NH 03766, USA
* Corresponding author.
E-mail address: Catherine.stanger@dartmouth.edu

Clinics Collections 9 (2020) 247–256
https://doi.org/10.1016/j.ccol.2020.07.037
2352-7986/20/© 2020 Elsevier Inc. All rights reserved.

CM programs (1) identify and specifically define target therapeutic behaviors, such as drug abstinence; (2) carefully monitor the target behavior(s) objectively on a prespecified schedule; and (3) deliver reinforcing or punishing events (eg, tangible rewards or incentives and loss of privileges) when the target behavior is or is not achieved. Often CM programs are managed and delivered directly by program staff. In addition, CM interventions for youth often guide parents in developing and implementing a CM program at home. The goals of CM interventions are to systematically weaken the influence of reinforcement derived from substance use and to increase the frequency and magnitude of reinforcement derived from healthier alternative activities, especially those that are incompatible with continued substance use.

PRINCIPLES OF CONTINGENCY MANAGEMENT

CM interventions are defined by the following metrics: the target behavior, the method of monitoring of the target behavior, the schedule used to deliver positive or negative consequences, the type of consequence, and the magnitude of the consequence. The most commonly selected target behavior used in CM programs has been drug abstinence. CM programs, however, also have targeted medication compliance, counseling attendance, and completion of prosocial activities or lifestyle changes. When choosing targets, it is important to be aware that successful change in one behavior may not result in change in another. For example, treatment attendance may improve by providing incentives for coming to sessions, but drug use might not be affected.[2] Thus, it is recommended that, if possible, abstinence should always be a target behavior, although other supplemental behaviors may be targeted as well provided they can be objectively defined and monitored, as described as follows.

Effective monitoring of the targeted behavior is essential to a CM program, because consequences (reinforcement or punishment) must be applied systematically in order to be effective. When abstinence is the target behavior, this typically involves some form of biochemical verification, usually via urinalysis testing. Such testing requires careful planning so that the schedule of testing (frequency) allows optimal detection of substance use and abstinence. For example, detection windows range from hours (for alcohol use) to many days (cannabis) and depend on the type of testing used (eg, breath, urine, and saliva). The importance of having a method for objectively and reliably verifying whether a target behavior occurred pertains as well to other target behaviors (eg, attending self-help meeting, going to the gym, attending an after-school program, and completing therapeutic practice assignments). Reliance on self-reports of drug use or completion of other therapeutic tasks is not adequate for effective delivery of a CM program.

The schedule of reinforcement or punishment refers to the temporal relation between the target behavior and the delivery of the consequence. Generally, efficacy is likely to improve as the temporal delay between the occurrence of the target behavior and delivery of the consequence decreases. For example, all else being equal, providing positive reinforcement for drug abstinence on the same day on which a youth submits a negative urine specimen likely is more effective than waiting a week before reinforcement is delivered. For this reason, the use of rapid drug tests in the clinic setting is preferred over laboratory tests that do not provide immediate results because they permit more immediate reinforcement of abstinence. In working with clinicians and researchers in diverse settings who are interested in using CM with their clients or patients, questions often arise about the need for and implementation of urine drug testing. Although it can be challenging to address positive urine drug test results in real time, it may help to think of such information as similar to many other health status indicators collected during a health visit that can guide the clinical interaction (eg, weight, blood pressure, and hemoglobin A_{1c}). Objective information about substance use is not only the most important target for CM but also a vital marker of problem severity and response to intervention.

Schedules with frequent opportunities for reinforcement (eg, at least weekly) are more likely to engender and strengthen abstinence. Once a behavior is established, less frequent schedules typically are considered for maintenance of behavior change. One schedule that has demonstrated efficacy across multiple substance abuse treatment studies is a fixed schedule with escalating rewards and a reset contingency (typically referred to as abstinence-based vouchers or incentives[3]). This schedule provides monetary rewards for each negative sample that can be held in a clinic account or loaded onto a reloadable credit card, with a small (usually financial) reward for the first negative sample and rewards increasing in value with each subsequent negative sample. Positive samples reset the reward value to the starting point, but a period of abstinence can reset the value back to the prior maximum. In addition, rewards can be provided according to an intermittent schedule using the fishbowl method,[4] in which negative samples earn the opportunity to complete draws that have a possibility of winning a reward, with rewards of varying values available.

The magnitude of reinforcement is also an important factor that can greatly affect the efficacy of CM interventions. For example, if the goal is drug abstinence, a $10 incentive for each negative drug test is likely to be more effective in increasing abstinence than an incentive worth $2.00. Multiple studies have demonstrated that greater magnitude schedules of reinforcement have resulted in better abstinence outcomes than lower magnitude.[5]

The type of reinforcers or punishers used in a CM program also can be critical to its success. Individuals vary greatly in terms of the types of goods and services that they value and hence that will serve as effective reinforcers/incentives. For example, a specific reinforcer (eg, pizza or movie theater passes) that serves as an effective incentive for one youth may not be reinforcing for another. Use of a range of incentives or allowing youth to choose their incentive can increase the probability that the incentive will be effective and facilitate the desired target behavior. Gift cards or reloadable credit cards often are used because they serve as flexible rewards, allowing youth to select personalized rewards that vary over time.

There are excellent resources available to assist clinicians and researchers in developing CM interventions. Examples include a National Institute on Drug Abuse and Substance Abuse and Mental Health Services Administration Blending Initiative, Promoting Awareness of Motivational Incentives,[6] online information and training (https://arenaebp.com/), and published manuals.[7,8]

RESEARCH ON CONTINGENCY MANAGEMENT WITH YOUTH

In 2 prior articles, the authors reviewed research on CM for substance use among youth prior to 2010[9] and from 2010 to 2016.[10] Since the publication of the latter article, the authors have become aware of 2 additional studies using CM with adolescents.[11,12] Most of these studies have involved youth whose primary or most frequent substance used is cannabis and have demonstrated efficacy of CM across highly diverse settings (school, clinic, juvenile justice, and continuing care), platform interventions using fixed (ie, vouchers) and intermittent (ie, fishbowl) incentive schedules, and incentive magnitude (approximately $25 to $725 total/ approximately $6 to $50 per week).

These studies fall into several distinct categories. First, there is a group of studies that used CM to target tobacco use among high school students.[13–16] Most of these studies were conducted in the school setting, but some also have been implemented remotely.[15,16] Across studies, 4-week abstinence rates generally were greater than 50%. One study also used a similar CM model to target substance use (primarily cannabis use) in the school setting, comparing brief motivational interviewing plus CM to brief motivational interviewing alone.[17] Results indicated greater reductions in cannabis use days per month when CM was added to motivational interviewing, with significant differences between conditions at the end of the 8-week intervention period but not at the 16-week follow-up assessment.

A series of studies has tested integration of family-based CM with juvenile drug court.[18] Incentives for abstinence were provided by both the clinic and parents, who also received instruction in setting up a home-based CM program. Youth receiving CM had decreased odds of a cannabis-positive urine test throughout the 9-month intervention (ie, documenting cannabis use) relative to control group youth who received drug court as usual. At the 9-month assessment, 20% of the youth in the CM condition versus 34% of the control youth tested positive for cannabis. This program has an excellent manual available[8] and is widely disseminated.[19]

CM also has been tested for adolescents stepping down from residential substance use treatment.[20] Youth receiving CM had more days of abstinence from cannabis through the 9-month post-treatment follow-up compared with usual continuing care.

The authors have conducted a series of 3 randomized clinical trials testing the impact of CM when added to an evidence-based individual counseling platform.[11,21,22] This 14-week CM intervention integrates clinic-delivered incentives (approximately $590 maximum for continuous abstinence) with home-based CM, in which parents receive instruction and weekly support in developing and implementing a substance monitoring contract (SMC) that specifies rewards for documented abstinence and consequences for substance use. Parents also earned incentives for session attendance and compliance with the SMC (maximum earnings approximately $270).

The home-based SMC specifies positive and negative consequences to be delivered by the parents in response to documented abstinence or use (based on clinic based urine drug test results) (**Fig. 1**). The consequences are determined via a collaborative process between therapist, parent, and adolescent and are revaluated each week during weekly counseling sessions. This contract uses the same target (abstinence), schedule (at least weekly), and monitoring method (urine drug testing) as the authors' clinic-based CM. Parents also are provided with disposable breathalyzers to test for alcohol use at home (see handout in **Fig. 2**). Parents personalize the type of consequence (monetary, voucher type system, or privileges) and the magnitude of the consequences, and these factors change throughout treatment in response to treatment success or failure. Examples of rewards have included earning a prespecified amount of money for each negative sample, family activities like going out to dinner or choosing the menu for dinner at home, and access to the family car or gas money. Examples of consequences have included restrictions on media/Internet/gaming/or phone use, grounding, and extra household chores. The procedures for working with parents to establish and implement their home contract were based on Adolescent Transitions,[23] an evidence-based parent training intervention. This model is now known as the Family Check-Up (https://reachinstitute.asu.edu/family-check-up), and diverse training options for providers plus information for families are available.

Substance Monitoring Contract

If _____ 's urine drug screen is negative (no drugs detected or reported) and there were no positive or refused alcohol breath tests since the last drug screen, I will:

1. Praise their progress!
2. Ask how I can help them keep up the good work.
3. Celebrate their progress by:

_____
_____
_____

If _____ 's urine drug screen is positive (drugs detected or reported) and/or there were positive or refused alcohol breath tests since the last drug screen, and/or the urine screen is refused, I will:

1. Remain calm!
2. Not give a lecture
3. Ask how I can help them
4. Express confidence that they can do better next time
5. Use the following consequence:

_____

_____
Parent Signature   Date

_____
Teen Signature   Date

_____
Therapist Signature   Date

Fig. 1. Substance monitoring contract for home-based contingency management.

Clinicians sometimes raise concerns about how parents might respond to test results indicating drug use. Working with parents to develop a home SMC can reduce conflict about test results, because parents and teens will have established a plan in advance for how to respond to the results—positive or negative. Moreover, reminders that the primary purpose of testing is to provide teens with an opportunity to demonstrate that they are abstinent and to earn rewards and privileges can help maintain a positive attitude toward the SMC and testing in general. Persistent positive test results indicating persistent substance use suggest the need for a higher level of care. **Fig. 3** provides a sample handout the authors have used with teens and parents to provide a rationale for and information about the urine monitoring program. If clinic-based urine testing is not available, parents can consider implementing these procedures at home, although the authors strongly recommend clinician support in implementing such a procedure because it has many challenges.

Across the 3 randomized clinical trials, there were consistent positive effects of CM during treatment. For example, in the first study,[22] CM enhanced continuous abstinence outcomes, engendering more weeks of continuous cannabis abstinence during treatment. More participants who received CM than those who did not achieve greater than or equal to 8 weeks (53% vs 30%) and greater than or equal to 10 weeks of continuous abstinence (50% vs 19%). There was, however, no significant between-condition difference in abstinence 9 months post-treatment. There was an increase in cannabis use from discharge to 9-month follow-up, that, although not returning to intake levels, was of significant concern. In the second study,[21] youth receiving CM were more likely to achieve 4 weeks of continuous cannabis abstinence during

Home Alcohol Testing Guidelines and Plan

Most urine drug tests do not test for alcohol use. Parents participating in this program will be given breathalyzers to use at home to tell if their teen has used alcohol recently. We will show you how to use them.

We want you to ask your teen to take the breath test every day, and especially when you think they might have used alcohol.

You should follow these steps:

Ask your teen if they have used alcohol that day.

> **If they say yes**, they used alcohol, you do not need to do the test.
> **If they say no**, they didn't use alcohol, ask them to take the test.
>
> > **If they refuse to take the test**, you should assume they used alcohol and follow the steps below.
> > **If they take the test, and it is negative** [indicates no alcohol use], thank them for taking the test and praise them for not using alcohol.
> > **If they take the test and it is positive** [indicates alcohol use], follow the steps below.

If your teen has used alcohol [breath test is positive, teen refuses to take test, or teen admits use], you should:

> Remain calm, don't yell or lecture
>
> *Not* help your teen get out of trouble [e.g., make excuses for them, protect them from the consequences of using]
>
> Express disappointment once
>
> Do what you need to do to ensure your teen's safety, **such as taking the keys to the car(s) so the teen cannot drive**
>
> Call your therapist the next day
>
> Use the following consequence:_____

Fig. 2. Alcohol testing guidelines and plan for home-based contingency management.

treatment (48%) than were those not receiving CM (30%). In addition, among youth with at least 1 negative urine drug test during treatment, those who received CM had significantly more weeks of continuous abstinence from cannabis than those who did not receive CM. They also were significantly more likely to be abstinent at the end of treatment, but rates of abstinence were comparable between conditions at post-treatment follow-up assessments, and significant relapse was observed. Self-reports of cannabis use frequency showed sustained decreases during treatment and post-treatment for all conditions. Thus, the effect of CM was greater when change in cannabis use was assessed as continuous abstinence and measured by urine drug tests than as days of use and measured by self-report. In the authors' most recent CM study,[11] which focused on youth with alcohol use problems with or without comorbid cannabis use, a similar percentage of youth maintained complete alcohol abstinence across the 36-week follow-up in both conditions. Among youth not entirely abstinent

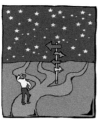

COMMON QUESTIONS ABOUT URINE TESTING

- **Why is urine monitoring an important part of this program?**

  – It helps decrease substance use

  – It keeps the focus of treatment on an important problem (substance use)

  – It gives us and your parents a chance to "catch you" *not* using drugs or alcohol

  – It gives us and your parents a chance to give you incentives, praise, or other kinds of positive support for abstinence

- It can help you and your therapist detect and work on relapse triggers – before use escalates

- It can help you overcome trying to hide substance use because of embarrassment, pride, or not wanting to get into trouble

- It can help you regain credibility with friends, parents, teachers, employers, etc. It can reassure everyone that you continue to do well

Remember - the primary reason for testing is an optimistic one. We want to know that you are not using!

- **WHAT DOES IT MEAN TO TEST "NEGATIVE"?**

  Testing NEGATIVE does not always mean that there is no trace of a substance(s) in your system. It means that you have a low level as a result of not using in the past few days.

- **WHEN I STOP USING DRUGS, HOW SOON WILL I TEST NEGATIVE?**

An average regular marijuana user will test negative after 2 weeks of no use. Other drugs and alcohol clear the body more quickly.

- **AFTER I START TO TEST NEGATIVE FOR MARIJUANA, WILL ALL MY TESTS BE NEGATIVE?**

The "washout period" is when your body is gradually ridding itself of marijuana. Because this "detoxification" can be influenced by your level of physical activity and certain bodily processes, it is possible that you may have a positive test in this period, even though you report not using marijuana, and have had a negative test before. Continue avoiding marijuana and you will see another negative reading at your next visit!

- **WHAT HAPPENS IF I USE MARIJUANA OR USE OTHER DRUGS AFTER TESTING NEGATIVE?**

If you use any marijuana or other drugs, it is likely that you will test positive on your next drug test.

- **PEOPLE SAY THAT THERE ARE METHODS AND PRODUCTS THAT CAN RID MY BODY OF MARIJUANA AND OTHER SUBSTANCES AND MAKE ME HAVE A NEGATIVE DRUG TEST. IS THIS TRUE?**

They don't work and they can be very expensive. Not using drugs is the way to guarantee a negative reading, and it will not empty your wallet.

- **PEOPLE SAY TO DRINK LOTS OF WATER TO GET A NEGATIVE READING, IS THIS TRUE?**

If you drink lots of water, the urine test may indicate that your sample is too dilute and cannot be read. At that point we may ask that you wait at least 4 hours and provide another urine sample within 24 hours. Even if you are not trying to "flush," drinking a lot can cause your urine to be too dilute. If you have a dilute sample on 2 consecutive days, your sample will be considered "positive."

- **IS THERE FOOD I SHOULD AVOID EATING?**

While you are receiving urine testing you should avoid eating poppy seeds. Foods that can contain poppy seeds include bagels, muffins, and other baked goods. Eating poppy seeds may give you an opiate-positive reading. It is your job to take the steps necessary to avoid any substance-positive readings!

- **WHAT DO I DO IF I THINK MY DRUG TEST IS WRONG?**

Please discuss this with your therapist.

Fig. 3. Handout addressing common questions about urine drug testing.

from alcohol, however, those receiving CM reported fewer alcohol use days during the 36 weeks after the end of treatment than those not receiving CM. Among youth who also used cannabis at baseline, results showed similar benefits of CM on cannabis use days.

PREDICTORS OF CONTINGENCY MANAGEMENT EFFICACY

Across all these studies with youth, no trial has tested the impact of CM magnitude (ie, compared different magnitudes or schedules) for substance using youth. To date, no trial has systematically tested the independent or combined efficacy of clinic-based CM versus parent-based CM. The best outcomes across studies were reported for youth with the lowest rates of baseline substance use, that is, those in juvenile drug court or those entering continuing care after residential treatment.[18,20] Intermediate, less enduring outcomes were reported for youth in outpatient and school-based settings.[17,21] Finally, across studies, long-term reduction in use or abstinence among youth remains a serious challenge, even among those who show better post-treatment outcomes. The one study focused on continuing care suggests that including additional targets of CM, such as engagement in specific types of prosocial activities, together with targeting abstinence might better facilitate enduring change.[20]

For the most part, studies have shown that although many baseline characteristics are associated with poorer treatment outcomes (eg, age, gender, ethnicity, and presence of comorbid mental health problems), there are not differential effects of CM across such groups.[18,24] Research is particularly limited, however, on moderation of CM efficacy by cognitive characteristics, such as delay discounting or other constructs related to executive function, including self-regulation or emotion regulation. The authors reported a post hoc analysis showing that youth with disruptive behavior disorder diagnoses (DBDs) in addition to cannabis use disorder had better outcomes when they received CM.[25] DBD-negative adolescents who received abstinence-based CM did not have significantly better cannabis use outcomes compared with counseling only. This may have been due to a ceiling effect; that is, DBD-negative adolescents receiving evidence-based individual counseling had good clinical outcomes, making it more difficult to demonstrate improved outcomes with abstinence-based CM. These findings highlight the importance of future research focused on testing CM and other treatment approaches tailored to pretreatment youth characteristics.

SUMMARY AND FUTURE DIRECTIONS

CM strategies can be effective for retaining youth in treatment, increasing treatment attendance, and promoting abstinence across multiple types of substance use problems. The growing acceptance of abstinence-based CM as one of the most efficacious interventions for youth SUD is evidenced by its recent use as a treatment platform in several clinical trials of new behavioral or pharmacological treatments that seek strategies to further enhance outcomes for adolescents.[26,27] That said, it is critical to attend to the defining components that make up each unique CM intervention, including the target, the monitoring method, the schedule of reinforcement, and the magnitude and type of rewards used, because each can influence intervention efficacy. Fortunately, evidence-based training and manuals are now available to guide research and practice. Avenues for future research include testing the efficacy of a solely parent-administered CM intervention without clinic-delivered CM incentives and developing CM models focused on maintaining treatment gains and preventing relapse. The authors also expect that the growing development and application of diverse technological devices and platforms to improve health behavior should provide a surplus of ideas and innovations for adapting and implementing CM-based programs to better address adolescent substance use problems.[28]

REFERENCES

1. Hogue A, Henderson CE, Becker SJ, et al. Evidence base on outpatient behavioral treatments for adolescent substance use, 2014-2017: outcomes, treatment delivery, and promising horizons. J Clin Child Adolesc Psychol 2018;47(4): 499–526.
2. Iguchi MY, Lamb RJ, Belding MA, et al. Contingent reinforcement of group participation versus abstinence in a methadone maintenance program. Exp Clin Psychopharmacol 1996;4:315–21.
3. Higgins ST, Heil SH, Lussier JP. Clinical implications of reinforcement as a determinant of substance use disorders. Annu Rev Psychol 2004;55:431–61.
4. Petry NM, Peirce JM, Stitzer ML, et al. Effect of prize-based incentives on outcomes in stimulant abusers in outpatient psychosocial treatment programs: a national drug abuse treatment clinical trials network study. Arch Gen Psychiatry 2005;62:1148–56.
5. Lussier JP, Heil SH, Mongeon JA, et al. A meta-analysis of voucher-based reinforcement therapy for substance use disorders. Addiction 2006;101(2):192–203.
6. Hamilton J, Kellogg S, Killeen T, et al. Promoting Awareness of Motivational Incentives (PAMI). 2009. Available at: http://pami.nattc.org/explore/priorityareas/science/blendinginitiative/pami/. Accessed September 29, 2009.
7. Petry N. Contingency management for substance abuse treatment: a guide to implementing this evidence-based practice. New York: Routledge; 2011.
8. Henggeler SW, Cunningham PB, Rowland MD, et al. Contingency management for adolescent substance abuse: a practitioner's guide. New York: Guilford Press; 2012.
9. Stanger C, Budney AJ. Contingency management approaches for adolescent substance use disorders. Child Adolesc Psychiatr Clin N Am 2010;19(3):547–62.
10. Stanger C, Lansing AH, Budney AJ. Advances in research on contingency management for adolescent substance use. Child Adolesc Psychiatr Clin N Am 2016; 25(4):645–59.
11. Stanger C, Scherer EA, Babbin SF, et al. Abstinence based incentives plus parent training for adolescent alcohol and other substance misuse. Psychol Addict Behav 2017;31(4):385–92.
12. Letourneau EJ, McCart MR, Sheidow AJ, et al. First evaluation of a contingency management intervention addressing adolescent substance use and sexual risk behaviors: risk reduction therapy for adolescents. J Subst Abuse Treat 2017;72: 56–65.
13. Cavallo DA, Cooney JL, Duhig AM, et al. Combining cognitive behavioral therapy with contingency management for smoking cessation in adolescent smokers: a preliminary comparison of two different CBT formats. Am J Addict 2007;16(6): 468–74.
14. Krishnan-Sarin S, Cavallo DA, Cooney JL, et al. An exploratory randomized controlled trial of a novel high-school-based smoking cessation intervention for adolescent smokers using abstinence-contingent incentives and cognitive behavioral therapy. Drug Alcohol Depend 2013;132(1–2):346–51.

15. Kong G, Goldberg AL, Dallery J, et al. An open-label pilot study of an intervention using mobile phones to deliver contingency management of tobacco abstinence to high school students. Exp Clin Psychopharmacol 2017;25(5):333–7.

16. Reynolds B, Dallery J, Shroff P, et al. A web-based contingency management program with adolescent smokers. J Appl Behav Anal 2008;41(4):597–601.

17. Stewart DG, Felleman BI, Arger CA. Effectiveness of motivational incentives for adolescent marijuana users in a school-based intervention. J Subst Abuse Treat 2015;58:43–50.

18. Henggeler SW, McCart MR, Cunningham PB, et al. Enhancing the effectiveness of juvenile drug courts by integrating evidence-based principles. J Consult Clin Psychol 2012;80(2):264–75.

19. Cunningham PB, Henggeler SW. The development and transportability of multi-systemic therapy-substance abuse: a treatment for adolescents with substance use disorders AU - Randall, Jeff. J Child Adolesc Subst Abuse 2018;27(2):59–66.

20. Godley MD, Godley SH, Dennis ML, et al. A randomized trial of assertive continuing care and contingency management for adolescents with substance use disorders. J Consult Clin Psychol 2014;82(1):40–51.

21. Stanger C, Ryan SR, Scherer EA, et al. Clinic- and home-based contingency management plus parent training for adolescent cannabis use disorders. J Am Acad Child Adolesc Psychiatry 2015;54(6):445–53.

22. Stanger C, Budney AJ, Kamon JL, et al. A randomized trial of contingency management for adolescent marijuana abuse and dependence. Drug Alcohol Depend 2009;105(3):240–7.

23. Dishion TJ, Kavanagh K. Intervening in adolescent problem behavior: a family-centered approach. New York: Guilford Press; 2003.

24. Kaminer Y, Burleson JA, Burke R, et al. The efficacy of contingency management for adolescent cannabis use disorder: a controlled study. Subst Abus 2014;35(4):391–8.

25. Ryan SR, Stanger C, Thostenson J, et al. The impact of disruptive behavior disorder on substance use treatment outcome in adolescents. J Subst Abuse Treat 2013;44:506–14.

26. Letourneau EJ, McCart MR, Asuzu K, et al. Caregiver involvement in sexual risk reduction with substance using juvenile delinquents: overview and preliminary outcomes of a randomized trial. Adolesc Psychiatry (Hilversum) 2013;3(4):342–51.

27. McCart MR, Sheidow AJ, Letourneau EJ. Risk reduction therapy for adolescents: targeting substance use and HIV/STI-risk behaviors. Cogn Behav Pract 2014;21(2):161–75.

28. Budney AJ, Marsch LA, Bickel WK. Computerized therapies in the treatment of substance use disorders: toward an addiction treatment technology test. In: el-Guebaly N, Carrà G, Galanter M, editors. Textbook of addiction treatment: international perspectives. Berlin: Springer-Verlag; 2014. p. 987–1006.

Prescription Stimulants
From Cognitive Enhancement to Misuse

Timothy E. Wilens, MD[a,b,*], Tamar Arit Kaminski, BS[c]

KEYWORDS

- Stimulant misuse • Nonmedical use of prescription stimulants
- Attention-deficit/hyperactivity disorder • ADHD • Transitional age youth
- College students

KEY POINTS

- Prescription stimulant misuse is associated with both short-term and long-term adverse outcomes.
- College students with fraternity affiliation, lower academic standing, and problematic substance use are at a higher risk for stimulant misuse.
- Recent studies examining the cognitive enhancing effects of prescription stimulants in healthy controls demonstrate stronger subjective relative to objective cognitive effects.
- Due to the correlates, impairments, and negative outcomes associated with stimulant misuse, providers are encouraged to closely monitor college students for stimulant misuse.

INTRODUCTION

Stimulant medications are among first-line agents in the treatment of attention-deficit/hyperactivity disorder (ADHD) across the life span. ADHD is prevalent in up to 9% of children,[1] with an estimated 8% of college students affected in the United States.[2] This neurobehavioral disorder is characterized by developmentally inappropriate levels of inattention, distraction, and/or hyperactivity and impulsivity. Although stimulants are considered safe and effective across age groups,[3] they are liable to misuse and diversion in adolescents and young adults, referred to in this article as transitional age youth (TAY) (for review, see Wilens and colleagues[4]). In this article, misuse is

This article originally appeared in *Pediatric Clinics*, Volume 66, Issue 6, December 2019.
Disclosure: See last page of the article.
[a] Child & Adolescent Psychiatry, Massachusetts General Hospital, Boston, MA 02114, USA;
[b] Department of Psychiatry, Harvard Medical School, Boston, MA 02114, USA; [c] Pediatric Psychopharmacology Program, Division of Child Psychiatry, Massachusetts General Hospital, Boston, MA 02114, USA
* Corresponding author. Child Psychiatry Service, Massachusetts General Hospital, 55 Fruit Street, YAW 6A, Boston, MA 02114.
E-mail address: twilens@partners.org

defined as using ADHD stimulants without a prescription or not following clinical guidelines when using a prescription (eg, nonmedical use). Misuse has increasingly been reported among TAY, particularly on college campuses, and has been associated with characteristics and behaviors distinct from other substance use.[5,6]

ATTENTION-DEFICIT/HYPERACTIVITY DISORDER

TAY are among the most vulnerable populations to the challenges that ADHD presents across academic, occupational, and interpersonal domains due to the increasing responsibility and independence associated with beginning work and college.[4] Managing and treating ADHD in this age group can be particularly difficult due to the emergence of comorbid psychopathologies, such as substance use disorder (SUD) and low rates of adherence to treatment.[4,7]

Although stimulant medications have a known potential for misuse, several recent, large studies have found a protective effect of therapeutic stimulant treatment of childhood ADHD on later SUD.[8,9] Ultimately, when treating TAY with ADHD with stimulants, it is necessary to carefully assess patients through psychiatric, addiction, social, cognitive, educational, medical, and family evaluations in order to mitigate increased liability for misuse at this age.[10]

PRESCRIPTION STIMULANT MISUSE AND DIVERSION
Prevalence and Sources

Stimulant misuse peaks in young adults, according to the "2017 National Survey on Drug Use and Health": 7.4% of young adults aged 18 years to 25 years reported past-year stimulant misuse compared with 1.8% of adolescents aged 12 years to 17 years and 1.7% of adults aged 26 and above.[11] Past-year prescription stimulant misuse in young adults has eclipsed past-year use of opioids as the most prevalent prescription misused.[11] The substantial rate of stimulant misuse among young adults is concerning due to the impairments, correlates, and associated perceptions.

The most common source of stimulants for adolescents[12] and young adults[13] has been consistently found to be peers, and, in accordance, a substantial proportion of individuals have been found to divert (sell, trade, or give away) their medication in high school[14] and college.[15] Furthermore, diversion has been found to be associated with misusing a prescription as well as using other substances in both age groups.[16,17]

Demographic Characteristics of Stimulant Misusers and High-Risk Groups

Certain demographic characteristics have been found associated with higher risk of stimulant misuse. For example, a higher incidence of misuse among whites and men has been reported.[18] The literature is inconsistent in regard to gender differences in motivations for and severity of stimulant misuse. Some studies have reported that women were more likely than men to use stimulants to lose weight[19] and may be at greater risk to develop dependence than male users.[20] Also, available demographic data on stimulant misuse are based on studies of college students due to the high prevalence in this population,[13,21] so these associations may not generalize to other groups.

Specifically, within college samples, certain characteristics have been reported to be linked to a higher risk of stimulant misuse (**Box 1**). Studies have found that misusers are more likely to have fraternity or sorority membership.[22] Additionally, several factors that predict low academic performance have been found to correlate with stimulant misuse, such as low grade point average (GPA), skipping class, and less time spent studying.[23,24]

Box 1
High-risk college groups for prescription stimulant misuse
White men
Attending colleges in the Northeast
Attending competitive colleges
Fraternity and sorority affiliation
Poor academic performance (low GPA, skipping class, etc.)
Substance use/SUD
Prominent ADHD symptoms and/or untreated ADHD
Poorer executive functioning and neuropsychological functioning

Comorbidity with Stimulant Misuse

Stimulant misuse in TAY has been found to be associated with psychopathology. Among psychiatric disorders reported in stimulant misusers, depression,[25] conduct disorder,[26] ADHD, and SUD are the most well documented in the literature.[21,24,26]

ADHD symptoms, such as higher levels of inattention and impulsivity, are more commonly reported among stimulant misusers compared with individuals who do not misuse stimulants.[27,28] Stimulant misusers have also been shown to exhibit greater deficits on subjective measures of executive functioning as well as objective tests of neuropsychological functioning.[29] Compared with controls, misusers demonstrate lower academic performance,[23,24] not unlike those found in ADHD. Punctuating the authors' previous work,[26] Benson and colleagues[30] found that students with increased ADHD symptomology were almost 3 times more likely to misuse stimulants, even when controlling for comorbidity. Although this evidence suggests that untreated ADHD could be directly associated with stimulant misuse, further analysis has also suggested that co-occurring conduct disorder and/or SUD may play an important role in the link between ADHD and stimulant misuse.[17,31]

One of the most replicated findings in the literature is the strong association between stimulant misuse and substance use and SUD. Stimulants often are misused in the context of alcohol, marijuana, or other drugs use.[24] For instance, in a sample of 12,431 high school seniors surveyed, McCabe and colleagues[32] found that among past-year stimulant misusers (n = 835), 64% co-ingested stimulants with other substances, primarily alcohol and marijuana. Not surprisingly, high school seniors who misuse stimulants have been reported to be at higher risk for increased substance use.[33] Similar results have been found in undergraduate populations, with 1 study showing 46% of stimulant misusers reporting co-use with alcohol[34] and others reporting that misusers were more likely to engage in other substance use and polydrug use.[35] Furthermore, those who engaged in co-ingestion of stimulants and alcohol were more likely to report lower GPAs, use of other substances, and worse consequences compared with peers who ingested either substance in isolation.[34] The authors also reported that more than one-third of college-aged stimulant misusers actually met *Diagnostic and Statistical Manual of Mental Disorders, fourth edition,* criteria for either subthreshold or full-threshold stimulant use disorder, and one-half met criteria for an SUD.[26] Stimulant misuse in college students may also lead to long-term adverse effects. In a 17-year follow-up study (mean age 35 years at follow-up) using a national survey of 8362 high schoolers, McCabe and colleagues[36] found a higher likelihood of substance use and substance-related problems in those who misused stimulants in high school compared with students with no use or appropriate use of stimulants. Thus, it is important to evaluate individuals with misuse for other comorbidities.

Motivations

There is increasing evidence that stimulants frequently are misused for academic reasons or as a study aid.[37–39] A majority of motivations for stimulant misuse have consistently been found to include achieving better grades, increasing productivity, and improving alertness or concentration.[26,27] In some cases, self-treating underlying ADHD symptoms also has been reported as a motivation for misuse.[26,35] Although less frequent, other motivations, such as getting high, partying, or enhancing other drugs, also have been reported in TAY.[26,35,37,38]

COGNITIVE ENHANCEMENT

Even though self-reported motivations for stimulant misuse frequently include performance enhancement and as an academic aid, data regarding measurable positive cognitive effects in healthy individuals using stimulants remain inconclusive (**Table 1**). For instance, some studies in healthy adult volunteers given stimulants have reported increased measured spatial working memory,[40] planning,[41] error detection,[42] declarative memory consolidation,[43] and 5-choice continuous performance test.[44] Additionally, others have shown that those healthy individuals who benefit most from stimulants also demonstrated lower baseline cognitive performance.[45]

Weighed against the aforementioned positive findings, recent work has reported a nil effect of stimulants on cognitive performance. Recent controlled studies have reported subjective differences in cognition rather than objective cognitive enhancement, suggesting perceived effects may play a large role in stimulant misuse as opposed to truly enhanced cognitive performance. For example, in a small controlled trial, 13 college students without ADHD were given mixed-salts amphetamine, 30 mg, and then underwent assessments of neurocognition, mood, activation, and perceived cognitive enhancement.[46] Weyandt and colleagues[46] found minimal associations with neurocognitive enhancements (decreased working memory and improved attention); however, significant increases in subjective drug experience, activated positive emotion, and autonomic activity (heart rate and diastolic and systolic blood pressure) were observed. Although participants did not perceive enhanced cognitive abilities after stimulant administration, they did report perceived reduced previous performance relative to placebo administration. Similarly, college students who endorsed high-risk behavior associated with misuse showed increased perceived mood but not improved enhanced performance when expecting to receive methylphenidate (MPH) and instead receiving placebo.[47] In a controlled crossover study, comparing mixed-amphetamine salt, 10 mg, versus placebo, participants on active medication did not demonstrate enhanced cognitive performance.[48] Instead, participants who believed they had taken placebo performed worse on cognitive tasks on both placebo and active medication, whereas, when participants received active medication and believed they had taken active medication, their cognitive performance improved.[48] These findings highlight the potential influence of expectancy or of placebo response in cognitive enhancement experienced with stimulant misuse. Alternatively, the enhancement could be motivational in nature rather than cognitive, as demonstrated in a pilot study that found that the strongest subjective effects misusers reported in a self-report survey were improvements in alertness and energy and not in other cognitive abilities.[49] These data support meta-analytic findings of inconsistent

Table 1
Representative studies of recent controlled studies of the cognitive enhancement effects of prescription stimulants

Study	Study Design	N	Age Range (y)	Stimulant	Dose	Cognitive Enhancement	Comments
Weyandt et al,[46] 2018	Double-blind, PBO-controlled, crossover	13	18–24	AMP	30 mg	Minimally improved attention performance (d = −0.17 – −0.73) and impaired working memory performance (d = 0.08–0.23)	Substantial effects on autonomic activity (d = 0.86–1.25; $P<.001$), subjective drug experience (d = 1.04–1.26; $P<.01$), and activated positive emotion (d = 0.71; $P<.05$)
MacQueen et al,[44] 2018	Double-blind, PBO-controlled, parallel	71	18–35	d-AMP	10 mg or 20 mg	Increased 5-choice continuous performance test for both doses in signal detection (d = 0.821, 0.758; $P<.05$) and response accuracy (d = 1.115 and 1.076; $P<.001$)	
Cropsey et al,[48] 2017	PBO-controlled, crossover	39	19–30	AMP	10 mg	None	Expecting medication was associated with cognitive enhancement and expecting placebo was associated with worse cognitive performance.
Agay et al,[45] 2014	PBO-controlled, crossover	39	20–40	MPH	0.3 mg/kg	Improved sustained attention ($P<.05$) and working memory ($P<.01$); no effects in decision making	Healthy individuals with lower baseline performance showed most improvement.
Linssen et al,[43] 2012	Double-blind, PBO-controlled, crossover	19	18–40	MPH	10 mg, 20 mg, or 40 mg	Dose-dependent improvement in memory consolidation ($P<.05$), set shifting ($P<.01$), and stopped signal performance ($P<.01$); no effects on spatial working memory or planning	

(continued on next page)

Table 1 (continued)							
Study	Study Design	N	Age Range (y)	Stimulant	Dose	Cognitive Enhancement	Comments
Looby & Earleywine,[47] 2011	Controlled, parallel (no active stimulant)	96	18–25	None	N/A	None	Expecting medication (blinded PBO) was associated with improved subjective mood (P<.01) vs no intervention.

All studies presented were randomized.
Abbreviations: AMP, mixed-salts amphetamine; d-AMP, dextroamphetamine; PBO, placebo.

neurocognitive enhancement effects of prescription stimulants in the literature, concluding that stimulants caused no effects on planning accuracy and optimal decision making and resulted only in potential improvements in processing speed in healthy adults.[50] Based on the literature, it seems that stimulant use in healthy individuals may produce mild cognitive enhancement, with the major confounds of expectations of cognitive enhancement with stimulants. Given the limited sample sizes, variability in outcome measures, and issues with differentiation of expectancy from objective outcomes, further research in this area is necessary.

CONSEQUENCES OF STIMULANT MISUSE

Nonmedical use of stimulants can lead to adverse short-term and longer-term outcomes. Besides common side effects of stimulants that also could occur in stimulant misuse, such as decreased appetite, insomnia, irritability, headaches, and stomachaches,[51] stimulants can cause an increase in heart rate and blood pressure, which may lead to adverse cardiovascular effects, especially in those with underlying conditions, such as high blood pressure, that are not screened as part of therapeutic administration. The lack of medical oversight during nonmedical use can lead to more severe outcomes due to risky behaviors, such as ingestion of high doses or with other substances, intranasal administration, or misuse by individuals with contraindications to stimulants.

The consequences of stimulant misuse are further demonstrated by the recent, significant increase in emergency department visits related to nonmedical stimulant misuse—tripling between 2005 and 2010[52]—and often linked to the use of stimulants and other substances simultaneously.[53] Mattson[54] found that in emergency department visits related to nonmedical stimulant use, other pharmaceutical drugs, illicit drugs, and alcohol were related in 45%, 21%, and 19% of visits respectively, highlighting the potential serious adverse effects of co-use of stimulant use and other substances.

Furthermore, when administered intranasally, prescription stimulants have been shown to have higher abuse liability and higher risk of cardiovascular effects[55] relative to oral administration. Although several studies have found that most students report oral use of stimulants,[38] a substantial minority of individuals use stimulants intranasally.[6] For instance, the authors recently reported that 38% of college students misused stimulants intranasally.[56] Intranasal administration has been found to be associated with co-ingestion of other substances and recreational motives compared with oral administration.[32] Additionally, the effects of intranasal stimulant misuse occur rapidly within minutes of administration compared with the slower onset (up to 1 hour) in oral administration, resulting in an increased abuse liability and similarities with the consequences of cocaine use (for review, see Sussman and colleagues[57]).

DISCUSSION: STRATEGIES TO MITIGATE AND PREVENT STIMULANT MISUSE AND DIVERSION

Because primary motivations for stimulant misuse are academic in nature and subjective cognitive enhancement seems to play a substantial role in stimulant misuse, it is important to portray accurate information about the potential consequences of misuse. Students misusing stimulants believe that taking stimulants will improve their grades,[27,39] and most misusers report perceiving misuse as widespread and not associated with negative consequences to physical or mental health.[58] Thus, individual prescribers and programs on college campuses that educate about these misperceptions and highlight the potential consequences of high-risk behavior and administration are necessary. Prevention efforts aimed at students who could be struggling academically should include accessible academic resources and support.

Additionally, when treating college-aged patients, it is helpful to consider behaviors and subgroups at risk for misuse and markers of more severe stimulant misuse. For example, evaluating methods of misuse may provide insight into the likelihood of other risky behavior and other substance use. Regarding treatment, practitioners may find that certain treatment plans could be enhanced, depending on any additional comorbidities identified. Stimulant misusers with ADHD symptoms may benefit from an evaluation and treatment of ADHD, increased academic support, and education on the risks of stimulant misuse. Misusers with SUD should be considered for full evaluation and treatment, including psychotherapy and/or pharmacotherapy, in order to evaluate and stabilize their SUD and accompanying comorbidities.

In cases of TAY patients presenting for ADHD, several guidelines have been posited that may reduce the likelihood of stimulant misuse and diversion. The provider must first consider if the patient is malingering to obtain medication. If there is any suspicion regarding a recent diagnosis, the provider can evaluate the patient in a more comprehensive, multistep process that includes requesting and assessing past records and lengthening the prescribing process, discouraging individuals seeking stimulants for nonmedical reasons.

If an ADHD diagnosis is confirmed and pharmacotherapy is initiated, conversations between the prescriber and patient should include clear instructions for proper administration and storage of medication and education regarding misuse and diversion. Providers should consider carefully which medication type and preparation are most appropriate when working with TAY. Prescribers are advised to screen adolescents and young adults with ADHD for substance use and SUD, because TAY who misuse alcohol, marijuana, or other substances are more likely to divert or misuse their own stimulant medication than non–substance-using peers.[59] For TAY patients with ADHD and comorbid SUD, nonstimulants, such as atomoxetine, bupropion, and tricyclic antidepressants, may be considered due to their lower abuse liability.[60] When considering stimulants, differences exist in abuse liability, with extended-release stimulants having lower abuse liability compared with equipotent doses of immediate-release stimulants,[61] resulting in less misuse and diversion of the extended-release compared with immediate-release preparations.[26] In addition to lower abuse liability, extended-release stimulants provide the benefit of consistent treatment to TAY throughout the day.[59]

When working with TAY with ADHD, providers should pay careful attention to possible misuse or diversion by monitoring pill counts, prescribing only the amount of medication necessary, and recognizing premature refill requests. Excess supplies of stimulant medication represent one of the largest sources of diverted, and subsequently misused, stimulants.[13] Querying about substance use and SUD should be considered at follow-up visits, with toxicology testing in those suspected of manifesting a SUD. Clinicians also are encouraged to provide patients and parents with instructions on safe storage (eg, not in medicine cabinets) and education regarding the medical, psychological, ethical, and legal consequences of misuse and diversion.

SUMMARY

Stimulants used to treat ADHD currently are the most common prescription medications used nonmedically in young people. Stimulant misuse is associated with other psychiatric comorbidities, such as ADHD and SUD, as well as academic underachievement, neuropsychological dysfunction, and continued impairment longer term. Due to the pervasive nature of stimulant misuse among adolescents and young adults, particularly on college campuses, prescribers should evaluate individuals for risk factors of misuse as well as educate and monitor for misuse or diversion. Young people with stimulant misuse should be evaluated for routes of misuse, behavioral disorders and SUD, and neuropsychological and academic dysfunction. Although the literature has not reached a consensus regarding the cognitive effects of ADHD stimulant use in healthy individuals, it seems that subjective effects might play a substantial role in perceived cognitive enhancement. Despite the wealth of information now available on stimulant misuse, additional research is necessary on prevention efforts to mitigate stimulant misuse, treatment strategies for those with stimulant misuse, and safer stimulant preparations.

DISCLOSURE

Dr T.E. Wilens is codirector of the Center for Addiction Medicine at Massachusetts General Hospital. He receives grant support from the following sources: NIH (NIDA). Dr T.E. Wilens has published a book, *Straight Talk about Psychiatric Medications for Kids* (Guilford Press), and coedited books, *Attention-Deficit Hyperactivity Disorder in Adults and Children* (Cambridge University Press), *Massachusetts General Hospital Comprehensive Clinical Psychiatry* (Elsevier), and *Massachusetts General Hospital Psychopharmacology and Neurotherapeutics* (Elsevier). Dr T.E. Wilens is co-owner of a copyrighted diagnostic questionnaire (Before School Functioning Questionnaire) and has a licensing agreement with Ironshore (BSFQ Questionnaire). He is or has been a consultant for Alcobra, KemPharm, Otsuka, and Ironshore and serves as a clinical consultant to the National Football League (ERM Associates), Minor/Major League Baseball, Gavin Foundation, and Bay Cove Human Services. T.A. Kaminski has no conflicts of interest to disclose.

REFERENCES

1. Merikangas KR, He JP, Burstein M, et al. Service utilization for lifetime mental disorders in U.S. adolescents: results of the National Comorbidity Survey-Adolescent Supplement (NCS-A). J Am Acad Child Adolesc Psychiatry 2011; 50(1):32–45.
2. Ascherman LI, Shaftel J. Facilitating transition from high school and special education to adult life: focus on youth with learning disorders, attention-deficit/hyperactivity disorder, and speech/language impairments. Child Adolesc Psychiatr Clin N Am 2017;26(2):311–27.
3. Stevens JR, Wilens TE, Stern TA. Using stimulants for attention-deficit/hyperactivity disorder: clinical approaches and challenges. Prim Care Companion 2013;15(2):1–12.
4. Wilens TE, Isenberg BM, Kaminski TA, et al. Attention-deficit/hyperactivity disorder and transitional aged youth. Curr Psychiatry Rep 2018;20(11):100.
5. McCabe SE, Teter CJ, Boyd CJ. Medical use, illicit use and diversion of prescription stimulant medication. J Psychoactive Drugs 2006;38(1):43–56.
6. Garnier-Dykstra LM, Caldeira KM, Vincent KB, et al. Nonmedical use of prescription stimulants during college: four-year trends in exposure opportunity, use, motives, and sources. J Am Coll Health 2012;60(3):226–34.
7. Miesch M, Deister A. Attention-deficit/hyperactivity disorder (ADHD) in adult psychiatry: data on 12-month prevalence, risk factors and comorbidity. Fortschr Neurol Psychiatr 2018;87(1):32–8 [in German].
8. McCabe SE, Dickinson K, West BT, et al. Age of onset, duration, and type of medication therapy for attention-deficit/hyperactivity disorder and substance

use during adolescence: a multi-cohort national study. J Am Acad Child Adolesc Psychiatry 2016;55(6):479–86.

9. Quinn PD, Chang Z, Hur K, et al. ADHD medication and substance-related problems. Am J Psychiatry 2017;174(9):877–85.

10. Wilens TE, McKowen J, Kane M. Transitional-aged youth and substance use: teenaged addicts come of age. Contemp Pediatr 2013;30(11):24–30.

11. Quality CfBHSa. 2017 National survey on drug use and health: detailed tables. Rockville (MD): Substance Abuse and Mental Health Services Administration; 2018.

12. Schepis TS, Wilens TE, McCabe SE. Prescription drug misuse: sources of controlled medications in adolescents. J Am Acad Child Adolesc Psychiatry 2019;58(7):670–80.e4.

13. McCabe SE, Teter CJ, Boyd CJ, et al. Sources of prescription medication misuse among young adults in the United States: the role of educational status. J Clin Psychiatry 2018;79(2) [pii:17m11958].

14. Epstein-Ngo QM, McCabe SE, Veliz PT, et al. Diversion of ADHD stimulants and victimization among adolescents. J Pediatr Psychol 2016;41(7):786–98.

15. Gallucci AR, Martin RJ, Usdan SL. The diversion of stimulant medications among a convenience sample of college students with current prescriptions. Psychol Addict Behav 2015;29(1):154–61.

16. McCabe SE, West BT, Cranford JA, et al. Medical misuse of controlled medications among adolescents. Arch Pediatr Adolesc Med 2011;165(8):729–35.

17. Wilens T, Gignac M, Swezey A, et al. Characteristics of adolescents and young adults with ADHD who divert or misuse their prescribed medications. J Am Acad Child Adolesc Psychiatry 2006;45(4):408–14.

18. Benson K, Flory K, Humphreys KL, et al. Misuse of stimulant medication among college students: a comprehensive review and meta-analysis. Clin Child Fam Psychol Rev 2015;18(1):50–76.

19. Cruz S, Sumstine S, Mendez J, et al. Health-compromising practices of undergraduate college students: Examining racial/ethnic and gender differences in characteristics of prescription stimulant misuse. Addict Behav 2017;68:59–65.

20. Wu LT, Schlenger WE. Psychostimulant dependence in a community sample. Subst Use Misuse 2003;38(2):221–48.

21. McCabe SE, Knight JR, Teter CJ, et al. Non-medical use of prescription stimulants among US college students: prevalence and correlates from a national survey. Addiction 2005;100(1):96–106.

22. Dussault CL, Weyandt LL. An examination of prescription stimulant misuse and psychological variables among sorority and fraternity college populations. J Atten Disord 2013;17(2):87–97.

23. Rabiner DL, Anastopoulos AD, Costello EJ, et al. Motives and perceived consequences of nonmedical ADHD medication use by college students: are students treating themselves for attention problems? J Atten Disord 2009;13(3):259–70.

24. Arria AM, Wilcox HC, Caldeira KM, et al. Dispelling the myth of "smart drugs": cannabis and alcohol use problems predict nonmedical use of prescription stimulants for studying. Addict Behav 2013;38(3):1643–50.

25. Poulin C. From attention-deficit/hyperactivity disorder to medical stimulant use to the diversion of prescribed stimulants to non-medical stimulant use: connecting the dots. Addiction 2007;102(5):740–51.

26. Wilens T, Zulauf C, Martelon M, et al. Nonmedical stimulant use in college students: association with attention-deficit/hyperactivity disorder and other disorders. J Clin Psychiatry 2016;77(7):940–7.

27. Peterkin AL, Crone CC, Sheridan MJ, et al. Cognitive performance enhancement: misuse or self-treatment? J Atten Disord 2011;15(4):263–8.
28. Looby A, Sant'Ana S. Nonmedical prescription stimulant users experience subjective but not objective impairments in attention and impulsivity. Am J Addict 2018;27(3):238–44.
29. Wilens TE, Carrellas NW, Martelon M, et al. Neuropsychological functioning in college students who misuse prescription stimulants. Am J Addict 2017;26(4):379–87.
30. Benson K, Woodlief DT, Flory K, et al. Is ADHD, independent of ODD, associated with whether and why college students misuse stimulant medication? Exp Clin Psychopharmacol 2018;26(5):476–87.
31. Brook JS, Balka EB, Zhang C, et al. ADHD, conduct disorder, substance use disorder, and nonprescription stimulant use. J Atten Disord 2017;21(9):776–82.
32. McCabe SE, West BT, Schepis TS, et al. Simultaneous co-ingestion of prescription stimulants, alcohol and other drugs: a multi-cohort national study of US adolescents. Hum Psychopharmacol 2015;30(1):42–51.
33. Teter CJ, DiRaimo CG, West BT, et al. Nonmedical use of prescription stimulants among US high school students to help study: results from a national survey. J Pharm Pract 2018. 897190018783887.
34. Egan KL, Reboussin BA, Blocker JN, et al. Simultaneous use of non-medical ADHD prescription stimulants and alcohol among undergraduate students. Drug Alcohol Depend 2013;131(1–2):71–7.
35. Rabiner DL, Anastopoulos AD, Costello EJ, et al. The misuse and diversion of prescribed ADHD medications by college students. J Atten Disord 2009;13(2):144–53.
36. McCabe SE, Veliz P, Wilens TE, et al. Adolescents' prescription stimulant use and adult functional outcomes: a national prospective study. J Am Acad Child Adolesc Psychiatry 2017;56(3):226–33.e4.
37. Teter CJ, McCabe SE, LaGrange K, et al. Illicit use of specific prescription stimulants among college students: prevalence, motives, and routes of administration. Pharmacotherapy 2006;26(10):1501–10.
38. Bavarian N, McMullen J, Flay BR, et al. A mixed-methods approach examining illicit prescription stimulant use: findings from a Northern California University. J Prim Prev 2017;38(4):363–83.
39. Arria AM, Geisner IM, Cimini MD, et al. Perceived academic benefit is associated with nonmedical prescription stimulant use among college students. Addict Behav 2018;76:27–33.
40. Mehta MA, Owen AM, Sahakian BJ, et al. Methylphenidate enhances working memory by modulating discrete frontal and parietal lobe regions in the human brain. J Neurosci 2000;20(6):RC65.
41. Elliott R, Sahakian BJ, Matthews K, et al. Effects of methylphenidate on spatial working memory and planning in healthy young adults. Psychopharmacology (Berl) 1997;131(2):196–206.
42. Hester R, Nandam LS, O'Connell RG, et al. Neurochemical enhancement of conscious error awareness. J Neurosci 2012;32(8):2619–27.
43. Linssen AM, Vuurman EF, Sambeth A, et al. Methylphenidate produces selective enhancement of declarative memory consolidation in healthy volunteers. Psychopharmacology (Berl) 2012;221(4):611–9.
44. MacQueen DA, Minassian A, Kenton JA, et al. Amphetamine improves mouse and human attention in the 5-choice continuous performance test. Neuropharmacology 2018;138:87–96.

45. Agay N, Yechiam E, Carmel Z, et al. Methylphenidate enhances cognitive performance in adults with poor baseline capacities regardless of attention-deficit/hyperactivity disorder diagnosis. J Clin Psychopharmacol 2014;34(2):261–5.
46. Weyandt LL, White TL, Gudmundsdottir BG, et al. Neurocognitive, autonomic, and mood effects of adderall: a pilot study of healthy college students. Pharmacy (Basel) 2018;6(3) [pii:E58].
47. Looby A, Earleywine M. Expectation to receive methylphenidate enhances subjective arousal but not cognitive performance. Exp Clin Psychopharmacol 2011;19(6):433–44.
48. Cropsey KL, Schiavon S, Hendricks PS, et al. Mixed-amphetamine salts expectancies among college students: Is stimulant induced cognitive enhancement a placebo effect? Drug Alcohol Depend 2017;178:302–9.
49. Ilieva IP, Farah MJ. Enhancement stimulants: perceived motivational and cognitive advantages. Front Neurosci 2013;7:198.
50. Marraccini ME, Weyandt LL, Rossi JS, et al. Neurocognitive enhancement or impairment? A systematic meta-analysis of prescription stimulant effects on processing speed, decision-making, planning, and cognitive perseveration. Exp Clin Psychopharmacol 2016;24(4):269–84.
51. Advokat CD, Guidry D, Martino L. Licit and illicit use of medications for Attention-Deficit Hyperactivity Disorder in undergraduate college students. J Am Coll Health 2008;56(6):601–6.
52. Substance Abuse and Mental Health Services Administration CfBHSaQ. The DAWN Report: emergency department visits involving attention deficit/hyperactivity disorder stimulant medications. Rockville, MD, January 24, 2013. 2013.
53. Chen LY, Crum RM, Strain EC, et al. Prescriptions, nonmedical use, and emergency department visits involving prescription stimulants. J Clin Psychiatry 2016;77(3):e297–304.
54. Mattson ME. Emergency department visits involving attention deficit/hyperactivity disorder stimulant medications. Rockville (MD): The CBHSQ report; 2013. p. 1–8.
55. Stoops WW, Glaser PE, Rush CR. Reinforcing, subject-rated, and hysiological effects of intranasal methylphenidate in humans: a dose-response analysis. Drug Alcohol Depend 2003;71(2):179–86.
56. Wilens TE, Martelon M, Yule A, et al. Disentangling the context of stimulant misuse in college students. 65th Annual Meetings of the Am Acad Child Adolesc Psychiatry. Seattle, Washington, October 22-27, 2018.
57. Sussman S, Pentz MA, Spruijt-Metz D, et al. Misuse of "study drugs:" prevalence, consequences, and implications for policy. Subst Abuse Treat Prev Policy 2006;1:15.
58. Kilmer JR, Geisner IM, Gasser ML, et al. Normative perceptions of non-medical stimulant use: associations with actual use and hazardous drinking. Addict Behav 2015;42:51–6.
59. Wilens T, Carrellas N, Biederman J. ADHD and substance misuse. In: Banaschewski T, editor. Oxford textbook of attention deficit hyperactivity disorder. New York: Oxford University Press; 2016. p. 215–26.
60. Colaneri N, Keim S, Adesman A. Physician practices to prevent ADHD stimulant diversion and misuse. J Subst Abuse Treat 2017;74:26–34.
61. Spencer TJ, Biederman J, Ciccone PE, et al. PET study examining pharmacokinetics, detection and likeability, and dopamine transporter receptor occupancy of short- and long-acting oral methylphenidate. Am J Psychiatry 2006;163(3):387–95.

Cocaine Use in Adolescents and Young Adults

Sheryl A. Ryan, MD*

KEYWORDS

- Cocaine • Crack cocaine • Cocaine use disorder • Neurobiology • Withdrawal
- Adolescents • Young adults

KEY POINTS

- Cocaine use, although less common than alcohol, tobacco, or marijuana use, continues to be used by significant numbers of adolescents and young adults.
- Cocaine is a potent stimulant with central nervous system effects through its ability to increase levels of neurotransmitters such as dopamine, norepinephrine and serotonin.
- Long-term heavy use of cocaine poses significant health effects on many organ systems mainly through its stimulation of the sympathetic nervous system.
- Diagnostic and Statistical Manual of Mental Disorders Fifth Edition criteria are used to determine whether individuals meet criteria of mild, moderate, or severe cocaine use disorders.
- Because there are no Food and Drug Administration–approved agents to treat cocaine use disorders, behavioral therapies are the mainstay of treatment.

INTRODUCTION

Cocaine has been estimated to be second only to heroin according to ranking scores that have used evidence-based data to assess drug "harmfulness."[1] Cocaine is a tropane ester alkaloid made from the leaves of the Erythroxylum coca plant, a bush that is native to the Andes Mountain regions of South America (chiefly Colombia, Peru, and Bolivia). It is an addictive stimulant drug and is used in 2 main forms: powder cocaine and crack. Common street names for cocaine and crack include snow, rock, flake, toot, candy, line, and blow.

Magnitude of Use by Adolescents and Young Adults

According to the Monitoring the Future study, in 2017, 2.7% of 12th graders reported annual use of cocaine, and 0.5% reported annual use of crack cocaine; 1.4% and

This article originally appeared in *Pediatric Clinics*, Volume 66, Issue 6, December 2019.
Disclosure Statement: The author has no financial conflicts to disclose.
Division of Adolescent Medicine, Department of Pediatrics, Milton S. Hershey Medical Center, Penn State Hershey Children's Hospital, Hershey, PA 17033, USA
* 500 University Drive, Hershey, PA 17033.
E-mail address: Sryan4@pennstatehealth.psu.edu

Clinics Collections 9 (2020) 269–281
https://doi.org/10.1016/j.ccol.2020.07.039
2352-7986/20/© 2020 Elsevier Inc. All rights reserved.

0.6% of 10th graders and 0.8% and 1.0% of 8th graders reported annual use of cocaine and crack cocaine, respectively.[2] Results from the 2017 National Survey of Drug Use and Health[3] indicate that an estimated 0.1% of 12 to 17 year olds (about 26,000 individuals) and 1.9% of 18 to 25 year olds (about 665,000 individuals) reported current cocaine (including crack cocaine) use. Significantly higher numbers of 18 to 25 year olds reported past-year rates than adolescents aged 12 to 17 years: 6.2% and 0.3% of 18 to 25 year olds reported past-year use of cocaine and crack cocaine, respectively, compared with 0.5% and 0.1% of 12 to 17 year olds. Finally, in 2017, 0.1% of the 12 to 17-year-old population and 0.7% of 18 to 25 year olds met Diagnostic and Statistical Manual of Mental Disorders Fourth Edition[3] criteria for a cocaine use disorder.[4]

Although peak ages for cocaine dependence are between 23 and 25 years of age, once use begins, cocaine dependence develops far more rapidly and "explosively" than what is seen with either marijuana or alcohol. For example, up to 5% to 6% of cocaine users will develop dependence within the first year of use.[5] Cocaine use is also highly associated with the use of other licit and illicit substances, and comorbid psychiatric conditions such as anxiety and depression.[6] Further, the earlier an adolescent begins using an illicit substance, including cocaine, the higher the risk of developing problems related to that use.[7]

EPIDEMIOLOGY

Cocaine use occurs among all demographic and socioeconomic groups.[4] Among those aged 12 to 17 years, past-year cocaine use was higher among Caucasians (0.6%), Latinos (0.5%), and those reporting 2 or more races (0.9%) compared with Blacks (0.1%), Native or Alaskan Americans (0.2%), or Asians (0.3%). For young adults aged 18 to 25 years, highest rates of past-year use were reported by Native/Alaskan Americans (10.6%) and those reporting 2 or more races (9.2%), followed by Caucasians (7.6%) and Latinos (6.2%), with Blacks (1.9%) and Asians (2.0%) reporting the lowest rates. For youth 12 to 17 years of age, no gender differences were seen with reported past-year use of cocaine; however, for 18 to 25 year olds, men reported higher rates than women. Results of the few studies investigating factors contributing to the use of cocaine by adolescents and young adults have found correlations between early onset of substance use and childhood history of behavioral, conduct, or antisocial behaviors, association with "deviant" peers, inadequate parental monitoring or supervision, and parental use of illicit substances.[8] Conversely, protective factors include role modeling of nonparent adults, development of social skills, participation in recreational activities, and religiosity.[9]

PHARMACOLOGY OF COCAINE

During the process of extraction of cocaine from the coca plant leaves, 2 forms are produced: a base form and a salt form. The base form is created by heating the salt form in an organic solvent that has a base pH, a process also knows as "freebasing" with the resulting formation of crack cocaine. This has a low melting point (98° C) and vaporizes readily before destruction of the active compound occurs. As a result, it can be smoked but cannot be injected because of its insolubility in water. In contrast, the salt form of cocaine, a white powder, cannot be smoked because it melts at a much higher temperature than the base form (195° C) and is destroyed before it vaporizes. However, it is readily injected or "snorted" through nasal mucosa and is highly water soluble, allowing for it to be easily dissolved and injected. Cocaine is readily absorbed through oral and nasal mucous membrane as well as from the respiratory, gastrointestinal, genitourinary tracts. Following ingestion, it is rapidly distributed and taken up into most organs including the brain, heart, kidney, adrenal glands, and liver. It can also be measured in blood, urine, hair, sweat, and breast milk; analysis of these fluids and tissues can be used for detection for legal, workplace, or treatment purposes.

The average purity of the salt form of cocaine powder is about 50%, and a variety of additives or adulterants are mixed with the powder. These additives can be inert and include lactose, dextrose, or starch, or active, such as benzocaine, procaine, hydroxyzine, diltiazem, phenacetin, or lidocaine. Psychoactive adulterants such as amphetamines, caffeine, phencyclidine, or ephedrine have been used and can potentially enhance or complicate the effects.

When cocaine is inhaled by smoking, or through injection, the onset and maximal peak effect occurs within minutes, and lasts for 15 to 30 minutes. When snorted intranasally, onset of action is slower, occurring within 30 to 45 minutes, with a longer peak effect and a more gradual decline to baseline—more than 60 to 90 minutes.[10]

Once ingested, cocaine undergoes metabolism via both liver and serum cholinesterases to 2 main metabolites, benzoylecgonine and ecgonine methyl ester. These substances are water soluble and readily excreted in the urine. The serum half-life of cocaine is between 45 and 90 minutes; thus, cocaine can be measured in either serum or urine only for several hours after ingestion. The metabolites can be detected in blood and urine up to 24 to 36 hours after use and toxicologic tests measuring the metabolites of benzoylecgonine and ecgonine provide evidence of recent use.[11]

MECHANISMS OF ACTION OF COCAINE IN THE CENTRAL AND PERIPHERAL NERVOUS SYSTEMS

The central neural circuit that has been the most studied and implicated in explaining the psychotropic and reinforcing effects of many addictive substances, including cocaine, is the mesocorticolimbic dopaminergic system.[12] This circuit includes brain structures integral for reward processing, impulse control, and inhibition[13]; it consists of dopaminergic cells in the ventral tegmental area located in the mesencephalon that project to structures in the forebrain such as the nucleus accumbens and the prefrontal cortex (**Fig. 1**). Studies using functional MRI (fMRI), PET, and single-photon emission computed tomography techniques have found that these brain regions show increased blood flow or activity in response to stimulants such as cocaine.[14]

Cocaine is similar to all stimulants in that it increases the extracellular and synaptic levels of monoamine neurotransmitters, such as dopamine, norepinephrine, and serotonin, which are integral to the normal functioning of the mesocorticolimbic circuit. Binding to the monoamine transporters located at nerve endings, dendrites, axons, and cell bodies, it blocks the reuptake of released monoamine neurotransmitters into neuronal cells. As a result, levels of synaptic dopamine are increased well above levels that are normally experienced through natural rewards, resulting in the acute euphoric effect experienced by cocaine users. This effect of cocaine on the reward circuit systems of the brain also lends support to observed difficulties with impulse control and cravings seen with cocaine use.[15] Several psychiatric disorders such as depression, anxiety, attention deficit disorder, and schizophrenia have been found to be associated with dysfunction of this system.

Dopamine Pathways   **Serotonin Pathways**

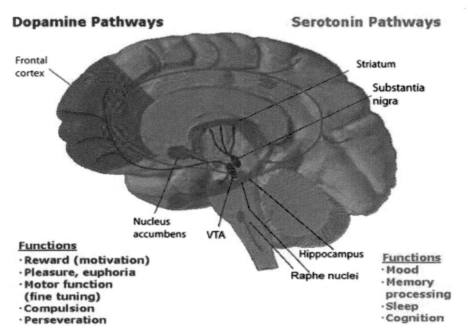

Fig. 1. Dopamine and serotonin pathways and functions. (*From* Deter, DT. Understanding the Disease of Addiction. Primary Care Clinics 38(1):1-7, DOI: 10.1016/j.pop.2010.11.001 with permission.)

CLINICAL MANIFESTATIONS
Acute Intoxication

The initial desired effect of cocaine use is euphoria. In addition, those using cocaine will experience increased energy, alertness, and sociability and decreased appetite and need for sleep. With increased duration of use, higher doses, or more efficient routes of administration, individuals may experience dysphoric effects such as anxiety, irritability, restlessness, and agitation; these may be especially prominent when the individual is coming down from a "high." Up to 30% of cocaine users report symptoms that include anxiety, depression, sleep problems, and weight loss.[16] **Table 1** lists the signs and symptoms commonly seen with acute intoxication, and **Table 2** lists adverse effects experienced with higher doses and more efficient methods of ingesting cocaine, such as through inhalation or intravenously.

Psychotic symptoms resembling acute schizophrenia can be experienced with higher doses and longer duration of use. Younger age is an independent risk factor for developing psychotic symptoms.[17] Compared with acute schizophrenia, patients with a cocaine use disorder may report more paranoia but fewer disordered thoughts and delusions. They may experience both auditory and tactile hallucinations, with fewer being visual.[18] A prominent tactile hallucination is formication or the sense of insects or parasites crawling under one's skin.

EFFECTS OF COCAINE ON SPECIFIC ORGAN SYSTEMS

With long-term and heavy use of cocaine, widespread and potentially lethal effects are seen throughout many organ systems. Many of these systemic effects result from the

Table 1
Signs and symptoms of acute cocaine intoxication

Symptoms	Signs
Euphoria—"Cocaine high"	Increased blood pressure
Intense pleasurable feelings	Elevated heart rate
Increased energy	Dilated pupils—mydriasis
Increased sociability	Diaphoresis
Decreased fatigue	Nausea/vomiting
Decreased need for sleep	Hyperventilation
Decreased appetite	Tremor
Restlessness	Acute coronary syndrome
	Seizures
	Rhabdomyolysis
	Hyperthermia
	Stroke

direct effect of cocaine's heightened stimulation of the sympathetic nervous system, causing peripheral vasoconstriction and organ ischemia. These effects can also be seen during intoxication or with first-time users.

Central Nervous System

Central nervous system effects include strokes, seizures, and movement disorders. A 5.7-fold increase in the risk of ischemic stroke was seen in a group of 15 to 49 year olds, even after adjusting for stroke risk factors such as tobacco use. In those reporting use immediately before the stroke, the greatest risk was within 6 hours of the reported cocaine use. It has been postulated that acute increases in blood pressure have contributed to the increased incidence in hemorrhagic types of stroke.[19]

Generalized, tonic-clonic, and partial seizures can be seen with first-time use and without any prior reports of seizure disorders. Most of these occur within the initial 60 minutes after ingestion when peak plasma concentrations are reached. These seizures are generally single, and do not require medication for control, although status epilepticus and repeat seizures have been reported.[20]

Cardiac

Cardiac symptoms are the most common symptoms reported by those seeking medical care as a result of their cocaine use, with chest pain being the most frequent complaint. Through its combined effects of being a powerful sympathomimetic agent

Table 2
Adverse psychological and behavioral effects of chronic cocaine use

Psychological	Behavioral
Anxiety, panic attacks	Agitation
Irritability	Restlessness
Dysphoria	Tremors
Paranoia	Dyskinesia
Hypervigilance	Stereotypical behaviors (ie, picking at skin)
Grandiosity	Impaired judgment
Psychotic symptoms	May result in involvement in high-risk behavior
Hallucinations—visual and tactile	

and through its adrenergic effects, it can acutely increase blood pressure, heart rate, and peripheral vascular resistance and stimulate coronary artery alpha-adrenergic receptors. The result may be coronary artery vasoconstriction with potential acute myocardial ischemia (MI) and/or infarction. The highest risk for ischemia is during the first 60 minutes after use, even in young individuals with no prior risk factors or small vessel disease,[21] and is independent of the amount used, the route of ingestion, or the frequency of use.[22] Cocaine use has been reported as the leading cause of death among young adults using illicit substances[23] and has been reported as a factor in 25% of nonfatal MIs in people younger than 45 years.[24] Long-term side effects on cardiac function are uncommon but have been reported.

Respiratory System

The respiratory effects of cocaine use are more likely to be seen with those who smoke and inhale crack cocaine. Fifty percent of users who smoke cocaine will experience acute shortness of breath, cough, wheezing, or hemoptysis; asthma exacerbation can also be seen.[25,26] When cocaine is insufflated (sniffed), both acute and chronic effects can be seen in the nasal and oral cavities.[27]

Renal System

Acute renal failure secondary to rhabdomyolysis can occur with acute cocaine use.[28]

Psychological and Cognitive Function

Several studies have reported that long-term cocaine use results in significant adverse effects on cognition, specifically in the areas of executive processing, attention, and working memory, and on social functioning and interactions.[29] In a recent systematic critical review of cognitive and neuroimaging studies done between 1999 and 2016 (N = 47) in cocaine users, Frazer and colleagues[30] found that "the current evidence does not support the view that chronic cocaine use is associated with broad cognitive deficits." They found no consistency among fMRI and imaging studies assessing the role of acute and chronic cocaine use on structural white or gray matter changes in brains of adults using cocaine and concluded that "converging evidence suggests that the compensatory neuroplastic changes associated with chronic cocaine exposure likely create conditions where cognitive performance is normalized during acute intoxication, declines during withdrawal, and recovers gradually over the course of abstinence".[30]

MANAGEMENT OF ACUTE INTOXICATION

When a teen or young adult presents to the emergency room with a constellation of symptoms that suggest acute intoxication (see **Table 1**), cocaine use should be considered, along with the use of other licit and illicit substances. It is also important to rule out other possible causes that may present similarly, such as hyperthyroidism, hypoglycemia, or psychiatric disorders such as panic attacks, mania from bipolar disorder, or acute schizophrenia. Toxicologic screens of both urine and blood are important, although it must be noted that blood concentrations are often not helpful prognostically, given that the blood concentrations generally do not correlate well with severity of symptoms.[31]

Initial management of acute intoxication presenting in the emergency department should be nonpharmacologic and focus on providing a safe and quiet environment for the teen or young adult, with as little stimulation as possible. Restraints should be avoided. The 2 major potential complications that need to be considered and are mentioned earlier include seizures and acute chest pain that may indicate cardiac ischemia. Both of these can be seen within the first hours of use, during acute ingestion and intoxication. The reader is referred to a comprehensive discussion of the management of cardiac complications.[32]

WITHDRAWAL

Hospitalization is rarely needed for medical reasons in those adolescents or young adults experiencing withdrawal, given that physical symptoms are less prominent than psychological symptoms and rarely life threatening. The individual may experience mild and transient nonspecific musculoskeletal pain or discomfort, chills, tremors, or involuntary muscle movements. MI has been reported to occur in the first week of withdrawal. Thus, any individual presenting during this time with chest pain or symptoms that suggest MI should be urgently evaluated.[32]

The psychological symptoms of withdrawal are more common and problematic. These include depression, anxiety, fatigue, difficulty concentrating, anhedonia, craving, increased appetite, and increased need for sleep.[10] In some cases, the depression and psychomotor retardation can be severe and debilitating and may be associated with suicidal ideation and attempts. Currently, there are no medications that have been found to be effective or approved specifically for cocaine withdrawal.

EVALUATION AND DIAGNOSIS OF COCAINE USE DISORDERS
Assessment/Screening

Several well-validated screening tools can be used with adolescents and young adults, such as the CRAFFT,[33] the S2BI,[34] and the 2-question National Institute on Alcohol Abuse and Alcoholism screener.[35] These generally identify whether there is any use of alcohol or drugs such as cocaine, for example, that warrants further investigation. Ask the teen or young adult directly about when the cocaine use started, how frequently it is used, whether this use has escalated, specific pattern of use, and methods of use. Asking about the use of other substances such as alcohol, tobacco, marijuana, or prescription opioids or stimulants is important, as cocaine use is most likely preceded by use of other substances. The provider should inquire about involvement in high-risk behaviors that may be linked to episodes of intoxication, such as driving while intoxicated or interpersonal violence. Unsafe sexual practices or the sharing of needles with injected substances can result in the acquisition of infections such as hepatitis B, C, or human immunodeficiency virus (HIV). Also query past or current history of medical and psychiatric conditions and treatment, family history of substance use/abuse, and psychiatric disorders and conduct a review of systems and complete psychosocial and developmental history.

A structured interview tool such as the HEEADSSS[36] screener allows assessment of social functioning and development in the areas of school or work, the home environment, and relationships with friends and family members. Noting both strengths as well as deficits is essential. Because the onset of significant substance use and abuse has been identified as a factor in the derailment of normative adolescent development,[37] it is important to identify whether the adolescent or young adult is achieving age-appropriate developmental milestones. Questions about progression through school, identification and progress toward future career, job, or life goals and demonstrated autonomy and responsibility for one's health and welfare are all important. A full review of all organ systems and mental health symptoms will identify whether the cocaine use or the concomitant use of other substances has caused any medical complications.

A full physical examination, focusing on vital signs and key organ systems such as the cardiac, pulmonary, and neurologic systems needs to be done. Looking for any stigmata of cocaine use, such as nasal irritation, oral lesions, or skin lesions secondary to injection should be included. A mental status examination can provide information about the youth's motivation around treatment as well as orientation, attention span, cognitive capacity, and mood. Laboratory tests can be guided by the information obtained through the history and the physical examination. These may include urine or blood toxicology tests, electrocardiogram, blood chemistries, or tests for sexually transmitted or blood-borne infections such as hepatitis B and C, HIV, Chlamydia trachomatis, and gonorrhea.

Outside of the emergency setting, urine testing for cocaine metabolites is limited because it provides information only about the most recent cocaine use and not about the onset of the substance use, recent pattern of use, or changes over time. These are all obtained through careful and nonjudgmental history taking with the youth in a confidential setting. Conversely, random urine testing can be helpful in monitoring adherence and abstinence during treatment.

At the completion of this initial assessment, a provider should be in a position to identify the extent of the youth's use of cocaine and other substances, the presence of concomitant mental health issues, and medical or psychosocial consequences of the cocaine use. The provider may determine that the teen or young adult has symptoms that indicate a cocaine use disorder or may determine that further evaluation is needed to confirm this diagnosis. With low levels of use, the provider may elect to do brief intervention in the office setting, using Screening, Brief Intervention, and Referral Treatment approaches.[38] The provider may also determine that the youth needs further assessment or referral for a higher level of care.

TREATMENT STRATEGIES FOR COCAINE USE AND ABUSE

The goals of treatment of any youth using cocaine, regardless of severity, should be complete abstinence of cocaine use. Given the strong cravings that may accompany cocaine use, and the high potential for medical consequences, there can be no support for "controlled use."[39] Additional goals for treatment should include abstinence from the use of any other licit or illicit substances; reduction in substance-associated high-risk behaviors; improvement in social functioning; and progress toward health, well-being, and age-appropriate developmental milestones. A substance use disorder is a chronic recurring disorder that requires continuing care, with expectations for periodic relapses during treatment that may require increasing the intensity of treatment. When resistance is seen during treatment, this may indicate the need to intensify or modify the treatment being provided.

A prominent hallmark that distinguishes cocaine use from other substance use is denial, given the highly reinforcing effect of the euphoria experienced with cocaine.[39] This results often in resistance to accepting the need for and referral to treatment and may also explain the high rates of relapse seen with cocaine use disorders.

In determining the most appropriate level of care that may be required, it is reasonable to start with individual or group outpatient sessions, when it has been determined that the youth has either cocaine use or mild cocaine use disorder. If the youth cannot adhere to treatment recommendations, or when there is a moderate cocaine use disorder, referral to an intensive outpatient program, augmented by either family-based therapy or contingency management components may be necessary. If there is continued inability to comply with recommendations, significant relapse, or a severe cocaine use disorder, residential treatment may be necessary. Unfortunately, in many communities treatment resources for youth with substance use disorders are limited, and this can pose significant barriers to accessing needed treatment. Evidence of this is the fact that juvenile justice programs, and not private or public insurers, are now the largest third-party payers for drug treatment programs for youth in the United States.[40]

Pharmacologic Therapy

There are currently no Food and Drug Administration–approved pharmacologic agents for the treatment of cocaine use disorders. Several experimental approaches are being studied, such as the use of Adderall, or the combination of naltrexone and bupropion, but these are strictly in the experimental stages. When an adolescent or young adult presents with a mental health disorder as well as a substance use disorder, it has been generally recommended that the disorder presenting the most problems for the youth be addressed initially and then the second disorder be addressed. However, there are those who also advocate for treating the substance use disorder initially, as this will enhance the youth's ability to engage in therapy aimed at the psychiatric disorder, such as depression, anxiety, or attention deficit disorder/attention-deficit hyperactivity disorder.

Behavioral Treatment Programs

Behavioral approaches are currently the mainstay of treatment of both cocaine use and cocaine use disorders, although very limited research has been done to evaluate the effectiveness of programs for the treatment of problematic stimulant use, including cocaine. Those that are available have been adapted from those developed specifically for tobacco and alcohol use. These include motivational interviewing, cognitive behavioral therapy programs, contingency management, and family-based treatment

---

Box 1
Behavioral treatment approaches for cocaine use disorders

Brief Interventions

Motivational interviewing[41]

Motivational enhancement therapy (METV)[42]

Cognitive Behavioral Therapy (CBT)[43,44]

Cognitive behavioral therapy with MET component[45]

Contingency Management

Voucher-based reinforcement therapy (VBRT)[46–49]

Family-Based Programs[42,50,51]

Multidimensional family therapy

Multisystemic family therapy

Functional family therapy

Family behavioral therapy
    Family behavioral therapy with MET/CBT component

Brief strategic family therapy

Adolescent community reinforcement approach (ACRA)

programs. Family-based programs have common elements that address parenting skills and family restructuring, such as positive communication, parental monitoring, and supervision, providing positive reinforcement and clear consequences tied to negative behaviors and clarifying expectations for substance-related behaviors. **Box 1** lists these and related references. Various types of individual- and group-oriented drug counseling have also been used. Many of these are grounded in the 12-step philosophy but may include cognitive, behavioral, insight-oriented, or supportive approaches.

SUMMARY

Cocaine use remains a significant public health problem for both adolescents and emerging adults. Its use and abuse can cause a wide range of significant medical and psychosocial effects and can disrupt normal psychosocial and psychological development. An understanding of the neurobiology of cocaine provides evidence for its acute intoxication effects as well as long-term physical effects. Few studies have focused on the treatment of cocaine use disorders, although behavioral techniques remain the mainstay of treatment. Further research needs to be done to provide information on better options for treatment and their effectiveness.

REFERENCES

1. Nutt D, King LA, Saulsbury W, et al. Development of a rational scale to assess the harm of drugs of potential misuse. Lancet 2007;369(9566):1047–53.
2. Johnston LD, Miech RA, O'Malley PM, et al. Monitoring the future national survey results on drug use: 1975-2017: overview, key findings on adolescent drug use. Ann Arbor (MI): Institute for Social Research, The University of Michigan; 2018. Available at: www.monitoringthefuture.org//pubs/monographs/mtf-overview2017.pdf. Accessed January 26, 2019.
3. American Psychiatric Association. Diagnostic and statistical manual of mental disorders, fifth edition. Arlington (VA): American Psychiatric Association; 2013.
4. Substance Abuse and Mental Health Services Administration. Key substance use and mental health indicators in the United States: results from the 2017 national survey on drug use and health. Rockville (MD): Center for Behavioral Health Statistics and Quality, Substance Abuse and Mental Health Services Administration; 2018 (HHS Publication No. SMA 18-5068, NSDUH Series H-53). Available at: https://www.samhsa.gov/data/.
5. Wagner FA, Anthony JC. From first drug use to drug dependence: developmental periods of risk for dependence upon marijuana, cocaine, and alcohol. Neuropsychopharmacology 2002;26(4):479–88.
6. Kandel DB, Huang FY, Davies M. Comorbidity between patterns of substance use dependence and psychiatric syndromes. Drug Alcohol Depend 2001; 64(2):233–41.
7. Anthony JC, Petronis KR. Early-onset drug use and risk of later drug problems. Drug Alcohol Depend 1995;40(1):9–15.
8. Chilcoat HD, Dishion TJ, Anthony JC. Parent monitoring and the incidence of drug sampling in urban elementary school children. Am J Epidemiol 1995; 141(1):25–31.
9. Latimer W, Zur J. Epidemiologic trends of adolescent use of alcohol, tobacco, and other drugs. Child Adolesc Psychiatr Clin N Am 2010;19(3):451–64.
10. Wilkins JN, Danovitch I, Gorelick DA. Management of stimulant, hallucinogen, marijuana, phencyclidine, and club drug intoxication and withdrawal. In:

Ries RK, Fiellin DA, Miller SC, et al, editors. The ASAM principles of addiction medicine. Philadelphia: Wolters Kluwer; 2014. p. 685–709.

11. Jeffcoat AR, Perez-Reyes M, Hill JM, et al. Cocaine disposition in humans after intravenous injection, nasal insufflation (snorting), or smoking. Drug Metab Dispos 1989;17(2):153–9.

12. Koob GF. Drugs of abuse: anatomy, pharmacology and function of reward pathways. Trends Pharmacol Sci 1992;13:177–84.

13. Volkow ND, Koob GF, McLellan AT. Neurobiologic advances from the brain disease model of addiction. N Engl J Med 2016;374(4):363–71.

14. Kalivas PW. Neurobiology of cocaine addiction: implications for new pharmacotherapy. Am J Addict 2007;16(2):71–8.

15. Volkow ND, Wang GJ, Fowler JS, et al. Addiction: beyond dopamine reward circuitry. Proc Natl Acad Sci U S A 2011;108(37):15037–42.

16. Williamson S, Gossop M, Powis B, et al. Adverse effects of stimulant drugs in a community sample of drug users. Drug Alcohol Depend 1997;44(2–3):87–94.

17. Smith MJ, Thirthalli J, Abdallah AB, et al. Prevalence of psychotic symptoms in substance users: a comparison across substances. Compr Psychiatry 2009; 50(3):245–50.

18. Roncero C, Ros-Cucurull E, Daigre C, et al. Prevalence and risk factors of psychotic symptoms in cocaine dependent patients. Actas Esp Psiquiatr 2012; 40(4):187–97.

19. Toosi S, Hess CP, Hills NK, et al. Neurovascular complications of cocaine use at a tertiary stroke center. J Stroke Cerebrovasc Dis 2010;19(4):273–8.

20. Neiman J, Haapaniemi HM, Hillbom M. Neurological complications of drug abuse: pathophysiological mechanisms. Eur J Neurol 2000;7(6):595–606.

21. Mittleman MA, Mintzer D, Maclure M, et al. Triggering of myocardial infarction by cocaine. Circulation 1999;99(21):2737–41.

22. Lange RA, Hillis LD. Cardiovascular complications of cocaine use. N Engl J Med 2001;345(5):351–8.

23. Substance Abuse and Mental Health Services Administration. Drug Abuse Warning Network, 2011: National Estimates of Drug-Related Emergency Department Visits. Rockville (MD): Substance Abuse and Mental Health Services Administration; 2013. HHS Publication No. (SMA) 13-4760 DAWN Series D-39.

24. Qureshi AI, Suri MF, Guterman LR, et al. Cocaine use and the likelihood of nonfatal myocardial infarction and stroke: data from the Third National Health and Nutrition Examination Survey. Circulation 2001;103(4):502–6.

25. Caponnetto P, Auditore R, Russo C, et al. Dangerous relationships: asthma and substance abuse. J Addict Dis 2013;32(2):158–67.

26. Tseng W, Sutter ME, Albertson TE. Stimulants and the lung. Clin Rev Allergy Immunol 2014;46(1):82–100.

27. Boghdadi MS, Henning RJ. Cocaine: pathophysiology and clinical toxicology. Heart Lung 1997;26(6):466–83.

28. Fernandez WG, Hung O, Bruno GR, et al. Factors predictive of acute renal failure and need for hemodialysis among ED patients with rhabdomyolysis. Am J Emerg Med 2005;23(1):1–7.

29. Spronk DB, Van Wel JHP, Ramaekers JG, et al. Characterizing the cognitive effects of cocaine: a comprehensive review. Neurosci Biobehav Rev 2013;37: 1838–59.

30. Frazer KM, Richards Q, Keith DR. The long-term effects of cocaine use on cognitive functioning: a systematic critical review. Behav Brain Res 2018;348:241–62.

31. Blaho K, Logan B, Winbery S, et al. Blood cocaine and metabolite concentrations, clinical findings and outcome of patients presenting to an ED. Am J Emerg Med 2000;18:593–8.
32. Schwartz BG, Rezkalla S, Kloner RA. Cardiovascular effects of cocaine. Circulation 2010;122(24):2558–69.
33. Knight JR, Sherritt L, Schrier LA, et al. Validity of the CRAFFT substance abuse screening test among adolescent clinic patients. Arch Pediatr Adolesc Med 2002;156:607–14.
34. Levy S, Weiss R, Sherritt L, et al. An electronic screen for triaging adolescent substance use by risk levels. JAMA Pediatr 2014;168(9):822–8.
35. National Institute on Alcohol Abuse and Alcoholism (US). Alcohol screening and brief intervention for youth: a practitioner's guide. Bethesda (MD): National Institute on Alcohol Abuse and Alcoholism, US Department of Health and Human Services, National Institutes of Health; 2011.
36. Goldenring J, Cohen E. Getting into adolescent heads: an essential update. Contemp Pediatr 2004;21(1):1–19.
37. Kandel DB, Davies M, Karus D, et al. The consequences in young adulthood of adolescent drug involvement: an overview. Arch Gen Psychiatry 1986;43(8):746–54.
38. Levy SJ, Williams JF, Ryan SA, et al. Substance use, brief intervention, and referral to treatment. Pediatrics 2016;138:e20161211.
39. Dackis CA, O'Brien CP. Cocaine dependence: a disease of the brain's reward centers. J Subst Abuse Treat 2001;21(3):111–7.
40. Caywood K, Riggs P, Novins D. Adolescent substance use disorder prevention and treatment. Colorado Journal of Psychiatry and Psychology: Child and Adolescent Mental Health 2015;1(1):42–9.
41. Miller WR, Rollnick S. Motivational interviewing: preparing people to change addictive behavior. New York: Guilford Press; 1991.
42. Strickland JC, Stoops WW. The prevention and treatment of adolescent stimulant and methamphetamine use. Adolescent substance abuse. Cham (Switzerland): Springer; 2018. p. 233–60.
43. Waldron HB, Turner CW. Evidence-based psychosocial treatments for adolescent substance abuse. J Clin Child Adolesc Psychol 2008;37(1):238–61.
44. Carroll KM, Ball SA, Nich C, et al. Computer-assisted delivery of cognitive-behavioral therapy for addiction: a randomized trial of CBT4CBT. Am J Psychiatry 2008;165(7):881–8.
45. Riggs P. Encompass: an integrated treatment intervention for adolescents with co-occurring psychiatric and substance use disorders. Scientific Proceedings of the American Academy of Child and adolescent Psychiatry 61st Annual Meeting (AACAP). San Diego, October 20, 2014.
46. Stanger C, Lansing AH, Budney AJ. Advances in research on contingency management for adolescent substance use. Child Adolesc Psychiatr Clin N Am 2016;25(4):645–59.
47. Farronato NS, Dursteler-Macfarland KM, Wiesbeck GA, et al. A systematic review comparing cognitive-behavioral therapy and contingency management for cocaine dependence. J Addict Dis 2013;32(3):274–87.
48. Yu CH, Tsao P, Jesuthasan JR, et al. Incentivizing health care behaviors in emerging adults: a systematic review. Patient Preference Adherence 2016;10:371.

49. Lott DC, Jencius S. Effectiveness of very low-cost contingency management in a community adolescent treatment program. Drug Alcohol Depend 2009;102(1–3): 162–5.
50. Baldwin SA, Christian S, Berkeljon A, et al. The effects of family therapies for adolescent delinquency and substance abuse: a meta-analysis. J Marital Fam Ther 2012;38(1):281–304.
51. Santisteban DA, Mena MP, McCabe BE. Preliminary results for an adaptive family treatment for drug abuse in Hispanic youth. J Fam Psychol 2011;25(4):610.

New and Emerging Illicit Psychoactive Substances

Ryan Graddy, MD, Megan E. Buresh, MD, Darius A. Rastegar, MD*

KEYWORDS

- Psychotropic drugs • Novel psychoactive substances • Designer drugs
- Cathinones • Cannabinoids

KEY POINTS

- Globalization and advances in neurochemistry have facilitated the development of novel substances which are often designed to circumvent regulations limiting access to psychoactive drugs.
- Most are in one of 4 broad categories: stimulant, cannabinoid, opioid, or benzodiazepine.
- Some novel stimulants and cannabinoids are potent and users may present with psychosis or seizures.
- Identification of use is hampered by lack of standardized rapid tests to identify these substances and clinicians must rely on history and clinical presentation.
- Treatment of toxicity is generally supportive; naloxone can be used for opioids and flumazenil for benzodiazepine toxicity.

INTRODUCTION

A 28-year-old man is evaluated by emergency medical technicians after a bystander calls 911 for concern about altered mental status. On arrival, the man is slow to respond to questions and has a blank stare. He is brought to the emergency department (ED) where he is lethargic but responds to tactile stimuli. His vital signs and oxygen saturation are within normal limits. On examination, the man has periods of zombielike groaning and moves his arms and legs slowly. Examination is otherwise notable for diffuse diaphoresis, without any focal neurologic deficits. Comprehensive laboratory analysis, including a standard urine immunoassay toxicology test and serum alcohol, is within normal limits without any toxins detected. Seven other patients with similar presentations evaluated in the same hospital on that day also had unremarkable laboratory tests. The patient is placed on an observation unit and his behavior normalizes after approximately 9 hours. On further history obtained later, he reports inhalation of a new substance he purchased recently before the episode.

This article originally appeared in *Medical Clinics*, Volume 102, Issue 4, July 2018.
Division of Chemical Dependence, Johns Hopkins University School of Medicine, 5200 Eastern Avenue, Suite D5W, Baltimore, MD 21224, USA
* Corresponding author.
E-mail address: drasteg1@jhmi.edu

Clinics Collections 9 (2020) 283–300
https://doi.org/10.1016/j.ccol.2020.07.040
2352-7986/20/© 2020 Elsevier Inc. All rights reserved.

Further analysis identifies a novel synthetic cannabinoid, methyl 2-(1-(4-fluorobenzyl)-1*H*-indazole-3-carboxamido)-3-methylbutanoate, in the serum of all 8 patients with similar symptoms.[1]

This case and others illustrate a new and growing phenomenon of individuals presenting with toxicity from psychoactive drugs that have not been seen before. Globalization and advances in neurochemistry have created conditions for the development and dissemination of novel psychoactive substances. Historically, psychoactive drugs have been obtained directly from natural sources (eg, cocaine from coca leaf) or derived from natural sources (eg, heroin derived from morphine in poppy bulbs), but the past few decades have seen the proliferation of drugs that are synthesized de novo without need to access regulated sources or precursors and that, for this reason, are sometimes referred to as designer drugs. Any review of this topic will be limited in that these drugs are new and rapidly evolving. The information on the clinical effects tends to focus on severe presentations and there is limited information on users' typical experience.

Although some of these drugs are brought to North America through traditional smuggling routes from Central and South America, many are marketed through the so-called dark Web (or cryptomarkets) and arrive through the mail.[2] Some arrive through legal channels and are labeled and marketed as not for human consumption or research chemicals to circumvent regulations.

This article provides a brief overview of these drugs, dividing them into 4 broad categories:

1. Stimulants
2. Cannabinoids
3. Opioids
4. Sedatives

Table 1 provides an overview of these substances and **Table 2** provides a summary of the clinical effects, detection, and treatment of exposure.

Stimulants

There are several novel stimulants that have been emerging in the past decades. These can be divided into 4 categories: synthetic cathinones, tryptamines, piperazines, and 2C (2 carbon) phenethylamines.

Synthetic cathinones

Pharmacology Synthetic cathinones are designed to mimic the primary psychoactive substance found in the leaves of the *Catha edulis* plant, colloquially referred to as khat.[3] They are derivatives of phenethylamine and are similar to amphetamines and 3,4-methylenedioxy-N-methylamphetamine (MDMA, or Ecstasy).[4] Cathinones have varying agonist activity on the dopamine, serotonin, and norepinephrine pathways through neurotransmitter reuptake inhibition and stimulation of neurotransmitter release.[5] Contrasting patterns of pathway activation contribute to the clinical effects observed with different compounds: dopamine agonism is associated with psychoactive effects and the addictive potential of cathinones, norepinephrine agonism with sympathomimetic effects, and serotonin agonism with paranoia and hallucinations.[6] The duration of effect is approximately 2 to 4 hours for many synthetic cathinones; 4-methylmethcathinone (mephedrone), the best-studied compound in the class, has a half-life of approximately 2 hours.[3,7]

Epidemiology Synthetic cathinones are often marketed as Bath Salts because of their white crystalline powder appearance. There are many nicknames for individual

Table 1
Overview of novel psychoactive substances

NPS Class	Selected Agents	Selected Street Names	Common Routes of Administration	Typical Duration of Effects (h)
Stimulants				
Cathinones	Mephedrone, methylone, MDPV	Bath Salts, Plant Food, research chemicals Meow-Meow, m-CAT, Bubbles, Bounce, Ivory Wave, Vanilla Sky, Energy-1	Nasal insufflation, oral, intravenous	2–4
Tryptamines	AMT, 5-MeO-DiPT	Foxy, Plant Food, research chemicals	Oral, nasal insufflation	6+
Piperazines	BZP, TFMPP	A2, Rapture, Frenzy, Bliss, Charge, herbal Ecstasy, Legal X, and Legal E	Oral	6–8
2C Phenylethylamines	2C-B	Nexus, Afro, Erox, Performax	Oral, nasal insufflation	8
Cannabinoids	Naphthoylindoles (JWH-018, JWH-073 and JWH-398), naphthylmethylindoles, naphthoylpyrroles, naphthylmethylindenes, phenylacetylindoles (ie, benzoylindoles, eg, JWH-250), cyclohexylphenols (eg, CP 47,497) classic cannabinoids (eg, HU-210)	Spice, K2, Scooby Snax, Mojo, Yucatan, Geeked Up, Smacked, Fake Weed, Trippy, Bad Guy, Green Giant, Ice Dragon, AK-47	Smoking, oral, liquid inhalation	2–5
Opioids	Carfentanil, ocfentanil, acetyl fentanyl, furanyl fentanyl, U-47700, AH-7921, and MT-45	Drop Dead, Serial Killer, Gray Death, Pink	Injection, nasal insufflation	2–8
Designer benzodiazepines	Clonazolam, diclazepam, etizolam, flubromazepam, flubromazolam, phenazepam, pyrazolam	Research chemicals	Oral	4–12

Abbreviations: AMT, alpha-methyltryptamine; BZP, N-benzylpiperazine; 2C-B, 4-bromo-2,5-dimethoxyphenethylamine; MDPV, methylenedioxypyrovalerone; 5-MeO-DiPT, 5-Methoxy-N,N-diisopropyltryptamine; JWH, John W. Huffman, an inventor of this class of compounds; NPS, novel psychoactive substances; TFMPP, 1-(3-trifluoromethyl-phenyl) piperazine.

Table 2
Overview of toxicity, testing, and treatment of novel psychoactive substances

NPS Class	Commonly Reported Toxicities	Urine Drug Testing	Treatment of Acute Toxicity
Stimulants			
Cathinones	Agitation, tachycardia, hypertension, restlessness, sweating, hyperthermia, paranoia, visual and auditory hallucinations, delusions, delirium, serotonin syndrome	Standard assay negative or false-positive for PCP	Supportive: benzodiazepines for agitation/anxiety; atypical antipsychotics for refractory agitation/psychosis
Tryptamines	Visual hallucinations, agitation, tachycardia, hyperthermia, delirium, flashbacks	Standard assay negative	Supportive: benzodiazepines for agitation/anxiety; atypical antipsychotics for refractory agitation/psychosis
Piperazines	Seizures, tachycardia, hypertension, hallucinations, insomnia, anxiety, headaches, nausea, tremors, diaphoresis, dizziness, palpitations, dyspnea, paranoia, hyponatremia, delirium, serotonin syndrome	Standard assay negative; BZP may cause false-positive for amphetamine	Supportive: benzodiazepines a mainstay because of high seizure risk
2C phenylethylamines	Hallucinations, tremor, diaphoresis, vision changes, nausea, vomiting, dizziness, seizures, serotonin syndrome, delirium	Standard assay negative	Supportive: benzodiazepines for agitation/anxiety; atypical antipsychotics for refractory agitation/psychosis
Cannabinoids	Agitation, nausea, tachycardia, lethargy, psychosis, seizures	Standard THC assay negative; specific assays for earlier-generation drugs available	Supportive: benzodiazepines for agitation/anxiety; atypical antipsychotics for refractory agitation/psychosis
Opioids	Sedation, respiratory depression	Fentanyl assay may be positive for related agents	Naloxone (2 mg IV/IM or 4 mg IN)
Designer benzodiazepines	Sedation, slurred speech, ataxia	Positive for benzodiazepines	Flumazenil (0.2 mg IV)

Abbreviations: BZP, N-benzylpiperazine; IV, intravenously; IM, intramuscularly; IN, intranasally; PCP, phencyclidine; THC, tetrahydrocannabinol.

compounds; some are listed in **Table 1**. Mephedrone was synthesized in 1929 but does not seem to have been used recreationally until the early 2000s when it reappeared among European dance club populations.[4] Slang terms for this compound include 4-MMC, Meow-Meow, m-CAT, Bubbles, and Bounce. Other synthetic cathinones used widely in the United States include 3,4-methylenedioxymethcathinone (methylone; bk-MDMA) and 3,4-methylenedioxypyrovalerone (MDPV; Ivory Wave, Vanilla Sky, Energy-1).[8,9]

Although synthetic cathinones were previously unregulated, a series of laws in the United Kingdom, United States, and elsewhere placed increasing restrictions on them in the early 2010s. The US Synthetic Drug Abuse Prevention Act of 2012 placed several synthetic cathinones, including mephedrone and MDPV, into the Schedule I category (no accepted medical use and high potential for misuse); subsequent Drug Enforcement Administration (DEA) regulations have expanded the number of synthetic cathinones in this category and no compounds in this class are approved for therapeutic use.[10]

Data on the prevalence of synthetic cathinone use are limited, but consumption seems to be around 1% or less among adults in the developed world.[11–13] Usage seems to be highest among adolescents and adults less than the age of 25 years. In some subpopulations, usage rates are substantially higher; for example, in the dance music scene in the United Kingdom, where rates of use may be higher than 40%, and among some men who have sex with men.[14,15]

Synthetic cathinones are often used with other psychoactive substances; one study found that 89% of mephedrone users also drank alcohol with their initial mephedrone use.[15] Use of other substances often occurs in an attempt to heighten the cathinone effects, alter the comedown, or enhance sexual performance. Common intentionally coadministered substances include heroin, cocaine, cannabis, ketamine, MDMA, methamphetamine, sildenafil, and gamma-hydroxybutyric acid (GHB).[4,6,15] In addition, many coadministered substances are ingested unintentionally, particularly among individuals using so-called party pills.[16]

The most common method of administration for synthetic cathinones is nasal insufflation. However, oral or intravenous use is common and there are reports of rectal, intramuscular, and subcutaneous administration as well.[6] Redosing at intervals of 1 to 2 hours is widespread given the short duration of action.[7]

Clinical effects Synthetic cathinones were initially developed as substitutes for other stimulants and MDMA, and have several shared clinical effects. The most common reason for presentation to EDs and poison control centers after ingestion is agitation.[11] Acute intoxication often presents with other signs and symptoms of sympathetic nervous system activation, including tachycardia, hypertension, restlessness, diaphoresis, and hyperthermia.[15,17,18] Psychiatric effects may include euphoria, paranoia, visual and auditory hallucinations, and delusions.[4,15,19] Serotonin syndrome has been reported in some cases,[19,20] as have seizures[21] and rhabdomyolysis.[22]

Data detailing the health effects of chronic cathinone use are limited; studies of long-term khat users suggest increased rates of psychiatric symptoms, including psychosis, as well as myocardial infarction.[23] Tolerance occurs with repeated use, and many users show behaviors meeting criteria for substance use disorder.[15,24] Withdrawal symptoms from cathinones are similar to those seen in other stimulants, including fatigue, nasal congestion, irritability, depression, anxiety, and insomnia.[15,24]

Causes of death associated with synthetic cathinones include metabolic acidosis, acute kidney injury, acute liver failure, disseminated intravascular coagulation, hyperthermia, arrhythmia, hyponatremia (possibly mediated by vasopressin release related to serotonin reuptake inhibition), and agitated delirium leading to injury.[11,25,26]

Evaluation Evaluation of suspected exposure must rely on the history and clinical presentation. Agitation, delirium, and sympathetic nervous system activation in the setting of unknown ingestion should heighten suspicion for cathinone exposure. Assessment for rhabdomyolysis is important in these scenarios given the apparent increased risk with cathinone ingestion.[22] Because of the frequency of simultaneous use of other psychoactive substances, suspicion for use should be high among individuals with other substance misuse as well.

There are no commercially available drug tests to identify synthetic cathinones.[27,28] Accurate techniques for identification of these compounds depend on liquid chromatography–mass spectrometry (LC-MS) testing but take too long to be clinically useful.[29,30] In some cases, cathinones may cross react with phencyclidine (PCP) enzyme-linked immunoassays (EIA) and result in false-positive results.[31]

Management Treatment of cathinone toxicity is supportive. In a 2011 US study of hospital evaluations for suspected synthetic cathinone toxicity, 49% of patients were treated in the ED and released, 21% admitted to an intensive care unit, 12% admitted to behavioral health or psychiatry, and 12% lost to follow-up.[32] Benzodiazepines are commonly used for management of agitation and seizures, and help with hyperthermia as well.[5] In some cases, cooling therapies are needed for hyperthermia; isotonic fluids for volume depletion, rhabdomyolysis, acute kidney injury, and disseminated intravascular coagulation; and fluid restriction and hypertonic saline to treat severe euvolemic hyponatremia.[11,30,33] Antipsychotics should be avoided in the setting of acute psychosis, because they are known to lower the seizure threshold and can exacerbate the danger of muscle injury and rhabdomyolysis because of the risk of extrapyramidal symptoms and neuroleptic malignant syndrome.[22,34,35] In 1 case, cathinone-induced serotonin syndrome was treated successfully with benzodiazepines and the serotonin antagonist cyproheptadine.[36]

Synthetic tryptamines

Pharmacology Tryptamine is a natural monoamine alkaloid found in plants, animals, fungi, and microbes. Serotonin is a natural derivative of tryptamine, and compounds in this class are typically serotonin receptor agonists.[37] Mushrooms containing psilocin and psilocybin, as well as ayahuasca, a tea containing naturally occurring dimethyltryptamine (DMT), contain tryptamines and are ingested for their hallucinogenic effects.[38,39]

Synthetic tryptamines have been used recreationally since at least the 1960s. Alpha-methyltryptamine (AMT) was initially developed as an antidepressant but was found to have limited medicinal value and intense hallucinogenic properties.[40] 5-Methoxy-N,N-diisopropyltryptamine (5-MeO-DiPT), commonly marketed as Foxy, has been used in the United States since 1999.[41] Both of these tryptamines have been listed as Schedule I substances since 2003.

All synthetic tryptamines are agonists at 5-hydroxytryptamine (5-HT) 2A receptors through serotonin reuptake inhibition, direct receptor agonism, or both.[42] Some tryptamines also interact with norepinephrine receptors, but they typically do not affect the dopaminergic system.[43]

Epidemiology The 2009 to 2013 US National Survey on Drug Use and Health identified psychedelic tryptamines as among the most commonly self-reported novel psychoactive substances used, with rates increasing from 12.9% to 28.8% of all novel psychoactive substances users over this 5-year period.[12] Users tend to be young and male; 1 US study found that 86% of patients seen at ED visits related to use were male, and 86% were less than 21 years of age.[44]

Administration is typically oral or by nasal insufflation, although smoking, injection, and rectal use have been reported.[45] Mixing with other substances for synergy or to avoid adverse effects is common, and concomitant administration of monoamine oxidase inhibitors seems to be widespread in order to potentiate the tryptamine effects.[45]

Clinical effects The onset of effects after oral tryptamine ingestion is typically rapid, within 30 minutes, and can last for 6 hours or more.[46] Visual hallucinations predominate, and many users describe a spiritual experience with euphoria and increased energy. Agitation, tachycardia, and hyperthermia have also been described.[40,41] No obvious tolerance or dependence has been documented with synthetic tryptamines.

Deaths related to synthetic tryptamines have been reported. In one case, a young man walked out into traffic after using N,N-diallyl-5-methoxytryptamine (5-MeO-DALT), and was fatally hit by a car.[37] In another case, fatal neurotoxicity and acute heart failure were attributed to rectal administration of Foxy.[47]

Evaluation and management Evaluation of suspected tryptamine toxicity must rely on clinical evaluation and history. Standard urine EIA drug tests do not detect synthetic tryptamines; individual compounds can be identified through LC-MS testing, but this takes too long to be clinically useful when acute toxicity is suspected.

Treatment of tryptamine toxicity is supportive. In some cases, sedation and intravenous hydration may be required. Benzodiazepines are often used to help with agitation. Activated charcoal may be helpful in the setting of oral ingestion.[45]

Piperazines
Pharmacology Piperazines are a class of compounds with stimulant and hallucinogenic properties with no naturally occurring counterpart. Two major structural groups exist: N-benzylpiperazine (BZP; a single drug) and N-phenylpiperazine [including several drugs, the best documented of which is 1-(3-trifluoromethyl-phenyl) piperazine (TFMPP)].

Piperazines are commonly marketed as alternatives to MDMA. BZP has been listed as a US Schedule I substance since 2002, and TFMPP is currently not assigned a controlled status by the DEA. BZP centrally stimulates dopamine and norepinephrine receptors, whereas TFMPP preferentially agonizes serotonin receptors and inhibits reuptake.[48]

Epidemiology Users of piperazines are predominantly young men[49–51] and use seems common in electronic dance clubs and raves. These drugs are almost exclusively used in combinations with other piperazines or other illicit and legal substances as so-called club drugs or party pills.[49,52]

There are limited data available on the prevalence of piperazine use. Evidence suggests that, in some countries with strict enforcement of laws prohibiting piperazines, rates of use have decreased substantially; in New Zealand, recent use of the piperazine BZP decreased from 15% to 3% following official prohibition in 2008.[53] However, the growth of the dark Web and other online markets for sale of illicit synthetic substances across international borders in recent years has likely contributed to an increase in use in some populations, including those without previous experience. A recent study of new psychoactive substances found in wastewater in major Chinese cities showed BZP (strictly illegal nationwide) detected at 100% of sewage treatment plants evaluated.[54]

Clinical effects Administration of piperazines is typically oral, although intravenous use has been reported.[52] The onset of effects can take up to 2 hours, and last for 6 to 8 hours. BZP ingestion has been associated with euphoria and sympathomimetic effects, described as 10 to 20 times less potent than amphetamine.[55] TFMPP ingestion commonly causes confusion and hallucinations.[51,56] Shared effects of piperazines and those seen with BZP/TFMPP simultaneous ingestion include insomnia, anxiety, headaches, nausea, tremor, diaphoresis, dizziness, palpitations, dyspnea, and paranoia.[49,55,56] Hyponatremia and serotonin syndrome have been described.[57] Seizures have also been associated with piperazine use; in one study of possible BZP-related poisonings at a New Zealand hospital, more than 18% of patients had seizures associated with use.[58] It is important to remember that piperazines are commonly used in party pills as combinations with other piperazines and often including other substances, including MDMA and cocaine.[49,52] Case reports of mortality related to piperazine ingestion have generally involved other drugs, including alcohol, and often result from accidental injuries.[59]

Evaluation and management As with other synthetic stimulants, evaluation of piperazine toxicity is based on history and clinical assessment. Standard urine EIA drug tests do not identify piperazines; however, BZP may trigger false-positives for amphetamines.[52] Treatment of piperazine toxicity is similar to management of synthetic cathinone toxicity, with general supportive measures, benzodiazepines for agitation or seizures, and blood pressure control with close monitoring.[57] Antipsychotic medications are second-line agents for agitation but should be given with caution because of the potential worsening of hyperthermia and cardiac arrhythmias.[48]

Two-carbon phenethylamines

Pharmacology The 2C drugs are a subgroup of phenethylamines, the class of compounds with the same basic structure as catecholamines, amphetamines, and cathinones. The name 2C is derived from the characteristic 2 carbon atoms between a benzene ring and a terminal amine group. Compounds in this class have an affinity for 5-HT2 receptors and occasionally alpha-adrenergic receptors as well, leading to hallucinogenic and sympathomimetic effects.[60] Metabolism occurs through monoamine oxidase, and monoamine oxidase inhibitors may potentiate or heighten the effects of 2C compounds. 2C compounds have been listed as US Schedule I substances since 1994. Although this class of substance has been in use for several decades, novel compounds continue to emerge.[61]

Epidemiology Users of 2C drugs are typically young men; raves and dance parties are common settings of use.[62] A nationally representative US survey found that self-reported lifetime use of psychedelic phenethylamines (of which the most commonly used compounds were from the 2C series) increased from 9.7% to 31.9% among individuals who had used any novel psychoactive substances from 2009 to 2013.[12] Lifetime prevalence of 2C series compounds in US adults was estimated at 0.2% in 2013.

2C compounds are commonly used in combination with other substances; one survey of recent users in Spain found that 69% had mixed MDMA with a 2C compound, and significant numbers also used alcohol and marijuana.[63] Administration is most commonly oral or by nasal insufflation.[58]

Clinical effects The onset of effects for 2C substances is rapid. The most widely studied compound in the 2C class, 4-bromo-2,5-dimethoxyphenethylamine (2C-B), produces effects approximately 30 minutes after oral ingestion, peaks around 2 hours, and lasts up to 8 hours.[64] Reported desirable effects include changes in tactile, auditory, and visual perception; euphoria; and hallucinations. Negative effects include trembling, sweating, difficulty seeing straight, nausea, vomiting, and dizziness.[65,66] The subjective experience of users seems similar to that of ayahuasca[39] (a hallucinogenic traditional brew used ritually in the northwest Amazon containing a $5-HT_{2A}$ agonist), salvia, and LSD (lysergic acid diethylamide). Seizures, serotonin syndrome, and agitated delirium have all been observed in the setting of use, and deaths have been reported.[66–68]

Evaluation and management As with the synthetic cathinones and other novel psychoactive substances, evaluation of suspected toxicity must rely on history and clinical assessment; standard urine EIA drug testing does not identify 2C compounds and LC-MS testing can be used for definitive detection. Timely diagnosis requires a high level of clinical suspicion in the appropriate setting. Treatment involves supportive care and may require rapid sedation, fluid resuscitation, and reduction of hyperthermia. Benzodiazepines are preferred agents for sedation given their antiepileptic activity; antipsychotics have also been used effectively.[59,69]

Synthetic Cannabinoids

Pharmacology

First developed in research laboratories in the 1960s to study the endocannabinoid system, synthetic cannabinoids emerged as drugs of illicit use in 2008.[69] These substances are structurally very different from Δ^9-tetrahydrocannabinol (Δ^9-THC), the cannabinoid found in marijuana. Synthetic cannabinoids are potent, full agonists of the cannabinoid type-1 (CB-1) receptors found in the central nervous system (CNS), lungs, liver, and kidneys,[70] and weaker agonists of CB-2 receptors found in immune system and at low levels in CNS.[71] They are 2 to 100 times more potent agonists of the CB-1 receptor than THC, which is only a partial agonist of CB-1.[72] Binding of CB-1 induces the classic cannabinoid tetrad of hypothermia, analgesia, cataplexy, and locomotor suppression[72] with psychoactive effects achieved via modulation of glutamate and GABA (gamma-aminobutyric acid) neurotransmitters.[2] Chronic activation of CB-2 in mice leads to dysregulation of $5-HT_{2A}$ receptors and has been associated with anxiety and psychosis, which are common side effects of synthetic cannabinoids not seen with THC.[73] The greater toxicity of synthetic cannabinoids compared with marijuana is thought to be caused by their greater agonist potency for CB-1 as well as lack of cannabidiol, terpenes, and other constituents of cannabis that may balance some effects.[71] They have multiple downstream metabolites that retain high affinity at CB-1 and CB-2, further potentiating their effects.[71,73]

Epidemiology

Often referred to as Spice and K2, synthetic cannabinoids are sold under hundreds of names; **Table 1** lists some of these.[2] They are dissolved in solvent and sprayed onto inert plant material, which is saturated and dried, leaving highly variable amounts of the substance.[69] They are marketed to consumers as safe and legal alternatives to marijuana, but are in fact much more potent.[69] They are sold in gas stations, convenience stores, marijuana paraphernalia stores, and over the Internet in addition to traditional black market dealers.[69] They are often labeled "Not for human consumption" to avoid government regulations. Synthetic cannabinoids are most commonly smoked or ingested,[74] but can also be administered by liquid inhalation and smoking liquid via refillable vaporizers.[75] As of July 2016, the DEA had banned 25 synthetic cannabinoids; however, laboratories quickly synthesize compounds with minor structural adjustments to evade scheduling laws.[69,76]

Synthetic cannabinoids increased in popularity as so-called legal highs, often viewed as safe and legal alternatives to marijuana.[70] Use is most common among young men and associated with cannabis, alcohol, and other illicit drugs.[72,77,78] It is also popular among military personnel and athletes seeking to avoid detection through drug tests.[72] In a survey of US high school students, use peaked at 11.9% in 2011 and has declined steadily since the 2012 DEA ban, to 4.8% in 2015, likely because of increased awareness of risk.[77,79] Despite the decline in reported use, clusters of synthetic cannabinoid intoxication (sometimes referred to as zombie outbreaks) seem to be increasing and have been reported in many US cities,[1,76,80,81] a likely result of the higher potency of later-generation compounds.

Clinical effects

Acute intoxication with synthetic cannabinoids produces cannabis-like effects that are more severe than those of marijuana.[70,82] Users are 30 times more likely to seek emergency services than marijuana users[83] and have higher rates of psychosis, agitation, and aggression.[84] Effects are seen within 10 minutes of smoking and peak at an average of 2 to 5 hours; most effects resolve in less than 24 hours,[70] although they may persist for days in severe cases.[85] In a systematic review of published cases, the most common effects were tachycardia (37%–77%), nausea (13%–94%), agitation (19%–32%), and lethargy (19%–32%).[86] Although most cases are mild, severe toxicity has been reported and includes seizures,[87] acute kidney injury,[88] rhabdomyolysis,[89] and ischemic stroke.[90] Adverse cardiac effects include myocardial ischemia,[91] bradycardia,[92] heart block,[93] and corrected QT prolongation.[94] Mortalities are 0.5% to 1% among US poison control calls.[73]

Little is known about the chronic effects of synthetic cannabinoid use in humans. Animal studies suggest that chronic exposure during adolescence can lead to behavioral deficits and increased anxiety as adults,[70] as well as increased vulnerability to substance use disorder and depression.[94] The withdrawal syndrome is marked by agitation, irritability, anxiety, mood swings, and tachycardia, and is more severe than withdrawal from marijuana.[95–97]

Evaluation

Evaluation of suspected exposure depends on history and clinical presentation. Synthetic cannabinoids are not detected in standard urine drug tests for THC metabolites. Although commercial testing for older synthetic cannabinoids is available, these tests do not detect most newer compounds.[98,99] LC-MS can detect a wider spectrum of synthetic cannabinoids, but it is too slow to be clinically useful and is limited by lack of reference samples. Exposure should be suspected in substance users who report marijuana use but present with more extreme psychosis and agitation.

Management

There is no reversal agent for synthetic cannabinoids and care for acute toxicity is supportive. Intravenous fluids should be given to prevent acute kidney injury and rhabdomyolysis. Benzodiazepines are first-line agents for management of anxiety and agitation. Atypical antipsychotics such as quetiapine may be used as second-line treatment of severe agitation and psychosis; however, caution should be used with medications that decrease seizure threshold because synthetic cannabinoids are associated with seizures.[83] Withdrawal may require inpatient treatment and can also be managed with benzodiazepines and antipsychotics.[97]

Opioids

Pharmacology
The past decade has seen an increase in the distribution and use of illicitly manufactured fentanyl and fentanyl-related compounds, including carfentanil, ocfentanil, acetyl fentanyl, and furanyl fentanyl.[100] There are several other synthetic opioids that have been reported, including U-47700, AH-7921, and MT-45.[101] The pharmacologic effects are similar to those of other opioids and the potency varies depending on the substance. Some are highly potent; compared with morphine, acetyl fentanyl is 16 times more potent, fentanyl and furanyl fentanyl are 50 to 100 times more potent, ocfentanil is 200 times more potent,[102] and carfentanil is 10,000 times more potent.[103] The potency of U-47700 is about 7.5 times that of morphine.[101]

Epidemiology
Fentanyl-related compounds are often sold as heroin (or mixed with heroin) or in the form of counterfeit pills, which resemble oxycodone, Xanax, or Norco.[100] Most of the epidemiologic data come from law enforcement seizures. In 2016, the DEA reported that the most commonly seized synthetic opioids were fentanyl, followed by furanyl fentanyl, acetyl fentanyl, and U-47700.[104]

Clinical effects
There are limited data on the clinical effects of these substances, but they seem to be similar to those of other opioids: euphoria, analgesia, and respiratory depression.[101] The main difference is the potency, which may lead to an increased risk of overdose, particularly when individuals are not aware of what they are using, because they are often sold as heroin.

Evaluation
Opioid exposure should be suspected in anyone presenting with the typical signs and symptoms: decreased level of consciousness, respiratory depression, and miosis. These substances are not detected in standard urine drug screens. Fentanyl can be detected by a separate EIA drug test and many of the fentanyl-related compounds cross react with this test, but they cannot be distinguished from fentanyl through this method.[101] They can be identified through LC-MS testing, but this takes more time and most laboratories do not have the reference materials needed to do this; these may become available in the future.

Management
The standard treatment of intoxication or overdose with these agents is the opioid antagonist naloxone, given intravenously (IV), intramuscularly (IM), or intranasally (IN). The usual dose for treatment of opioid overdose is 0.4 mg IV/IM; however, it has been reported that overdoses with the more potent agents often require higher doses of naloxone and it is recommended that 2 mg IV/IM or 4 mg IN be used.[101] Among patients who have an opioid use disorder, the most effective treatment is opioid agonist therapy with buprenorphine or methadone; the opioid antagonist naltrexone is another option.

Sedatives

Pharmacology
There are several so-called designer benzodiazepines that have become available in illicit drug markets in recent years. Some of these are available by prescription in other

countries; others are classified as research chemicals. **Table 1** provides a list of some of these drugs.

Epidemiology

There is very little information on the epidemiology of use of these drugs. The DEA "Emerging Threat Report" from the first quarter of 2017 identified 7 instances of etizolam contributing to drug seizures, which is significantly lower that of many other novel psychoactive substances.[105] In an analysis of blood samples from drugged drivers and suspected drug offenders in Norway, designer benzodiazepines were detected in 0.3% of cases.[106]

Clinical effects

There is very little information on the clinical effects of these drugs. It would be expected that they would have many of the same effects of other benzodiazepines, but there may be differences in relative anxiolytic or hypnotic effects, as well as onset and duration of action.

Evaluation and management

Benzodiazepine toxicity should be suspected in anyone presenting with a decreased level of consciousness or confusion and concern for ingestion. Designer benzodiazepines may be detected in standard EIA drug tests but cannot be differentiated from other benzodiazepines.[107]

The standard treatment of benzodiazepine toxicity is supportive measures, including intravenous fluids and ventilator support, if needed. A benzodiazepine antagonist, flumazenil, can be given IV in serious cases. There are limited data on its use for designer benzodiazepine overdose, but it has been reported to be effective in some case reports.[108]

FUTURE CONSIDERATIONS/SUMMARY

Novel psychoactive substances are a growing problem and require ongoing vigilance to deal with the adverse consequences of use. Clinicians need to be aware of the substances being used in their community; the National Institute of Drug Abuse (NIDA) publishes a periodic update on emerging trends that is available online (https://www.drugabuse.gov/drugs-abuse/emerging-trends-alerts). Clinicians also need to question patients about use of these substances, particularly among young people who use other drugs and those presenting with agitation, seizures, or other possible complications. Rapid tests are needed to identify these drugs and to aid in the evaluation and treatment of acutely ill patients. Counseling users on the realistic risks of these substances is likely the best initial approach; more research is needed on effective management strategies.

ACKNOWLEDGMENTS

The authors wish to thank Paul Christopher, Brown University, for providing a critical review of this article.

REFERENCES

1. Adams AJ, Banister SD, Irizarry L, et al. "Zombie" outbreak caused by the synthetic cannabinoid AMB-FUBINACA in New York. N Engl J Med 2017;376(3): 235–42.

2. Kemp AM, Clark MS, Dobbs T, et al. Top 10 facts you need to know about synthetic cannabinoids: not so nice spice. Am J Med 2016;129:240–4.
3. Valente MJ, Guedes De Pinho P, De Lourdes Bastos M, et al. Khat and synthetic cathinones: a review. Arch Toxicol 2014;88:15–45.
4. Papaseit E, Molto J, Muga R, et al. Clinical pharmacology of the synthetic cathinone mephedrone. Curr Top Behav Neurosci 2017;32:313–32.
5. Schifano F, Orsolini L, Duccio Papanti G, et al. Novel psychoactive substances of interest for psychiatry. World Psychiatry 2015;14:15–26.
6. Zawilska JB. Mephedrone and other cathinones. Curr Opin Psychiatry 2014;27:256–62.
7. Capriola M. Synthetic cathinone abuse. Clin Pharmacol Adv Appl 2013;5:109–15.
8. 3,4-Methylenedioxypyrovalerone (MDPV). (2013). [online] Drug Enforcement Administration Office of Diversion Control. Available at: https://www.deadiversion.usdoj.gov/drug_chem_info/mdpv.pdf. Accessed July 18, 2017.
9. 3,4-Methylenedioxymethcathinone (Methylone). (2013). [online] Drug Enforcement Administration Office of Diversion Control. Available at: https://www.deadiversion.usdoj.gov/drug_chem_info/methylone.pdf. Accessed July 18, 2017.
10. 112th Congress. Synthetic Drug Control Act of 2012, S3190. Senate, Washington, DC, May 16, 2012.
11. Karila L, Megarbane B, Cottencin O, et al. Synthetic cathinones: a new public health problem. Curr Neuropharmacol 2015;13:12–20.
12. Palamar JJ, Martins SS, Su MK, et al. Self-reported use of novel psychoactive substances in a US nationally representative survey: prevalence, correlates, and a call for new survey methods to prevent underreporting. Drug Alcohol Depend 2015;156:112–9.
13. Patrick ME, O'Malley PM, Kloska DD, et al. Novel psychoactive substance use by US adolescents: characteristics associated with use of synthetic cannabinoids and synthetic cathinones. Drug Alcohol Rev 2016;35(5):586–90.
14. Winstock AR, Mitcheson LR, Deluca P, et al. Mephedrone, new kid for the chop? Addiction 2011;106:154–61.
15. Winstock A, Mitcheson L, Ramsey J, et al. Mephedrone: use, subjective effects and health risks. Addiction 2011;106:1991–6.
16. Palamar JJ, Salamone A, Vincenti M, et al. Detection of "bath salts" and other novel psychoactive substances in hair samples of ecstasy/MDMA/"Molly" users. Drug Alcohol Depend 2016;161:200–5.
17. Dargan PI, Sedefov R, Wood DM. The pharmacology and toxicology of the synthetic cathinone mephedrone (4-methylmethcathinone). Drug Test Anal 2011;3:454–63.
18. Papaseit E, Pérez-Mañá C, Mateus J-A, et al. Human pharmacology of mephedrone in comparison with MDMA. Neuropsychopharmacology 2016;41:2704–13.
19. Joksovic P, Mellos N, van Wattum PJ, et al. "Bath salts"–induced psychosis and serotonin toxicity. J Clin Psychiatry 2012;73:1125.
20. Miotto K, Striebel J, Cho AK, et al. Clinical and pharmacological aspects of bath salt use: a review of the literature and case reports. Drug Alcohol Depend 2013;132:1–12.
21. Wood DM, Greene SL, Dargan PI. Clinical pattern of toxicity associated with the novel synthetic cathinone mephedrone. Emerg Med J 2011;28:280–2.

22. O'Connor AD, Padilla-Jones A, Gerkin RD, et al. Prevalence of rhabdomyolysis in sympathomimetic toxicity: a comparison of stimulants. J Med Toxicol 2015; 11(2):195–200.
23. Al-Habori M. The potential adverse effects of habitual use of *Catha edulis* (khat). Expert Opin Drug Saf 2005;4(6):1145–54.
24. Carhart-Harris RL, King LA, Nutt DJ. A web-based survey on mephedrone. Drug Alcohol Depend 2011;118:19–22.
25. Karila L, Billieux J, Benyamina A, et al. The effects and risks associated to mephedrone and methylone in humans: a review of the preliminary evidences. Brain Res Bull 2016;126:61–7.
26. Banks ML, Worst TJ, Rusyniak DE, et al. Synthetic cathinones ("Bath salts"). J Emerg Med 2014;46:632–42.
27. Ellefsen KN, Anizan S, Castaneto MS, et al. Validation of the only commercially available immunoassay for synthetic cathinones in urine: Randox Drugs of Abuse V Biochip Array Technology. Drug Test Anal 2015;6:728–38.
28. Moeller KE, Kissack JC, Atayee RS, et al. Clinical interpretation of urine drug tests: what clinicians need to know about urine drug screens. Mayo Clin Proc 2016;92:774–96.
29. Concheiro M, Anizan S, Ellefsen K, et al. Simultaneous quantification of 28 synthetic cathinones and metabolites in urine by liquid chromatography-high resolution mass spectrometry. Anal Bioanal Chem 2013;405:9437–48.
30. Swortwood MJ, Boland DM, Decaprio AP. Determination of 32 cathinone derivatives and other designer drugs in serum by comprehensive LC-QQQ-MS/MS analysis. Anal Bioanal Chem 2013;405:1383–97.
31. Penders TM, Gestring RE, Vilensky DA, et al. Intoxication delirium following use of synthetic cathinone derivatives. Am J Drug Alcohol Abuse 2012;38:616–7.
32. Spiller HA, Ryan ML, Weston RG, et al. Clinical experience with and analytical confirmation of "bath salts" and "legal highs" (synthetic cathinones) in the United States. Clin Toxicol 2011;49:499–505.
33. Boulanger-Gobeil C, St-Onge M, Laliberté M, et al. Seizures and hyponatremia related to ethcathinone and methylone poisoning. J Med Toxicol 2012;8:59–61.
34. Jerry J, Collins G, Streem D. Synthetic legal intoxicating drugs: the emerging "incense" and "bath salt" phenomenon. Cleve Clin J Med 2012;79:258–64.
35. Kersten BP, McLaughlin ME. Toxicology and management of novel psychoactive drugs. J Pharm Pract 2015;28:50–65.
36. Mugele J, Nañagas KA, Tormoehlen LM. Serotonin syndrome associated with MDPV use: a case report. Ann Emerg Med 2012;60:100–2.
37. Corkery JM, Durkin E, Elliott S, et al. The recreational tryptamine 5-MeO-DALT (N,N-diallyl-5-methoxytryptamine): a brief review. Prog Neuropsychopharmacol Biol Psychiatry 2012;39:259–62.
38. Tittarelli R, Mannocchi G, Pantano F, et al. Recreational use, analysis and toxicity of tryptamines. Curr Neuropharmacol 2015;13:26–46.
39. dos Santos RG, Bouso JC, Hallak JEC. Ayahuasca, dimethyltryptamine, and psychosis: a systematic review of human studies. Ther Adv Psychopharmacol 2017;7:141–57.
40. Boland DM, Andollo W, Hime GW, et al. Fatality due to acute alpha-methyltryptamine intoxication. J Anal Toxicol 2005;29:394–7.
41. Drug Enforcement Administration Office of Diversion Control. 3,4-Methylenedioxypyrovalerone (MDPV). (2013). [online] Drug Enforcement Administration Office of Diversion Control. Available at: https://www.deadiversion.usdoj.gov/drug_chem_info/methylone.pdf. Accessed July 18, 2017.

42. Scherbaum N, Schifano F, Bonnet U. New psychoactive substances (NPS) - a challenge for the addiction treatment services. Pharmacopsychiatry 2017; 50(3):116–22.
43. Rickli A, Moning OD, Hoener MC, et al. Receptor interaction profiles of novel psychoactive tryptamines compared with classic hallucinogens. Eur Neuropsychopharmacol 2016;26(8):1327–37.
44. Maxwell JC. Psychoactive substances—some new, some old: a scan of the situation in the U.S. Drug Alcohol Depend 2014;134:71–7.
45. Araujo AM, Carvalho F, Bastos Mde L, et al. The hallucinogenic world of tryptamines: an updated review. Arch Toxicol 2015;89:1151–73.
46. Meyer MR. New psychoactive substances: an overview on recent publications on their toxicodynamics and toxicokinetics. Arch Toxicol 2016;90:2421–44.
47. Tanaka E, Kamata T, Katagi M. A fatal poisoning with 5-methoxy-N,N-diisopropyltryptamine, foxy. Forensic Sci Int 2006;163:152–4.
48. Schep LJ, Slaughter RJ, Vale JA, et al. The clinical toxicology of the designer "party pills" benzylpiperazine and trifluoromethylphenylpiperazine. Clin Toxicol 2011;49:131–41.
49. Wilkins C, Sweetsur P, Girling M. Patterns of benzylpiperazine/trifluoromethylphenylpiperazine party pill use and adverse effects in a population sample in New Zealand. Drug Alcohol Rev 2008;27:633–9.
50. Drug Enforcement Administration Office of Diversion Control. N-benzylpiperazine. Available at: https://www.deadiversion.usdoj.gov/drug_chem_info/bzp.pdf. Accessed July 18, 2017.
51. 1-[3-(Trifluoro-methyl)-phenyl]piperazine. (2013). [online] Drug Enforcement Administration Office of Diversion Control. Available at: https://www.deadiversion.usdoj.gov/drug_chem_info/tfmpp.pdf. Accessed July 18, 2017.
52. Arbo M, Bastos M, Carmo H. Piperazine compounds as drugs of abuse. Drug Alcohol Depend 2012;122(3):174–85.
53. Wilkins C, Sweetsur P. The impact of the prohibition of benzylpiperazine (BZP) 'legal highs' on the prevalence of BZP, new legal highs and other drug use in New Zealand. Drug Alcohol Depend 2013;127(1–3):72–80.
54. Gao T, Du P, Xu Z, et al. Occurrence of new psychoactive substances in wastewater of major Chinese cities. Sci Total Environ 2017;575:963–9.
55. Lin JC, Jan RK, Kydd R, et al. Subjective effects in humans following administration of party pill drugs BZP and TFMPP alone and in combination. Drug Test Anal 2011;3:582–5.
56. Musselman ME, Hampton JP. "Not for human consumption": a review of emerging designer drugs. Pharmacotherapy 2014;34:745–57.
57. Gee P, Richardson S, Woltersdorf W, et al. Toxic effects of BZP-based herbal party pills in humans: a prospective study in Christchurch, New Zealand. N Z Med J 2005;118:35–44.
58. Gee P, Gilbert M, Richardson S, et al. Toxicity from the recreational use of 1-benzylpiperazine. Clin Toxicol 2008;46:802–7.
59. Elliott S, Smith C. Investigation of the first deaths in the United Kingdom involving the detection and quantitation of the piperazines BZP and 3-TFMPP. J Anal Toxicol 2008;32:172–7.
60. Dean BV, Stellpflug SJ, Burnett AM, et al. 2C or not 2C: phenethylamine designer drug review. J Med Toxicol 2013;9:172–8.
61. Nikolau P, Papoutsis I, Stefanidou M, et al. 2C-I-NBOMe, an "N-bomb" that kills with "smiles". Drug Chem Toxicol 2015;38(1):113–9.

62. Nelson ME, Bryant SM, Aks SE. Emerging drugs of abuse. Emerg Med Clin North Am 2014;32:1–28.
63. Caudevilla-Gálligo F, Riba J, Ventura M, et al. 4-Bromo-2,5-dimethoxyphenethyl-amine (2C-B): presence in the recreational drug market in Spain, pattern of use and subjective effects. J Psychopharmacol 2012;7:1026–35.
64. 4-Bromo-2,5-Dimethoxyphenethylamine. (2013). [online] Drug Enforcement Administration Office of Diversion Control. Available at: https://www.deadiversion.usdoj.gov/drug_chem_info/bromo_dmp.pdf. Accessed July 18, 2017.
65. Sanders B, Lankenau SE, Bloom JJ, et al. "Research chemicals": tryptamine and phenethylamine use among high-risk youth. Subst Use Misuse 2008;43:389–402.
66. Hill SL, Thomas SHL. Clinical toxicology of newer recreational drugs. Clin Toxicol 2011;49:705–19.
67. Curtis B, Kemp P, Choi C, et al. Postmortem identification and quantitation of 2,5-dimethoxy-4-n-propylthiophenethylamine using GC-MSD and GC-NPD. J Anal Toxicol 2003;27:493–8.
68. Bosak A, Lovecchio F, Levine M. Recurrent seizures and serotonin syndrome following "2C-I" ingestion. J Med Toxicol 2013;9:196–8.
69. Auwarter V, Dresen S, Weinmann W, et al. 'Spice' and other herbal blends: harmless incense of cannabinoid designer drugs? J Mass Spectrom 2009;44:832–7.
70. White CM. The pharmacologic and clinical effects of illicit synthetic cannabinoids. J Clin Pharmacol 2017;57:297–304.
71. Castaneto MS, Gorelick DA, Desrosiers NA, et al. Synthetic cannabinoids: epidemiology, pharmacodynamics, and clinical implications. Drug Alcohol Depend 2014;144:12–41.
72. Fantegrossi WE, Moran JH, Radominska-Pandyab A, et al. Distinct pharmacology and metabolism of K2 synthetic cannabinoids compared to Δ9-THC: mechanism underlying greater toxicity? Life Sci 2014;97:45–54.
73. Tai S, Fantegrossi WE. Pharmacological and toxicological effects of synthetic cannabinoids and their metabolites. Curr Top Behav Neurosci 2017;32:249–62.
74. Law R, Schier J, Martin C, et al. Centers for Disease Control (CDC). Notes from the field: increase in reported adverse health effects related to synthetic cannabinoid Use - United States, January-May 2015. MMWR Morb Mortal Wkly Rep 2015;64:618–9.
75. Springer YP, Gerona R, Scheunemann E, et al. Increase in adverse reactions associated with use of synthetic cannabinoids - Anchorage, Alaska, 2015-2016. MMWR Morb Mortal Wkly Rep 2016;65:1108–11.
76. DEA, Controlled Substances Act, 1308.11 Schedule I. Available at: https://www.deadiversion.usdoj.gov/21cfr/cfr/1308/1308_11.htm. Accessed July 31, 2017.
77. Palamar JJ, Acosta P. Synthetic cannabinoid use in a nationally representative sample of US high school seniors. Drug Alcohol Depend 2015;149:194–202.
78. Caviness CM, Tzilos G, Anderson BJ, et al. Synthetic cannabinoids: use and predictors in a community sample of young adults. Subst Abus 2015;36:368–73.
79. Keyes KM, Rutherford C, Hamilton A, et al. Age, period, and cohort effects in synthetic cannabinoid use among US adolescents, 2011-2015. Drug Alcohol Depend 2016;166:159–67.
80. Monte AA, Bronstein AC, Cao DJ, et al. An outbreak of exposure to a novel synthetic cannabinoid. N Engl J Med 2014;370:389.

81. Kasper AM, Ridpath AD, Arnold JK, et al. Severe illness associated with reported use of synthetic cannabinoids - Mississippi, April 2015. MMWR Morb Mortal Wkly Rep 2015;64(39):1121–2.
82. Gunderson EW, Haughey HM, Ait-Daoud N, et al. "Spice" and "K2" herbal highs: a case series and systematic review of the clinical effects and biopsychosocial implications of synthetic cannabinoid use in humans. Am J Addict 2012;21: 320–6.
83. Winstock A, Lynskey M, Borschmann R, et al. Risk of emergency medical treatment following consumption of cannabis or synthetic cannabinoids in a large global sample. J Psychopharmacol 2015;29:698–703.
84. Bassir Nia A, Medrano B, Perkel C, et al. Psychiatric comorbidity associated with synthetic cannabinoid use compared to cannabis. J Psychopharmacol 2016;30:1321–30.
85. Hermanns-Clausen M, Kneisel S, Szabo B, et al. Acute toxicity due to the confirmed consumption of synthetic cannabinoids: clinical and laboratory findings. Addiction 2013;108:534–44.
86. Tait RJ, Caldicott D, Mountain D, et al. A systematic review of adverse events arising from the use of synthetic cannabinoids and their associated treatment. Clin Toxicol (Phila) 2016;54:1–13.
87. Courts J, Maskill V, Gray A, et al. Signs and symptoms associated with synthetic cannabinoid toxicity: systematic review. Australas Psychiatry 2015;24:598–601.
88. Zarifi C, Vyas S. Spice-y kidney failure: a case report and systematic review of acute kidney injury attributable to the use of synthetic cannabis. Perm J 2017; 21. https://doi.org/10.7812/TPP/16-160.
89. Adedinsewo DA, Odewole O, Todd T. Acute rhabdomyolysis following synthetic cannabinoid ingestion. N Am J Med Sci 2016;8:256–8.
90. Bernson-Leung ME, Leung LY, Kumar S. Synthetic cannabis and acute ischemic stroke. J Stroke Cerebrovasc Dis 2014;23:1239–41.
91. Mir A, Obafemi A, Young A, et al. Myocardial infarction associated with use of the synthetic cannabinoid K2. Pediatrics 2011;128:e1622–7.
92. Andonian DO, Seaman SR, Josephson EB. Profound hypotension and bradycardia in the setting of synthetic cannabinoid intoxication - A case series. Am J Emerg Med 2017;35:940.e5-6.
93. Von Der Haar J, Talebi S, Ghobadi F, et al. Synthetic cannabinoids and their effects on the cardiovascular system. J Emerg Med 2016;50:258–62.
94. Seely KA, Lapoint J, Moran JH, et al. Spice drugs are more than harmless herbal blends: a review of the pharmacology and toxicology of synthetic cannabinoids. Prog Neuropsychopharmacol Biol Psychiatry 2012;39:234–43.
95. Nacca N, Vatti D, Sullivan R, et al. The synthetic cannabinoid withdrawal syndrome. J Addict Med 2013;7:296–8.
96. Zimmermann US, Winkelmann PR, Pilhatsch M, et al. Withdrawal phenomena and dependence syndrome after the consumption of "spice gold". Dtsch Arztebl Int 2009;106:464–7.
97. Macfarlane V, Christie G. Synthetic cannabinoid withdrawal: a new demand on detoxification services. Drug Alcohol Rev 2015;34:147–53.
98. Franz F, Angerer V, Jechle H, et al. Immunoassay screening in urine for synthetic cannabinoids - an evaluation of the diagnostic efficiency. Clin Chem Lab Med 2017;55(9):1375–84.
99. Namera A, Kawamura M, Nakamoto A, et al. Comprehensive review of the detection methods for synthetic cannabinoids and cathinones. Forensic Toxicol 2015;33:175–94.

100. Centers for Disease Control and Prevention. Influx of fentanyl-laced counterfeit pill and toxic fentanyl-related compounds further increases risk of fentanyl-related overdose and fatalities. Atlanta (GA): CDC HAN; 2016. p. 00395. Available at: https://emergency.cdc.gov/han/han00395.asp.
101. Prekupec MP, Mansky PA, Baumann MH. Misuse of novel synthetic opioids: a deadly new trend. J Addict Med 2017;11(4):256–65.
102. Dussy FE, Hangartner S, Hamberg C, et al. An acute ocfentanil fatality: a case report with postmortem concentrations. J Anal Toxicol 2016;40:761–6.
103. George AV, Lu JJ, Pisaon MV, et al. Carfentanil–an ultra potent opioid. Am J Emerg Med 2010;28:530–2.
104. Emerging threat report: Annual 2016. (2017). [online] Drug Enforcement Administration. Available at: https://ndews.umd.edu/sites/ndews.umd.edu/files/emerging-threat-report-2016-annual.pdf. Accessed June 4, 2017.
105. Drug Enforcement Administration. Emerging threat report: first quarter 2017.
106. Høiseth G, Skogstad S, Karinen R. Blood concentrations of new designer benzodiazepines in forensic cases. Forensic Sci Int 2016;268:35–8.
107. O'Connor LC, Torrance HJ, McKeown DA. ELISA detection of phenazepam, etizolam, pyrazolam, flubormazepam, diclazepam, and delorazepam in blood using Immunalysis benzodiazepine kit. J Anal Toxicol 2016;40:159–61.
108. O'Connell CW, Sadler CA, Tolia VM, et al. Overdose of etizolam: the abuse and risk of a benzodiazepine analog. Ann Emerg Med 2015;65:465–6.

Sleep Management Among Patients with Substance Use Disorders

Subhajit Chakravorty, MD[a],*, Ryan G. Vandrey, PhD[b],
Sean He, BS[c,d], Michael D. Stein, MD[e]

KEYWORDS

- Sleep initiation and maintenance disorders • Substance-related disorders
- Alcoholism • Cocaine-related disorders • Marijuana abuse
- Opioid-related disorders

KEY POINTS

- Insomnia is linked with substance use and withdrawal.
- Cognitive behavioral therapy for insomnia has shown promise as an intervention for insomnia in individuals with alcohol and possibly other drug use disorders.
- Sleep-disordered breathing should be considered in the differential diagnosis of sleep maintenance insomnia, especially for patients misusing opioids and alcohol.
- Abstinence from substance use should be recommended for those with short-term insomnia.
- A referral to a sleep medicine clinic should be considered for insomnia disorder or other intrinsic sleep disorders, especially during abstinence.

This article originally appeared in *Medical Clinics*, Volume 102, Issue 4, July 2018.
Disclosure Statement: Dr S. Chakravorty has received research support from AstraZeneca and Teva Pharmaceuticals. Dr R.G. Vandrey is a paid consultant or serves on the advisory board of Zynerba Pharmaceuticals, Insys Therapeutics Inc, Battelle Memorial Institute, and several small US businesses engaged in state medicinal cannabis programs. The study was supported by VA grant IK2CX000855 (S. Chakravorty), U01 DA031784 (R.G. Vandrey), R01 DA034261, R01 NR015977 R34 DA032800 R21 DA031369 (M.D. Stein). The content of this publication does not represent the views of the Department of Veterans Affairs or any other institution.
[a] Department of Psychiatry, Perelman School of Medicine, Corporal Michael J. Crescenz VA Medical Center, MIRECC, 2nd Floor, Postal Code 116, 3900 Woodland Avenue, Philadelphia, PA 19104, USA; [b] Behavioral Pharmacology Research Unit, Johns Hopkins University School of Medicine, 5510 Nathan Shock Drive, Baltimore, MD 21224, USA; [c] Post-baccalaureate studies program, College of Liberal Arts and Professional Studies, University of Pennsylvania, 3440 Market Street Suite 100, Philadelphia, PA 19104, USA; [d] Department of R & D, Corporal Michael J. Crescenz VA Medical Center, 3900 Woodland Avenue, Philadelphia, PA 19104, USA; [e] Department of Health Law, Policy and Management, Boston University School of Public Health, 715 Albany Street, Talbot Building, Boston, MA 02118, USA
* Corresponding author.
E-mail address: Subhajit.Chakravorty@uphs.upenn.edu

INTRODUCTION: SLEEP AND ITS ASSOCIATION WITH SUBSTANCE USE DISORDERS

A disturbance of sleep continuity has effects on next-day functioning and behavior. One such behavior is the use of psychoactive substances. Disturbed sleep is also a frequent complaint among persons using alcohol and illicit drugs. Further, sleep dysfunction in the context of substance misuse may contribute to increased severity of substance use disorder (SUD), impaired quality of life, comorbid psychiatric complaints, suicidal behavior, and psychosocial problems.[1,2] This narrative review focuses on the identification and treatment of sleep disorders in persons with comorbid SUDs.

ASSESSMENT AND DIAGNOSIS OF SUBSTANCE USE AND SLEEP DISORDERS
Substance Use and Substance Use Disorder

Various aspects of substance use are relevant to sleep. Drugs can have an acute impact on sleep by either increasing or decreasing arousal. Pharmacologically specific sleep-related withdrawal symptoms may occur on cessation or reduction of heavy, sustained periods of substance use.[3] Problematic patterns of substance use also may lead to distress, which may in turn impact sleep via nonpharmacological mechanisms. Commonly used substances in the context of sleep-related problems include alcohol, cocaine, cannabis (marijuana), opioids, and sedative-hypnotic-anxiolytic medications.

APPROACH TO THE ASSESSMENT OF PATIENTS WITH SLEEP DISORDERS

Patient complaints related to sleep most often consist of difficulty falling asleep, difficulty staying asleep, or impaired daytime functioning. Symptoms of impaired daytime functioning may include mood disturbance, fatigue, problems with concentration, or daytime sleepiness. The common sleep-related disorders evaluated in the context of substance use include the following:

1. Insomnia
2. Circadian rhythm disorder–delayed sleep phase type (CRSD-DSP)
3. Sleep-related breathing disorder (SRBD)

   Fig. 1 explains a strategy for screening patients in a clinical setting, especially in the context of a primary care setting when substance use is suspected or confirmed.

Insomnia

Insomnia is a disorder characterized by complaints of poor sleep continuity (ie, difficulty falling asleep and/or staying asleep), early morning awakening, and impairment of daytime functioning.[4] Insomnia may be assessed using a structured rating instrument, such as the Insomnia Severity Index or a sleep diary. The sleep diary should be prospectively completed for a week or more and yields multiple indices, see **Table 1**. Acute insomnia denotes a recent onset of insomnia, less than 3 months in duration and commonly precipitated by a psychosocial stressor, that may be treated with reassurance, close monitoring, or with medications. Acute insomnia also is common in the acute withdrawal phase from substances. However, most of the hypnotic medications approved by the Food and Drug Administration (FDA), such as temazepam or zolpidem, may be contraindicated in patients with SUD. For those with chronic insomnia (≥3 months in duration), behavioral interventions, such as cognitive behavioral therapy for insomnia (CBT-I), are the recommended first-line intervention. Insomnia comorbid with active substance use is optimally treated in a substance misuse program or primary care setting staffed by clinicians with experience in

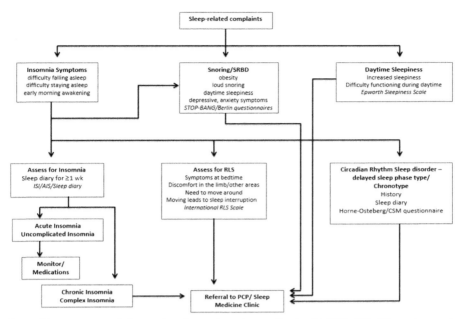

Fig. 1. Management of sleep-related symptoms in a patient with SUD. AIS, Athens insomnia scale; CSM questionnaire, composite scale of morningness questionnaire; ISI, Insomnia Severity Index scale; PCP, primary care provider; STOP-BANG questionnaire, a screening questionnaire for OSA.

substance-related problems. In contrast, chronic insomnia in patients with remitted SUD are best treated by referral to a sleep medicine clinic (see **Fig. 1**).

Circadian Rhythm Sleep Disorder–Delayed Sleep Phase Type

CRSDs are generated as a consequence of a mismatch between the individual's internal (biological) rhythm and the required environmental schedule. CRSD-DSP is a particular subtype of CRSD that is characterized by going to bed later in the night and awakening later in the morning. This later sleep-wake timing may interfere with daily activities, and patients may present with complaints of insomnia, sleepiness, and impaired daytime functioning. CRSDs may be easily assessed in a clinic setting using sleep diaries, actigraphy, or with the help of rating scales that evaluate the patient's propensity for sleep at a particular time during the 24-hour period. Prior research has linked alcohol use with the blunting of circadian rhythms in healthy adults,[5] and, alcohol use disorder (AUD) with insomnia and a nocturnal delay in the rise of melatonin level (a marker of circadian activity).[6,7]

Sleep-Related Breathing Disorder

SRBDs are characterized by disruption of sleep by respiratory events. An individual may be screened for SRBD either using an in-laboratory clinical polysomnogram or home sleep monitoring using a portable sleep monitor. Obstructive sleep apnea (OSA) is condition characterized by loud snoring, breath interruptions, and polysomnographic evidence of obstructive apneas and/or obstructive hypopneas, see **Table 1**. Central sleep apnea (CSA) syndrome may present similarly, but mostly

Table 1
Commonly used terminologies in sleep medicine

Acronym	Term	Description
SE	Sleep efficiency (%)	The proportion of time spent sleeping through the night
NREM	NREM sleep	The initial stages of sleep (N1 + N2 + SWS); approximately 80% of sleep
N1	Stage 1 sleep	Characterized by low eye movements, waves with low amplitude, and, mostly 4–7-Hz frequency
N2	Stage 2 sleep	The sleep stage that demonstrates sleep spindles and K complexes
N3/SWS	Slow-wave sleep (stages 3 + 4)	The presence of high amplitude and low frequency (0.5–2.0 Hz), $\geq$20% of the epoch
REM	Rapid eye movement sleep	Sleep with sawtooth waveforms, rapid eye movements, and low muscle tone
SOL	Sleep-onset latency (min)	Time from "lights out" until the onset of sleep in the reading pane
REM-L	REM-onset latency (min)	Interval of time from onset of sleep to the appearance of the first epoch of REM sleep
S1	Stage 1 (%)	The fraction of sleep that is spent in N1 (total Stage 1 sleep/TST $\times$ 100); usually approximately 4%–5%
S2	Stage 2 (%)	The fraction of sleep that is spent in N2 (total Stage 2 sleep/TST $\times$ 100); usually approximately 45%–55%
SWS	Slow-wave sleep (%)	The percentage of sleep that is spent in SWS (total SWS sleep/TST $\times$ 100); usually approximately 16%–21%
REM	REM (%)	The percentage of sleep that is spent in REM (total REM sleep/TST $\times$ 100); usually approximately 20%–25%
Apnea	(polysomnography or home sleep test)	A complete cessation of airflow for $\geq$10 s
Hypopnea	(polysomnography or home sleep test)	A partial cessation of airflow for $\geq$10 s, and either a $\geq$4% drop in SpO_2, or, an arousal (as seen on electroencephalogram)
AHI	Apnea Hypopnea Index (events/h)	Total number of apneas and hypopneas per hour of sleep; that is, total number of apneas and hypopneas/TST
Advance	Phase advance	Shift of the sleep cycle to an earlier time during a circadian period (24 h)
Delay	Phase delay	Shift of the sleep cycle to a later time during a circadian period (24 h)
SRBD	Sleep-related breathing disorder	Abnormalities of respiration during sleep; include OSA, CSA, and obesity hypoventilation and hypoventilation syndromes
OSA	Obstructive sleep apnea	A syndrome with symptoms (loud snoring and breathing interruptions)/cardio-metabolic syndrome + AHI $\geq$5 events/h of sleep
CSA	Central sleep apnea	A syndrome with symptoms (sleepiness, insomnia, snoring, and witnessed apneas)/atrial fibrillation/CHF + $\geq$5 central events/h of sleep
CPAP	Continuous positive airway pressure	A machine delivering air at a continuous pressure to prevent collapse of the air passage during sleep

(continued on next page)

Table 1 (continued)		
Acronym	Term	Description
BiPAP	Bi-level positive airway pressure	A machine delivering air at 2 pressures: a higher pressure during inspiration and a lower pressure during expiration
ASV	Adaptive servo-ventilation	A specialized form of positive airway pressure support in which the delivered pressure changes when respiratory events are detected
CBT-I	Cognitive behavioral therapy for insomnia	A manualized behavioral treatment for insomnia, consisting of sleep restriction, stimulus control, and cognitive therapy, for ≤8 wk

Abbreviation: CHF, congestive heart failure; NREM, non–rapid eye movement; TST, total sleep time.
  Data from American Academy of Sleep Medicine (AASM). The AASM manual for the scoring of sleep and associated events. 2007; and American Academy of Sleep Medicine (AASM). 2012. Available at: http://www.sleepnet.com/definition.html. Accessed October 28, 2017.

consists of events with complete cessation of airflow along with cessation of thoracic and abdominal wall movements for ≥10 seconds. **Fig. 1** elaborates on ways to screen for SRBD in an outpatient setting. The management of SRBD requires referral to a sleep medicine service.

Limb Movement Disorders in Sleep

This category of sleep disorders includes restless leg syndrome (RLS) and periodic limb movement disorder. A patient with RLS presents with "an urge to move the legs usually accompanied by or thought to be caused by uncomfortable and unpleasant sensation in the legs," which in turn leads to difficulty falling asleep at bedtime.[4] Patients in whom these disorders are suspected also should be referred to a sleep center.

It should be noted that an individual might have multiple comorbid sleep and/or SUDs. Complex case presentations may require cotreatment in substance use and sleep medicine clinics.

ALCOHOL AND SLEEP DISORDERS
Alcohol and Insomnia

Acute alcohol use has sedating effects, particularly on the descending limb of the blood-alcohol concentration curve, and is sometimes used for its sleep-promoting effects. However, alcohol may disrupt sleep by interfering with homeostatic and circadian balance, disrupting local sleep mechanisms, and distorting the electrophysiology of sleep.[1]

Risky alcohol use and AUD have been associated with subjective insomnia as well as objective sleep continuity disturbance. In those with AUD, the prevalence of insomnia ranges from 36% to 91% as compared with the 10% prevalence in the general population, and is prevalent in all stages of AUD.[1] The prevalence of insomnia decreases once alcohol-dependent individuals transition from active drinking to abstinence, with persisting insomnia possibly being a risk factor for relapse.[1] However, in heavy drinkers with AUD, sleep dysfunction may persist up to 2 years into recovery in a subset of individuals and is a risk factor for relapse.[8] Those who screen positive for AUD should be educated about the association of insomnia with AUD.

Behavioral and pharmacologic interventions for insomnia in AUD have been studied. Behavioral interventions have consistently demonstrated efficacy in treating insomnia among individuals with AUD.[1] CBT-I is the recommended first-line treatment for insomnia.[9] Prior studies have demonstrated conflicting results with gabapentin and trazodone.[1] Other drugs that have demonstrated an improvement in insomnia among alcohol-dependent patients have included acamprosate, agomelatine, and quetiapine.[1]

If insomnia persists despite continued abstinence, patients should be referred to a sleep medicine clinic. If a behavioral sleep medicine specialist is unavailable in the sleep clinic, bibliotherapy, online sleep treatment programs, or evidence-based psychopharmacologic interventions should be considered, such as gabapentin or ramelteon.

Most of the currently approved hypnotic medications, such as zolpidem or eszopiclone, are contraindicated in those with current AUD due to the potential risk of dependence and drug-drug interactions secondary to polypharmacy in this population. Therefore, gabapentin may be an alternative for those who continue to drink, although risks and benefits should be carefully reviewed.

Alcohol and Sleep-Related Breathing Disorder

Alcohol relaxes the musculature of the upper airway and impairs protective arousal response during sleep. These effects may lead to an aggravation of snoring, fragmentation of sleep, and worsening of preexisting SRBD. Treatment-seeking persons with AUD have a higher intensity of sleep-disordered breathing during alcohol withdrawal and a high prevalence of SRBD.[1] Continuous positive airway pressure (CPAP) is the first-line treatment modality, although alternatives to CPAP are also available depending on severity.

OPIOIDS AND SLEEP DISORDERS

Opioid prescriptions for chronic pain analgesia, along with opioid morbidity, have increased dramatically over the past 2 decades. Hassamal and colleagues[10] demonstrated that prescription opioid receipt and increasing opioid dose were associated with greater self-reported sleep disturbance among individuals with chronic pain, suggesting opioids worsen sleep beyond the disruptive sleep effects of pain. Insomnia and SRBD are the primary sleep disorders reported in those using opioids. Because pain and respiratory control are mediated by the endogenous opioid system, opioid-induced impairment in breathing must be a central concern of clinical evaluation in sleep-impaired persons.

Opioids and Insomnia

Most persons receiving opioids for chronic pain have insomnia, and approximately three-quarters of persons receiving methadone maintenance treatment (MMT) or buprenorphine for opioid use disorder (OUD) have sleep complaints. Acute dosing of opioids for the treatment of pain appears to improve aspects of sleep quality.[11] But as use continues, there appears to be a significant association between prescription opioid dose and self-reported sleep dysfunction. The most frequent complaints include increased sleep latency and increased time awake after sleep onset.[12]

Among individuals with OUD, sleep gradually improves during the first 90 days after initiating treatment with buprenorphine/naltrexone.[13] Factors contributing to persisting sleep complaints in opioid users are pain, depression,[14] benzodiazepine (BZD) use, and cigarette smoking. It should be noted that use of medications in the BZD class is common in this population and is associated with longer sleep time estimates by patients than is demonstrated during sleep studies. Still, many opioid users will use BZDs to facilitate sleep,[15] increasing their risk for overdose, as both substances suppress respiration.[16,17]

CBT-I treatment has been shown to improve sleep-related outcomes,[18-20] including patients who had previously been prescribed medications for sleep[21] and among patients whose impaired sleep was secondary to pain.[22] Trazodone has failed to show efficacy in one study,[23] and no data exist on other medications like doxepin or suvorexant.

Opioids and Sleep-Related Breathing Disorder

Opioid-induced impairment of breathing includes central depression of the respiratory rate, amplitude and reflex responses, reduced brain arousal, and upper airway dysfunction.[24] SRBDs occur in most chronic opioid users.[25] OSA was observed in 39% of 140 patients with chronic pain taking opioids,[26] whereas the prevalence of OSA in the general population is estimated at 9% in women and 24% in men.[27] Risk factors for SRBD in patients with OUD include smoking, female gender, and increased body weight.[10] OSA in this population is likely due to opioid-induced reductions in airway muscle activation.[28] CSA may arise from depression of hypoxic and hypercapnic ventilatory drives, which are already reduced during sleep.[24] This effect has been reported to occur in 0% to 60% of MMT patients,[10] although it is rarely observed in the general population. CSA has been associated with methadone dose and concomitant BZD use, and with higher methadone blood concentration.[10] Cases in which CSA reverses after discontinuation of opioid treatment have been reported.[10] Although very little information exists on SRBD associated with buprenorphine/naloxone, 1 study demonstrated incidence rates of 63% for mild, 16% for moderate, and 17% for severe OSA.[29]

Treatment recommendations for opioid-induced SRBD are limited by a lack of research on the topic. As a first step, the option of discontinuing opioids should be considered in the context of risks and benefits with this decision. When long-term treatment with opioid therapy is continued, and SRBD is identified, treatment options include CPAP, adaptive servo-ventilation, and bi-level spontaneous timed therapy.[24] An alternative option is switching to an injectable formulation of depot-Naltrexone, a mu-opioid receptor antagonist.

CANNABIS AND SLEEP DISORDERS

Acute cannabis or tetrahydrocannabinol (THC) administration is associated with reduced latency to sleep onset, a decrease in rapid eye movement sleep and an increase in Stage 3 sleep.[30] The hypnotic properties of cannabis are often reported as a reason for use of cannabis, and may drive sustained use patterns among individuals with underlying sleep dysfunction.[2] However, there is evidence of tolerance developing to the hypnotic effects of cannabis use, likely due to neurobiological changes in the endocannabinoid system.[30]

Daily cannabis users self-report greater sleep disturbance compared with nonusers and less-frequent users, and treatment-seeking cannabis users have high rates of disordered sleep.[31,32] However, it remains unclear whether increased sleep problems among daily and treatment-seeking cannabis users reflects a direct impact of heavy cannabis use or that the sleep dysfunction in this population is due to an underlying psychiatric or sleep pathology that predated, and possibly contributed to the development of cannabis use disorder (CUD). Notably, one of the defining features of CUD is a cannabis withdrawal syndrome, in which sleep difficulty and an increase in vivid/strange dreams are hallmark features.[33] Sleep difficulty typically lasts 2 to 3 weeks before returning to baseline levels, but the increase in vivid/strange dreams appears to persist indefinitely, suggesting that cannabis suppresses the recall or vividness of dreams rather than this being a true withdrawal effect.[33]

Sleep difficulty during cannabis abstinence is a commonly reported barrier to cessation, with individuals reporting relapse to cannabis use, increased alcohol use, or use of sedative/hypnotic drugs to mitigate abstinence-induced sleep problems.[33] Treatment-seeking cannabis users often exhibit clinically significant sleep dysfunction, and poor sleep at the beginning of treatment predicts relapse early in a quit attempt.[32,34] Pilot studies suggest that behavioral and pharmacologic interventions that can improve sleep during treatment for CUD may improve cannabis use outcomes.[35,36]

The medicinal use of cannabis in the treatment of pain, multiple sclerosis, or post-traumatic stress disorder (PTSD) can result in improved sleep. In some cases, the sleep improvement may contribute to better clinical outcomes and an improved quality of life. However, long-term use of cannabis or THC primarily as a hypnotic agent is not recommended due to the development of tolerance to its hypnotic properties, risk of long-term sleep disturbance, and subsequent withdrawal symptoms on abrupt cessation, which can exacerbate symptoms of certain illnesses (eg, PTSD).

COCAINE AND ITS ASSOCIATED SLEEP DISORDERS

Acute cocaine use increases arousal, and binge use often occurs when the individual does not sleep. Persons with cocaine use disorder (CoUD) seldom seek help for insomnia; however, recent studies that included objective measures indicate sleep dysfunction is common during cocaine withdrawal.[33]

In a controlled trial of CoUD, modafinil (an FDA-approved medication for sleepiness in adequately treated OSA, narcolepsy, and shift work sleep disorder) was superior to placebo in improving the total sleep time, Stage 3 sleep, and abstinence from cocaine.[33] Other medications investigated for sleep continuity disturbance in individuals with CoUD have included lorazepam, tiagabine, and mirtazapine. In a comparative efficacy trial of lorazepam and tiagabine, both drugs decreased sleep latency, but tiagabine increased slow-wave sleep in recently abstinent persons with CoUD.[37] Mirtazapine, compared with placebo, transiently improved sleep-onset latency in depressed subjects with CoUD after 4 weeks of treatment, but did not reduce cocaine consumption.[38]

SEDATIVE-HYPNOTIC-ANXIOLYTIC DRUGS AND SLEEP DISORDERS

Sedative-hypnotic-anxiolytic medications include BZD medications and newer non-BZD Z-drugs. Long-term use of BZDs may lead to dependence and characteristic withdrawal symptoms on discontinuation that include autonomic hyperactivity, insomnia, anxiety, and agitation. Similarly, reports also exist for unhealthy use of non-BZD Z-drugs, although the rate of misuse of these medications is lower than for BZDs.

BZD use has been associated with other SUDs, including alcohol and opioid use, conditions that are also independently linked with insomnia symptoms.[39–41] Abrupt cessation of these medications has been associated with sleep complaints, such as decreased total sleep time and a poor sleep quality. Among the sedative-hypnotic medications, the intensity of withdrawal-induced insomnia is higher in those using BZD-class drugs as compared with the newer Z-drugs. In fact, withdrawal insomnia may be mild or nonexistent after cessation of use of these Z-drugs. Sleep disturbances following abstinence from hypnotic medications typically improve over time during recovery, suggesting it is a true withdrawal effect.[42]

There is scant literature on the treatment of sleep problems in patients with sedative-hypnotic use disorder. Pregabalin has shown promise in decreasing insomnia and the use of BZDs and to bolster abstinence.[43,44] In addition to medications, behavioral interventions, such as relaxation therapy and CBT-I, have demonstrated promise in treating the insomnia.[45]

SUMMARY AND FUTURE DIRECTIONS

Sleep and SUDs are commonly comorbid conditions. Use of psychoactive substances often leads to the development of complaints of disturbed sleep, insomnia disorder, or circadian rhythm sleep disorders. Abrupt cessation of substances of unhealthy use commonly results in sleep disruption, which may be treated with behavioral or pharmacologic interventions as a means of improving cessation attempt outcomes. Other sleep disorders, such as SRBD should be considered in the differential diagnosis for insomnia, especially in those with opioid use or AUD. When chronic insomnia or another intrinsic sleep disorder is suspected, a referral to the local sleep center is recommended. Chronic insomnia may be optimally treated with CBT-I. Acute insomnia or insomnia in the context of active substance use may be best treated in an addiction medicine or a primary care setting in which the preliminary focus should be to target abstinence.

ACKNOWLEDGMENTS

The editors thank Deirdre A. Conroy, University of Michigan, and Bhanu Prakash Kolla, Mayo Clinic, Rochester, MN, for providing a critical review of this article.

REFERENCES

1. Chakravorty S, Chaudhary NS, Brower KJ. Alcohol dependence and its relationship with insomnia and other sleep disorders. Alcohol Clin Exp Res 2016;40(11): 2271–82.
2. Vandrey R, Babson KA, Herrmann ES, et al. Interactions between disordered sleep, post-traumatic stress disorder, and substance use disorders. Int Rev Psychiatry 2014;26(2):237–47.
3. DSM-5. Diagnostic and statistical manual of mental disorders, 5th edition. Arlington (VA): American Psychiatric Publishing; 2013.
4. International classification of sleep disorders - 3rd edition. Darien (IL): American Academy of Sleep Medicine; 2014.
5. Danel T, Libersa C, Touitou Y. The effect of alcohol consumption on the circadian control of human core body temperature is time dependent. Am J Physiol Regul Integr Comp Physiol 2001;281(1):R52–5.
6. Kuhlwein E, Hauger RL, Irwin MR. Abnormal nocturnal melatonin secretion and disordered sleep in abstinent alcoholics. Biol Psychiatry 2003;54(12):1437–43.
7. Conroy DA, Hairston IS, Arnedt JT, et al. Dim light melatonin onset in alcohol-dependent men and women compared with healthy controls. Chronobiol Int 2012;29(1):35–42.
8. Brower KJ. Insomnia, alcoholism and relapse. Sleep Med Rev 2003;7(6):523–39.
9. Schutte-Rodin S, Broch L, Buysse D, et al. Clinical guideline for the evaluation and management of chronic insomnia in adults. J Clin Sleep Med 2008;4(5): 487–504.

10. Hassamal S, Miotto K, Wang T, et al. A narrative review: the effects of opioids on sleep disordered breathing in chronic pain patients and methadone maintained patients. Am J Addict 2016;25(6):452–65.

11. Dimsdale JE, Norman D, DeJardin D, et al. The effect of opioids on sleep architecture. J Clin Sleep Med 2007;3(1):33–6.

12. Peles E, Schreiber S, Adelson M. Variables associated with perceived sleep disorders in methadone maintenance treatment (MMT) patients. Drug Alcohol Depend 2006;82(2):103–10.

13. Zheng WH, Wakim RJ, Geary RC, et al. Self-reported sleep improvement in buprenorphine MAT (Medication Assisted Treatment) population. Austin J Drug Abuse Addict 2016;3(1) [pii: 1009].

14. Tsuno N, Besset A, Ritchie K. Sleep and depression. J Clin Psychiatry 2005; 66(10):1254–69.

15. Stein MD, Kanabar M, Anderson BJ, et al. Reasons for benzodiazepine use among persons seeking opioid detoxification. J Subst Abuse Treat 2016;68: 57–61.

16. Li L, Sangthong R, Chongsuvivatwong V, et al. Lifetime multiple substance use pattern among heroin users before entering methadone maintenance treatment clinic in Yunnan, China. Drug Alcohol Rev 2010;29(4):420–5.

17. Stein MD, Herman DS, Bishop S, et al. Sleep disturbances among methadone maintained patients. J Subst Abuse Treat 2004;26(3):175–80.

18. Backhaus J, Hohagen F, Voderholzer U, et al. Long-term effectiveness of a short-term cognitive-behavioral group treatment for primary insomnia. Eur Arch Psychiatry Clin Neurosci 2001;251(1):35–41.

19. Montgomery P, Dennis J. Cognitive behavioural interventions for sleep problems in adults aged 60+. Cochrane Database Syst Rev 2003;(1):CD003161.

20. Trauer JM, Qian MY, Doyle JS, et al. Cognitive behavioral therapy for chronic insomnia: a systematic review and meta-analysis. Ann Intern Med 2015;163(3): 191–204.

21. Dolan DC, Taylor DJ, Bramoweth AD, et al. Cognitive-behavioral therapy of insomnia: a clinical case series study of patients with co-morbid disorders and using hypnotic medications. Behav Res Ther 2010;48(4):321–7.

22. Currie SR, Wilson KG, Pontefract AJ, et al. Cognitive-behavioral treatment of insomnia secondary to chronic pain. J Consult Clin Psychol 2000;68(3):407–16.

23. Stein MD, Kurth ME, Sharkey KM, et al. Trazodone for sleep disturbance during methadone maintenance: a double-blind, placebo-controlled trial. Drug Alcohol Depend 2012;120(1–3):65–73.

24. Van Ryswyk E, Antic NA. Opioids and sleep-disordered breathing. Chest 2016; 150(4):934–44.

25. Correa D, Farney RJ, Chung F, et al. Chronic opioid use and central sleep apnea: a review of the prevalence, mechanisms, and perioperative considerations. Anesth Analg 2015;120(6):1273–85.

26. Webster LR, Choi Y, Desai H, et al. Sleep-disordered breathing and chronic opioid therapy. Pain Med 2008;9(4):425–32.

27. Young T, Palta M, Dempsey J, et al. The occurrence of sleep-disordered breathing among middle-aged adults. N Engl J Med 1993;328(17):1230–5.

28. Hajiha M, DuBord MA, Liu H, et al. Opioid receptor mechanisms at the hypoglossal motor pool and effects on tongue muscle activity in vivo. J Physiol 2009;587(Pt 11):2677–92.

29. Farney RJ, McDonald AM, Boyle KM, et al. Sleep disordered breathing in patients receiving therapy with buprenorphine/naloxone. Eur Respir J 2013;42(2): 394–403.

30. Schierenbeck T, Riemann D, Berger M, et al. Effect of illicit recreational drugs upon sleep: cocaine, ecstasy and marijuana. Sleep Med Rev 2008;12(5):381–9.

31. Conroy DA, Kurth ME, Strong DR, et al. Marijuana use patterns and sleep among community-based young adults. J Addict Dis 2016;35(2):135–43.

32. Pacek LR, Herrmann ES, Smith MT, et al. Sleep continuity, architecture and quality among treatment-seeking cannabis users: an in-home, unattended polysomnographic study. Exp Clin Psychopharmacol 2017;25(4):295–302.

33. Angarita GA, Emadi N, Hodges S, et al. Sleep abnormalities associated with alcohol, cannabis, cocaine, and opiate use: a comprehensive review. Addict Sci Clin Pract 2016;11(1):9.

34. Babson KA, Boden MT, Bonn-Miller MO. The impact of perceived sleep quality and sleep efficiency/duration on cannabis use during a self-guided quit attempt. Addict Behav 2013;38(11):2707–13.

35. Babson KA, Ramo DE, Baldini L, et al. Mobile app-delivered cognitive behavioral therapy for insomnia: feasibility and initial efficacy among veterans with cannabis use disorders. JMIR Res Protoc 2015;4(3):e87.

36. Mason BJ, Crean R, Goodell V, et al. A proof-of-concept randomized controlled study of gabapentin: effects on cannabis use, withdrawal and executive function deficits in cannabis-dependent adults. Neuropsychopharmacology 2012;37(7): 1689–98.

37. Morgan PT, Malison RT. Pilot study of lorazepam and tiagabine effects on sleep, motor learning, and impulsivity in cocaine abstinence. Am J Drug Alcohol Abuse 2008;34(6):692–702.

38. Afshar M, Knapp CM, Sarid-Segal O, et al. The efficacy of mirtazapine in the treatment of cocaine dependence with comorbid depression. Am J Drug Alcohol Abuse 2012;38(2):181–6.

39. Kroll DS, Nieva HR, Barsky AJ, et al. Benzodiazepines are prescribed more frequently to patients already at risk for benzodiazepine-related adverse events in primary care. J Gen Intern Med 2016;31(9):1027–34.

40. Hackman DT, Greene MS, Fernandes TJ, et al. Prescription drug monitoring program inquiry in psychiatric assessment: detection of high rates of opioid prescribing to a dual diagnosis population. J Clin Psychiatry 2014;75(7):750–6.

41. Manthey L, Lohbeck M, Giltay EJ, et al. Correlates of benzodiazepine dependence in the Netherlands Study of Depression and Anxiety. Addiction 2012; 107(12):2173–82.

42. Lichstein KL. Behavioral intervention for special insomnia populations: hypnotic-dependent insomnia and comorbid insomnia. Sleep Med 2006;7(Suppl 1): S27–31.

43. Oulis P, Konstantakopoulos G. Efficacy and safety of pregabalin in the treatment of alcohol and benzodiazepine dependence. Expert Opin Investig Drugs 2012; 21(7):1019–29.

44. Cho YW, Song ML. Effects of pregabalin in patients with hypnotic-dependent insomnia. J Clin Sleep Med 2014;10(5):545–50.

45. Beaulieu-Bonneau S, Ivers H, Guay B, et al. Long-term maintenance of therapeutic gains associated with cognitive-behavioral therapy for insomnia delivered alone or combined with zolpidem. Sleep 2017;40(3).